CASE STUDIES

Stahl's Essential Psychopharmacology

Volume 4

"In today's complex and burdened healthcare environment, this essential psychopharmacology for child and adolescent psychiatry gives the busiest clinicians readily available tools to navigate complex scenarios with clear, sequential, and logical guidance. The clinical pearls are written in pragmatically and with adult learning principles in mind. Thank you, Dr's Stahl and Strawn, for capitulating the wisdom of our field in such an accessible and engaging way."

Manpreet Kaur Singh, MD, MS
Associate Professor of Psychiatry and Behavioral Sciences
Stanford University, Stanford, CA, USA

"Dr's Strawn and Stahl have really done it! The case-based teaching format and dozens of easy-to-read graphs and illustrations, walks clinicians of all levels through the complex world of pediatric psychopharmacology. Using easy-to-follow color-coded backgrounds and icons, the cases illustrate the evolution of each patient's treatment, the interplay of science and clinical wisdom, and the common pitfalls in the practice of pediatric psychopharmacology. In this era of rapidly advancing knowledge, this book provides a foundation rooted in the latest clinical pharmacology literature; it is a must-read for anyone practicing pediatric psychopharmacology."

John T. Walkup, MD
Margaret C. Osterman Professor of Psychiatry
Chair, Pritzker Department of Psychiatry and Behavioral Health
Ann and Robert H. Lurie Children's Hospital of Chicago, IL, USA
President-Elect, American Academy of Child & Adolescent Psychiatry

"This collection of case studies is the most comprehensive and clinically relevant that I have ever read. As a practicing Child and Adolescent Psychiatrist, I have come face to face with many of the same clinical presentations and found Dr Strawn's review of the management thoughtful and integrative.

The way the text is written provides a unique framework for how to approach these difficult interactions and gives a glimpse into how to combine science with the art of psychopharmacology when the evidence base is lacking.

I wholeheartedly believe this text is a must have for any Child and Adolescent Psychiatrist's library. I will certainly use it when teaching my residents and fellows and in my own practice as well."

Nicole M. Ballinger, DO, MPH, FAPA
Adult, Child and Adolescent Psychiatrist
Medical Staff President/ Director Child and Adolescent Psychiatry Partial Hospital
Program/Site Director, Child and Adolescent Psychiatry Fellows and Residents for
Aurora Psychiatric Hospital, Wauwatosa, WI, USA
Clinical Associate Professor, Department of Psychiatry and Behavioral Medicine,
Medical College of Wisconsin and Affiliated Hospitals

CASE STUDIES: Stahl's Essential Psychopharmacology

Children and Adolescents
Volume 4

Jeffrey R. Strawn
University of Cincinnati, Cincinnati, Ohio

Stephen M. Stahl
University of California, San Diego, California

With illustrations by
Nancy Muntner

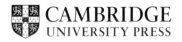
CAMBRIDGE
UNIVERSITY PRESS

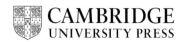

Shaftesbury Road, Cambridge CB2 8EA, United Kingdom

One Liberty Plaza, 20th Floor, New York, NY 10006, USA

477 Williamstown Road, Port Melbourne, VIC 3207, Australia

314–321, 3rd Floor, Plot 3, Splendor Forum, Jasola District Centre,
New Delhi – 110025, India

103 Penang Road, #05–06/07, Visioncrest Commercial, Singapore 238467

Cambridge University Press is part of Cambridge University Press & Assessment,
a department of the University of Cambridge.

We share the University's mission to contribute to society through the pursuit of
education, learning and research at the highest international levels of excellence.

www.cambridge.org
Information on this title: www.cambridge.org/9781009048965

DOI: 10.1017/9781009049719

First published 2024

Printed in Mexico by Litográfica Ingramex, S.A. de C.V.

A catalogue record for this publication is available from the British Library.

Library of Congress Cataloging-in-Publication Data
Names: Strawn, Jeffrey R., 1977– author. | Stahl, Stephen M., 1951– author. |
    Stahl, Stephen M., 1951– Case studies.
Title: Case studies : Stahl's essential psychopharmacology. Volume 4,
    Children and adolescents / authored by Jeffrey R. Strawn, Stephen M. Stahl.
Other titles: Case studies (Strawn) | Children and adolescents
Description: Cambridge, United Kingdom ; New York, NY : Cambridge University Press, 2024. |
    Preceded by Case studies : Stahl's essential psychopharmacology / Stephen M. Stahl. 2011. |
    Includes bibliographical references and index.
Identifiers: LCCN 2023018486 | ISBN 9781009048965 (paperback) | ISBN 9781009049719 (ebook)
Subjects: MESH: Mental Disorders – drug therapy | Child | Adolescent | Psychotropic Drugs – therapeutic use |
    Psychopharmacology – methods | Case Reports | Examination Questions
Classification: LCC RC483 | NLM WS 18.2 | DDC 616.89/18–dc23/eng/20230605
LC record available at https://lccn.loc.gov/2023018486

ISBN 978-1-009-04896-5 Paperback

Contents

Introduction   xi
List of icons   xv
Abbreviations   xix

1   **The Case:** The salutatorian who couldn't speak: selective serotonin
    reuptake inhibitor (SSRI)-refractory anxiety in an adolescent   1
    The Question: What do you do when anxiety fails to respond to multiple
    SSRIs and cognitive–behavioral therapy (CBT)?
    The Psychopharmacological Dilemma: Whether and when to add
    adjunctive benzodiazepines remains unclear for many clinicians

2   **The Case:** From anxious to activated: selective serotonin reuptake
    inhibitor (SSRI)-related activation   17
    The Question: How can clinicians predict side effects associated with
    SSRIs in children and adolescents?
    The Psychopharmacological Dilemma: Balancing side effects,
    side-effect management, and efficacy is challenging

3   **The Case:** The girl who couldn't sleep: posttraumatic stress
    disorder (PTSD) in a young girl   35
    The Question: When should adjunctive medications be used in
    pediatric PTSD?
    The Psychopharmacological Dilemma: Randomized clinical trials of
    first-line medications, such as selective serotonin reuptake inhibitors
    (SSRIs), in adults with PTSD generally fail to show benefit in children
    and adolescents with PTSD

4   **The Case:** Depressed and still depressed: major depressive disorder
    (MDD) in an adolescent   49
    The Question: When should adjunctive medications be used in adolescents
    with treatment-resistant MDD?
    The Psychopharmacological Dilemma: There is uncertainty regarding
    how and when to "change course" in managing treatment-resistant MDD
    in adolescents, and adjunctive medications may have unique tolerability
    concerns related to primary pharmacotherapy in this age group

5   **The Case:** A 13-year-old adolescent who feels "amazing": selective
    serotonin reuptake inhibitor (SSRI)-induced mania in an adolescent   65
    The Questions: What medications should be used in an adolescent who
    develops mania when treated with an SSRI? Does SSRI-related mania
    represent bipolar disorder?
    The Psychopharmacological Dilemma: How to treat patients who are at
    "high risk" for developing bipolar disorder but are experiencing depressive
    and/or anxiety symptoms presents a challenge for many clinicians,
    particularly as SSRIs are the first-line pharmacotherapy for adolescents
    with depressive and anxiety disorders

6   **The Case:** Counting on a cure: obsessive compulsive disorder (OCD)
    in an adolescent   77
    The Question: When should medications other than selective serotonin
    reuptake inhibitors (SSRIs) be used, and how should clomipramine be
    dosed and monitored in pediatric OCD?
    The Psychopharmacological Dilemma: The decision to move beyond
    SSRIs in treating adolescents with OCD is difficult for many clinicians.
    In addition, some clinicians experience trepidation about initiating
    clomipramine and using therapeutic drug-monitoring strategies

7   **The Case:** Struggles in the second grade: attention-deficit hyperactivity
    disorder (ADHD) in a child   95
    The Question: When should nonstimulant medications be used in
    pediatric patients with ADHD?
    The Psychopharmacological Dilemma: When to add nonstimulants
    to stimulant medications in children with ADHD is unclear for many
    clinicians. Furthermore, how to choose a nonstimulant, based on the
    mechanism of action, is a source of uncertainty

8   **The Case:** From prodrome to psychosis: early-onset schizophrenia   119
    The Question: What constitutes an evidence-based work-up for children
    and adolescents who have prodromal psychotic symptoms or are
    experiencing a first psychotic episode?
    The Psychopharmacological Dilemma: The approach to the young patient
    with a possible psychotic disorder is unclear for many clinicians, and
    varies considerably in practice. How specific factors should be considered
    and what interventions should be used are common questions for
    clinicians

9   **The Case:** Too much, too little, or just right? Lithium dosing in
    an adolescent   137
    The Question: How is lithium dosed differently in adolescents
    compared with adults?

The Psychopharmacological Dilemma: Approaches to monitoring and dosing lithium in pediatric patients differ substantially from the strategies used in adults. This confusion often complicates lithium use and monitoring in adolescents, and represents a significant barrier to using lithium

10 **The Case:** Tic, tic, tic: motor and vocal tics in a boy   155
The Question: What is the role of pharmacotherapy in Tourette syndrome?
The Psychopharmacological Dilemma: Although tics can be common in children and adolescents, choosing among pharmacological approaches to management of Tourette syndrome is complex

11 **The Case:** How slow can you go? Selective serotonin reuptake inhibitor (SSRI) withdrawal and discontinuation in an adolescent   173
The Questions: When should SSRIs be discontinued in adolescents? How should SSRIs be discontinued in adolescents? What are the strategies for managing SSRI-related discontinuation symptoms?
The Psychopharmacological Dilemma: Stopping SSRIs after remission is certainly a goal of treating adolescents with depressive and anxiety disorders, although clinicians vary in their thresholds for discontinuing these medications, and disagree about approaches to discontinuation of SSRIs

12 **The Case:** The adolescent who doesn't eat: anorexia nervosa in an adolescent   185
The Questions: What is the "medical" workup in a child or adolescent with an eating disorder? When should a child or adolescent with anorexia nervosa be hospitalized? What is the psychopharmacological approach to treating eating disorders and related behaviors in children and adolescents?
The Psychopharmacological Dilemma: Eating disorders can create anxiety for many clinicians as a result of confusion related to the medical workup for these patients, treatment decisions, and special considerations related to using pharmacotherapy in this population

13 **The Case:** High or higher antidepressant concentrations? Cannabis-related drug interactions in an adolescent   203
The Questions: How does cannabis affect outcomes in adolescents with depressive disorders? What is the impact of cannabis on selective serotonin reuptake inhibitor (SSRI) pharmacokinetics in adolescents?
The Psychopharmacological Dilemma: Cannabis use is increasingly common in adolescents, yet the pharmacological implications are unclear for many clinicians

14   **The Case:** The boy whose bed was always wet: nocturnal enuresis
     in a child   223
     The Question: What is the role of pharmacotherapy in managing
     nocturnal enuresis in children?
     The Psychopharmacological Dilemma: Views on when and how to use
     pharmacotherapy in children with nocturnal enuresis vary considerably
     among clinicians

15   **The Case:** Counting sheep and counting treatment trials: insomnia
     disorder in an adolescent   233
     The Question: What is the evidence-based approach to addressing
     insomnia in adolescents?
     The Psychopharmacological Dilemma: Managing sleep-related
     problems in adolescents – particularly in those with anxiety and/or
     depressive disorders – is complicated and requires an understanding of
     developmental and pharmacological principles

16   **The Case:** Second-generation antipsychotics/mixed dopamine–serotonin
     receptor agonists (SGAs), side effects, and the autism spectrum:
     SGA-related side effects in a boy with autism spectrum disorder (ASD)   259
     The Questions: What is the evidence-based workup for a child with
     ASD? Which SGAs have evidence for specific symptoms in children and
     adolescents with ASD and how should they be diagnosed? How should
     tolerability of SGAs be monitored in children and adolescents with ASD?
     The Psychopharmacological Dilemma: Managing SGAs in children
     and adolescents with ASD can be complicated, but awareness of
     pharmacological/pharmacogenetic principles can help to predict specific
     tolerability concerns

17   **The Case:** The "standard treatment" is earning a "D": treatment-resistant
     schizophrenia   279
     The Question: When and how should clozapine be used in older
     adolescents with treatment-resistant schizophrenia?
     The Psychopharmacological Dilemma: When to use clozapine and how
     to dose and monitor its use is a source of debate and uncertainty for
     many clinicians, yet the evidence – largely based on decades of studies in
     adults – suggests that this agent has response rates substantially higher
     than those for other second-generation antipsychotics (SGAs) in patients
     with treatment-resistant schizophrenia

18   **The Case:** Symptoms, side effects, or both? Selective serotonin
     reuptake inhibitor (SSRI) tolerability and physical symptoms in an
     anxious adolescent   301

The Questions: How should SSRIs be cross-titrated in adolescents? What is mechanism-based inhibition, and how does it relate to the pharmacokinetics of some SSRIs in adolescents?

The Psychopharmacological Dilemma: SSRIs are commonly associated with tremendous improvement in adolescents with anxiety and depressive disorders; however, they may be associated with side effects that require medication changes. Cross-titrating SSRIs requires an understanding of both pharmacodynamic and pharmacokinetic principles

Appendices   323
Index of case studies   333
Index of drug names   343

Introduction

Following the success of the third volume of *Case Studies* in 2021, we are very pleased to present a fourth collection of new clinical cases. This collection of cases comes from Dr. Strawn's clinics and consultations, from his research in clinical pharmacology, and from discussions with his talented collaborators, including pharmacologists, nurse practitioners, psychologists, and fellow child and adolescent psychiatrists. *Stahl's Essential Psychopharmacology* started in 1996 as a textbook (currently in its fifth edition) on how psychotropic medications work. It expanded to a companion Prescriber's Guide in 2005 (currently in its seventh edition) on how to prescribe psychotropic medications. In 2008, a website was added (**stahlonline.cambridge.org**) with both of these books available online in combination with several more, including an illustrated series of books covering specialty topics in psychopharmacology. The *Case Studies* show how to apply the concepts presented in these previous books to real patients in a clinical practice setting.

Why a case book? For practitioners, it is necessary to know the science and application of psychopharmacology – namely, both the mechanism of action of psychotropic medications and the evidence-based data on how to prescribe them – but this is not sufficient to become a master clinician. Many patients are beyond the data and are excluded from randomized controlled trials. Thus, a true clinical expert also needs to develop the art of psychopharmacology: namely, how to listen, educate, destigmatize, mix psychotherapy with medications, and use intuition to select and combine medications. The art of psychopharmacology is especially important when confronting the frequent situations where there is no evidence on which to base a clinical decision.

What do you do when there is no evidence? The short answer is to combine the science with the art of psychopharmacology. Being able to combine science and art and to adapt findings from studies in adults is critical for clinicians treating children and adolescents. However, the successful psychiatric clinician working with children and adolescents must not only integrate science and art but also do so with a strong background in developmental pharmacology, attention to development, learning disorders, and family dynamics. The best way to learn this approach is probably by seeing individual patients and their families. Here we hope you will join us and peer over our shoulders to observe these complex cases from our child and adolescent psychiatric clinics and consultations. Each case is anonymized in identifying details, but incorporates real case outcomes that are not fictionalized. Sometimes more than one case is combined into a single case. Hopefully, you will recognize many of these patients as similar to those you have seen in your own practice (although they will not be exactly the same patient, as the identifying historical details are changed here to comply with disclosure standards, and many patients can look very much like many other patients you know, which is why you may find this teaching approach effective for your clinical practice).

We have presented cases from our clinical practice for many years and in courses (especially at the annual Neuroscience Education Institute Psychopharmacology Congress). Over the years, we have been fortunate to have many young child and adolescent psychiatrists and other trainees from our universities, and indeed from all over the world, sit in on our practices to observe these cases, and now we attempt to bring this information to you in the form of a fourth case book.

The cases are presented in a novel written format in order to follow consultations over time, with different categories of information designated by different background colors and explanatory icons. For those of you familiar with *The Prescriber's Guide*, this layout will be recognizable. Included in the case book, however, are many unique sections as well; for example, presenting what was on our minds at various points during the management of the case, and also questions along the way for you to ask yourself in order to develop an action plan. Additionally, these cases incorporate ideas from the recent changes in the maintenance of certification standards by the American Board of Psychiatry and Neurology, for those of you interested in recertification in psychiatry. Thus, there is a section on Performance in Practice (called here "Confessions of a psychopharmacologist"). There is a short section at the end of several cases looking back and seeing what could have been done better in retrospect. Another section of most cases is a short psychopharmacology lesson or tutorial, called the "Two-minute tutorial," with background information, tables, and figures from literature relevant to the case in hand. Medications are listed by their generic and brand names for ease of learning. Indexes are included at the back of the book for your convenience. Lists of icons and abbreviations are provided in the front of the book. Finally, this fourth collection updates the reader on the newest psychotropic medications and their uses, and adopts the language of *DSM-5*.

The case-based approach is how this book attempts to complement "evidence-based prescribing" from other books in the *Essential Psychopharmacology* series, plus the literature, with "prescribing-based evidence" derived from empiric experience. It is certainly important to know the data from randomized controlled trials, but after knowing all this information, case-based clinical experience supplements those data. The old saying that applies here is that wisdom is what you learn *after* you know it all, and the same can be said for studying cases after seeing the data.

A note of caution: we are not so naïve as to think that there are not potential pitfalls to the centuries-old tradition of case-based teaching. Thus, we think it is a good idea to point some of them out here in order to try to avoid these traps. Do not ignore the "law of small numbers" by basing broad predictions on narrow samples or even a single case.

Do not ignore the fact that if something is easy to recall, particularly when associated with a significant emotional event, we tend to think it happens more often than it does.

Do not forget the recency effect, namely, the tendency to think that something that has just been observed happens more often than it does.

According to editorialists,[1] when moving away from evidence-based medicine to case-based medicine, it is also important to avoid:
- eloquence- or elegance-based medicine
- vehemence-based medicine
- providence-based medicine
- diffidence-based medicine
- nervousness-based medicine
- confidence-based medicine.

We have been counseled by colleagues and trainees that perhaps the most important pitfall for us to try to avoid in this book is "eminence-based medicine," and to remember specifically that:
- radiance of gray hair is not proportional to an understanding of the facts
- eloquence, smoothness of the tongue, and sartorial elegance cannot change reality
- qualifications and past accomplishments do not signify privileged access to the truth
- experts almost always have conflicts of interest
- clinical acumen is not measured in frequent flier miles.

Thus, it is with all humility as practicing psychiatrists that we invite you to walk a mile in our shoes; experience the fascination, the disappointments, the thrills, and the learnings that result from observing cases in the real world.

Jeffrey R. Strawn, MD

Stephen M. Stahl, MD, PhD

[1] Isaccs, D. and Fitzgerald, D. Seven alternatives to evidence-based medicine. *British Medical Journal* 1999; 319: 1618.

List of icons

	Pre- and post test self-assessment question; question
	Patient evaluation on intake
	Psychiatric history
ABC	Social and personal history
	Medical history
	Family history
Rx	Medication history
	Current medications

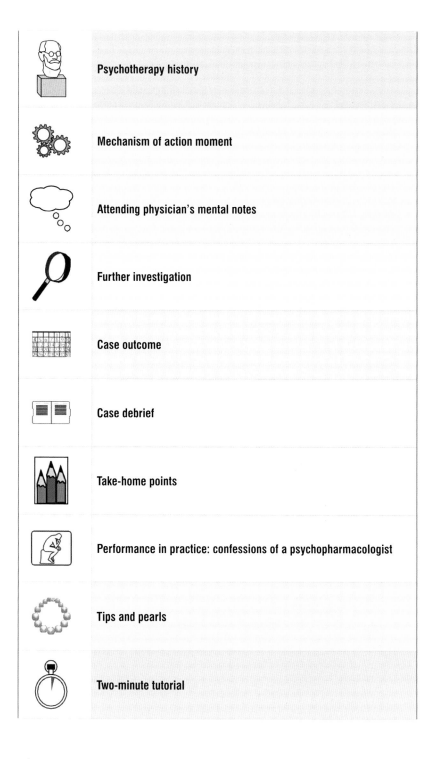

Psychotherapy history

Mechanism of action moment

Attending physician's mental notes

Further investigation

Case outcome

Case debrief

Take-home points

Performance in practice: confessions of a psychopharmacologist

Tips and pearls

Two-minute tutorial

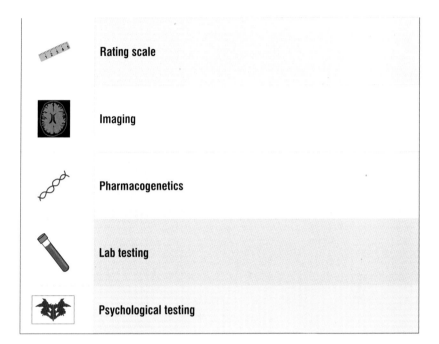

Rating scale

Imaging

Pharmacogenetics

Lab testing

Psychological testing

Abbreviations

2-AG	2-arachidonoylglycerol	BED	binge eating disorder
5-HT	serotonin	BMI	body mass index
AACAP	American Academy of	BN	bulimia nervosa
	Child and Adolescent	BUN	blood urea nitrogen
	Psychiatry	BZD	benzodiazepine
AAP	American Academy of	cAMP	cyclic adenosine
	Pediatrics		monophosphate
ABA	applied behavioral	$CB_{1/2}$	cannabinoid-1/-2
	analysis		receptors
ACh	acetylcholine	CBC	complete blood count
ACMG	American College of	CBD	cannabidiol
	Medical Genetics	CBT	cognitive behavior
ACR	albumin to creatinine		therapy
	ratio	CBT-I	cognitive behavior
ACTH	adrenocorticotropic		therapy for insomnia
	hormone	CBIT	Comprehensive
ADH	antidiuretic hormone		Behavioral Intervention
ADHD	attention-deficit		for Tics
	hyperactivity disorder	CKD	chronic kidney disease
ADOS	Autism Diagnostic	CNS	central nervous
	Observation Scale		system
AIMS	Abnormal Involuntary	COPD	chronic obstructive
	Movement Scale		pulmonary disease
AMPA	α-amino-3-hydroxy-	CPT	Cognitive Processing
	5-methyl-4-		Therapy
	isoxazolepropionic acid	CRF	corticotropin-releasing
AN	anorexia nervosa		factor
ANC	absolute neutrophil	CRH	corticotropin-releasing
	count		hormone
AN-P	anorexia nervosa binge	CRHQ	Children's Sleep Habits
	purge type		Questionnaire
AP	advanced placement	CSSRS	Columbia–Suicide
ASD	autism spectrum		Severity Rating Scale
	disorder	CT	computed tomography
AUC	area under the curve	CY-BOCS	Children's Yale-Brown
AV	atrioventricular		Obsessive-Compulsive
AVP	arginine vasopressin		Scale
BD	Block Design	DA	dopamine

dACC	dorsal anterior cingulate cortex	HIV	human immunodeficiency virus
DAT	dopamine transporter	HPA	hypothalamic–pituitary–adrenal
DD	developmental disabilities	HPG	hypothalamic–pituitary–gonadal
DDAVP	desmopressin	HRT	Habit Reversal Therapy
DHA	docosahexaenoic acid	ICSD	International Classification of Sleep Disorders
DLPFC	dorsolateral prefrontal cortex		
DMDD	disruptive mood dysregulation disorder	IEP	Individualized Education Plan
DSM-5	*Diagnostic and Statistical Manual of Mental Disorders*, 5th edn.	IPT	Interpersonal Psychotherapy
		IPT-A	Interpersonal Psychotherapy for Adolescents
EKG	electrocardiogram		
EEG	electroencephalogram	IUGR	in-utero growth restriction
eGFR	estimated glomerular filtration rate	IV	intravenous
EMUO	early morning urine osmolality	LDT	laterodorsal tegmentum
EPS	extrapyramidal symptoms	MAOI	monoamine oxidase inhibitor
FDA	U.S. Food and Drug Administration	MAP	mean arterial blood pressure
FIR	fluid intake record		
FRI	Fluid Reasoning Index	MBT-A	Mindfulness-Based Therapy for Adolescents
FSIQ	Full-scale Intelligence Quotient	mCPP	methylchloropiperazine
GABA	γ-aminobutyric acid	MDD	major depressive disorder
GAD	generalized anxiety disorder		
GAI	General Ability Index	MECP2	methyl CpG binding protein-2
GERD	gastroesophageal reflux disease	MGH	Massachusetts General Hospital
GFR	glomerular filtration rate		
GLP-1	glucagon-like peptide-1	mGluR	metabotropic glutamate receptor
glu/Glu	glutamine		
GnRH	gonadotropic releasing hormone	MMPI-A	Minnesota Multiphasic Personality Inventory-Adolescent version
GPA	grade point average		
H_1	histamine-1 receptor	MPH	methylphenidate
HA	histamine	MRI	magnetic resonance imaging
HCN	hyperpolarization-activated cyclic nucleotide-gated		
		mTOR	mammalian target of rapamycin

NAC	*N*-acetylcysteine	PSG	polysomnography
NAMI	National Alliance on Mental Health	PSI	Processing Speed Index
NSAID	nonsteroidal anti-inflammatories	PTEN	phosphatase and tensin homolog
NDRI	norepinephrine–dopamine reuptake inhibitor	PTSD	posttraumatic stress disorder
NE	norepinephrine	QIDS	Quick Inventory of Depressive Symptomatology
NET	norepinephrine transporter	QIDS-SR	Quick Inventory of Depressive Symptomatology – Self-Report
NICU	neonatal intensive care unit		
NMDA	*N*-methyl-ᴅ-aspartate	QTc	corrected QT interval
NSF	National Sleep Foundation	SCARED	Screen for Child Anxiety-Related Emotional Disorders
OCD	obsessive compulsive disorder	SCN	suprachiasmatic nucleus
ODD	oppositional defiant disorder	SERT	serotonin transporter
OGT	oxygenated glycerol triester	SGA	second-generation antipsychotic/mixed dopamine–serotonin receptor agonist
OROS	osmotic controlled-release oral delivery system	SNRI	serotonin–norepinephrine reuptake inhibitor
PAI-A	Personality Assessment Inventory for Adolescents	SRI	serotonin reuptake inhibition
		SSRI	selective serotonin reuptake inhibitor
PANSS	Positive and Negative Symptoms of Schizophrenia	T_3	triiodothyronine
		T_4	thyroxine
PET	positron emission tomography	TAT	Thematic Apperception Test
PFC	prefrontal cortex	TCA	tricyclic antidepressant
PHQ-9	Patient Health Questionnaire-9	TF-CBT	trauma-focused cognitive behavior therapy
PLM	periodic limb movement	THC	Δ9-tetrahydrocannabinol
PLMi	Periodic Limb Movement Index	TMS	transcranial magnetic stimulation
PMDD	premenstrual dysphoric disorder	TORDIA	Treatment of SSRI-Resistant Depression in Adolescents study
PO	oral		
PPT	pedunculopontine tegmentum	TSH	thyroid-stimulating hormone

UCLA	University of California Los Angeles	VP	Visual Puzzles
V_2	vasopressin-2 receptor	VSCC	voltage-sensitive calcium channel
VCI	Verbal Comprehension Index	VSI	Visual-Spatial Index
		VTA	ventral tegmental area
VEGF	vascular endothelial growth factor	WISC(-IV/V)	Wechsler Intelligence Scale for Children (4th/5th edition)
VLPFC	ventrolateral prefrontal cortex	WMI	Working Memory Index
VMAT2	vesicular monoamine transporter-2	YMRS	Young Mania Rating Scale

Case 1: The salutatorian who couldn't speak: selective serotonin reuptake inhibitor (SSRI)-refractory anxiety in an adolescent

The Question: What do you do when anxiety fails to respond to multiple SSRIs and cognitive–behavioral therapy (CBT)?

The Psychopharmacological Dilemma: Whether and when to add adjunctive benzodiazepines remains unclear for many clinicians

Pretest self-assessment question

Which of the following represents an evidence-based intervention for a patient with treatment-resistant anxiety?

A. Duloxetine (Cymbalta)
B. High-dose escitalopram (Lexapro)
C. Adjunctive clonazepam (Klonopin)
D. Guanfacine (Tenex, Intuniv)
E. All of the above

Answer: C (Adjunctive clonazepam, Klonopin)

Patient evaluation on intake

- A 17-year-old African American high-school senior with severe social anxiety
- Severe social anxiety disorder and possible generalized anxiety disorder
- Her social anxiety symptoms have led to significant avoidance, and this avoidance and anticipation of catastrophic social criticism has perpetuated her anxiety, thus creating a vicious cycle
- There are concerns that family factors may galvanize her anxiety; these concerns include accommodation
- She readily acknowledges the excessive nature of these fears, yet still has some degree of belief in them and certainly experiences subjective fear about them
- She recognizes that her chronic anxiety interferes with her life, is preventing her from enjoying her senior year and her time with friends, and could threaten her success at college

Psychiatric history

- Social anxiety symptoms began when the patient was in the fifth grade
- In middle school, she struggled to do group work, was anxious about going out with friends, and could not spend the night at friends' houses

- In high school, her social anxiety intensified. She dreaded being called on in class, or having to give presentations, and she felt so uncomfortable in the cafeteria that she ate her lunch in the school guidance counselor's office. She avoided going with her family to restaurants, and could not order her own food because she feared that she might say something incorrectly or that she would embarrass herself
- Despite her anxiety, she excelled academically and was the class salutatorian. However, she would often think about the salutatorian's public address at graduation, and this caused her significant distress
- Initial insomnia with a sleep latency of 1–2 hours, which is worse on school nights. She feels fatigued and has difficulty concentrating, but denies depressed mood
- When the family goes to restaurants, her parents frequently order her food. At larger family events, such as Christmas at her aunt's home, her parents arrange for her to sit in the car or to go to a quiet room, away from the family, if her anxiety becomes overwhelming
- Her parents are very concerned about her anxiety and about her being able to attend college. Of note, she has been accepted at three colleges, including her "dream school," which is located 5 hours away from her parents' home

Social and personal history

- Lives with her mother and father
- She is in the 12th grade at an all-girls high school and excels academically, although her anxiety makes some engagement with teachers difficult
- She is not currently in a relationship
- There is no history of abuse or trauma

Medical history

- Delivered at 40 weeks to a 37-year-old mother and 40-year-old father
- Normal developmental milestones, although separation anxiety persisted until age 8–9
- Seasonal allergies for which she takes cetirizine 10 mg daily
- Chronic recurrent abdominal pain, which is worse on school days

Family history

- Father with panic disorder and generalized anxiety disorder
- Mother with social anxiety and major depressive disorder
- Maternal grandmother with anxiety, posttraumatic stress disorder (PTSD), and depression

Medication history

- Currently treated with escitalopram (Lexapro) 20 mg daily (3 months)
- No response to sertraline, which was titrated to 200 mg daily (4 months)
- Bupropion extended-release formulation (Wellbutrin SR) 100 mg twice daily worsened her anxiety and initial insomnia as a tremor was associated with it; it was discontinued within 2 weeks of initiation
- Fluoxetine 10 mg daily was discontinued after 2 weeks secondary to feeling "jittery," worsening anxiety, and two symptom-limited panic attacks
- Divalproex extended-release formulation (Depakote ER) 500 mg twice daily was discontinued because of nausea
- Quetiapine (Seroquel) 50 mg every night at bedtime, which was associated with sedation

Current medications

- Cetirizine (Zyrtec) 10 mg every morning
- Escitalopram (Lexapro) 20 mg every morning

Psychotherapy history

- She worked with an "art therapist" weekly for 2–3 months when she was a junior in high school. She enjoyed this therapy, but her anxiety failed to improve
- Thereafter, she transitioned to a cognitive–behavioral therapist and worked primarily on her thoughts and "anticipation of what might happen"
- Her anxiety persisted despite both therapies

Further investigation

Is there anything else that you would like to know about the patient? What about details related to her prior medication trials? What are the side effects that she experienced with fluoxetine (Prozac) and bupropion SR (Wellbutrin SR)?

- She experienced both symptoms of activation (e.g. restlessness, worsening anxiety, "jitteriness") with fluoxetine, and a tremor as well as worsening insomnia with low-dose bupropion extended-release formulation (100 mg twice daily)
- Side effects of both medications emerged relatively early during treatment

What about additional physical symptoms and vital signs?

- No reports of depressed mood, guilt, anhedonia, or suicidal ideation
- Vital signs are within normal limits; her body mass index (BMI) is in the 75th percentile for age and sex
- There is no heat or cold intolerance, recent weight loss, or dysmenorrhea
- She denies cardiac symptoms, including palpitations

Attending physician's mental notes: initial psychiatric evaluation

- This patient has severe social anxiety disorder and some features of generalized anxiety disorder
- Her symptoms are in the severe range, and there is a suggestion of medication resistance
- There are also concerns related to *accommodation*
  - Her parents find it difficult not to attend to their daughter's anxiety and inadvertently reinforce her anxiety and catastrophic reactions. Over time, this has actively reduced her distress by facilitating avoidance. This is intuitively understandable, as accommodation (i.e. attention to anxious behavior and facilitating avoidance) perpetuates anxiety
  - From a family standpoint, effective interventions will require not only treating the patient's anxiety but also helping her parents to re-engage their daughter in life activities, rather than reinforcing avoidance, as well as reinforcing coping and tolerance of anxiety distress rather than dysregulated and anxious behavior
- Regarding side effects of prior medication trials, it is noteworthy that this patient had poor tolerability – within a very short time – with two medications that are metabolized primarily by CYP2D6. The side effects (activation with fluoxetine, and anxiety/tremor with bupropion) may be related to blood levels (i.e. exposure). This raises the possibility that the patient is a poor CYP2D6 metabolizer. Also, consistent with this notion, side effects from both medications emerged early during treatment

Question

This patient has had two psychotherapy trials and trials of several SSRIs, although her social anxiety symptoms have persisted and are severe. Which of the following would be your next step?

- Discontinue escitalopram (Lexapro) and begin duloxetine (Cymbalta)
- Titrate escitalopram (Lexapro) from 20 mg daily to 30 mg daily

- Begin adjunctive clonazepam (Klonopin)
- Reattempt a trial of an adjunctive mixed dopamine serotonin receptor antagonist
- Initiate a trial of high-frequency left dorsolateral prefrontal cortex transcranial magnetic stimulation (TMS) for 6 weeks

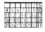

Case outcome: first interim follow-up (week 4)

- At the patient's last visit, escitalopram was increased from 20 mg to 30 mg daily
- She reports excellent adherence and no side effects
- There has been a slight decrease in her anxiety, but overall this is only about a 20% improvement

Attending physician's mental notes: first interim follow-up (week 4)

- Given the patient's minimal response to two SSRIs that are metabolized by CYP2C19 (sertraline and escitalopram), and the fact that she is African American, there is a reasonable chance that she is an ultra-rapid metabolizer (i.e. she has one or two *17 alleles for the *CYP2C19* gene)
- Therefore, the decision was made to increase escitalopram from 20 mg to 30 mg. If she is an ultra-rapid metabolizer, this would produce blood levels comparable to those in a normal metabolizer treated with 20 mg daily (Strawn et al. 2018b)
- However, this failed to produce significant improvement in her anxiety symptoms

Question

This patient has had two psychotherapy trials and also trials of several SSRIs. Titration of escitalopram to 30 mg produced a mild improvement, but her social anxiety symptoms have persisted and are severe. Which of the following would be your next step?

- Discontinue escitalopram (Lexapro) and begin duloxetine (Cymbalta)
- Begin adjunctive clonazepam (Klonopin)
- Re-attempt a trial of an adjunctive mixed dopamine serotonin receptor antagonist
- Initiate a trial of high-frequency left dorsolateral prefrontal cortex TMS for 6 weeks

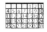

Case outcome: second interim follow-up (week 8)

- After beginning clonazepam 0.5 mg twice daily, the patient's anxiety rapidly improved
- She re-engaged in psychotherapy with a new therapist
- Following a brief scheduled phone check-in, clonazepam (Klonopin) was titrated to 0.5 mg every morning and every afternoon, with 1 mg every night at bedtime

Attending physician's mental notes: second interim follow-up (week 8)

- After beginning clonazepam, the patient's anxiety rapidly improved and there were no tolerability concerns
- Increasing the evening dose to address her persistent initial insomnia is a reasonable option, although the prudent psychopharmacologist will monitor for early-morning sedation, especially if the patient drives herself to school, and also depending on whether she has an attentionally demanding first-period class
- The fact that the patient re-engaged in psychotherapy is important, although the psychopharmacologist will need to collaborate closely with the psychotherapist. There is concern that the earlier psychotherapeutic strategies were too cognitively focused and did not include sufficient exposure work. Exposure work is the key ingredient for child and adolescent anxiety (Peris et al. 2015, 2017)
- The psychotherapist will also need to work with the patient's family to address accommodation within the family, which can perpetuate adolescent anxiety (Peris et al. 2012)

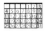

Case outcome: third interim follow-up (week 12)

- The patient's sleep has normalized, and her anxiety symptoms are in remission
- Psychotherapy is going well, although she notes that the exposures, such as ordering her own food at a drive-thru, have been difficult from time to time
- Her psychotherapist further reports that she is doing well with session homework, following session structure, and has developed an exposure hierarchy. The psychotherapist shared with the treating psychiatrist that during the patient's last session they completed two in-session exposure tasks which involved calling several restaurants for directions. They discussed the patient's expectation that she is "inconveniencing others" and the fact that these exposures have been associated with a clear violation of expectations, which were discussed

- She feels increasingly motivated and committed to taking better care of herself, and denies side effects
- She is exercising regularly and has begun a "metabolism-boosting diet" that was featured on a national talk show
  - Her diet consists of unlimited vegetables at lunch and dinner, a serving of protein at two meals per day, and half a grapefruit at every meal
- However, over the past 3–4 weeks she has been feeling tired, and she fell asleep twice while at school, after lunch

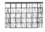

Attending physician's mental notes: third interim follow-up (week 12)

- The psychopharmacologist was initially concerned about non-adherence, given the abrupt onset of symptoms; however, a careful history revealed the cause of these new side effects to be grapefruit
- Grapefruit significantly affects the pharmacokinetics of most benzodiazepines (and other medications that are metabolized by CYP3A4). In fact, grapefruit increases peak benzodiazepine blood levels (C_{MAX}) by almost 60%, increases the time to maximum concentration (t_{MAX}) by 80%, and boosts absorption by up to 50%
- The psychopharmacologist also considered the possibility that the patient's tiredness was related to antihistaminergic effects, which can occur at high doses with escitalopram. However, this was less likely given that these were not present previously
- The psychopharmacologist enquired too about the possible addition of a proton pump inhibitor for the patient's indigestion, which could have affected escitalopram levels, resulting in a "new" escitalopram-related side effect

Case outcome: fourth interim follow-up (week 16)

- The patient is encouraged by her weight loss and feels better; she wishes to continue the "Grapefruit Diet." Therefore her clonazepam dose is reduced by 50%, with a contemporaneous improvement in tiredness
- She agrees to speak with her psychopharmacologist when she changes her diet, so that her benzodiazepine regimen can be re-evaluated

Take-home points

- Anxiety disorders often begin in childhood and, if untreated, can result in accumulated impairment that puts adolescents and young adults at risk for poor adaptation and maladaptive behaviors

- In children and adolescents, anxiety behavior may be reinforced and may thus recur when it leads to successful avoidance of anxiety triggers. This cycle worsens when parents inadvertently reinforce this behavior by accommodating avoidance behavior
- Benzodiazepines, although not first-line treatments for anxiety, have an important adjunctive role, particularly in patients with a partial response to "first-line" interventions
- When selecting benzodiazepines, consider risk factors for substance use disorders and the pharmacology of the benzodiazepine (e.g. lipophilicity, half-life, etc.)
- Interactions, especially CYP3A4 interactions, are particularly important for benzodiazepines

Performance in practice: confessions of a psychopharmacologist

- A benzodiazepine might have been tried earlier, particularly given that the patient is an adolescent, there is a lack of risk factors for abuse, and she has previously had a trial of another CYP2C19-metabolized SSRI (sertraline) at a high dose
- Since drinking grapefruit juice in significant quantities is uncommon in this age group, the patient's clinician did not discuss it with her. If such a discussion had taken place earlier on it could have prevented this interaction

Tips and pearls

- SSRIs and psychotherapy remain the mainstay of treatment of pediatric anxiety disorders (Locher et al. 2017; Strawn et al. 2018b, 2021)
- Meta-analyses reveal that SSRIs produce greater and faster improvement compared with serotonin–norepinephrine reuptake inhibitors (SNRIs) in children and adolescents with generalized, separation, and social anxiety disorders (Figure 1.1). Additionally, in these meta-analyses, SSRI-related improvement occurs early in the course of antidepressant treatment (week 2 for both SSRIs and SNRIs). In fact, approximately 50% of the treatment-related improvement, at week 12, occurred by week 4 of treatment (Strawn et al. 2018b)
- For adolescents with social anxiety disorder, some suggest treatment with an SSRI prior to initiating psychotherapy, based on

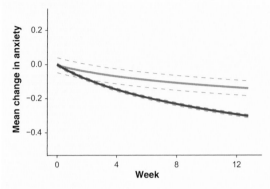

Figure 1.1 Response trajectory in antidepressant-treated pediatric patients with generalized, separation, and social anxiety disorders. Green and blue lines represent SNRIs and SSRIs. *Reproduced from* Strawn et al. (2018b).

> data from the Child/Adolescent Anxiety Multimodal Study (Compton et al. 2014; Walkup et al. 2008)

- Benzodiazepines are often forgotten, but they represent a powerful tool for adjunctively managing anxiety, particularly in the "right" patient

Mechanism of action moment

- All benzodiazepines share a common mechanism of action but vary in their pharmacological characteristics (Strawn and Stimpfl 2023)
- Benzodiazepines are positive allosteric modulators of γ-aminobutyric acid A (GABA$_A$) receptors. The combination of benzodiazepines and GABA increases the frequency of opening of the inhibitory chloride channels (although it does not increase either the conductance of chloride across the individual channels or the length of time for which the channel is open) (Figure 1.2)
- It has been hypothesized that benzodiazepines modulate excessive amygdala output during fear responses in patients with anxiety disorders. This amygdala activity is theoretically reduced by enhancing the phasic inhibitory actions of benzodiazepine positive allosteric modulators at postsynaptic GABA$_A$ receptors within the amygdala to blunt fear outputs (Stahl et al. 2021)
- Benzodiazepines can be categorized based on their lipophilicity, and these differences affect their clinical profile (Figure 1.3)

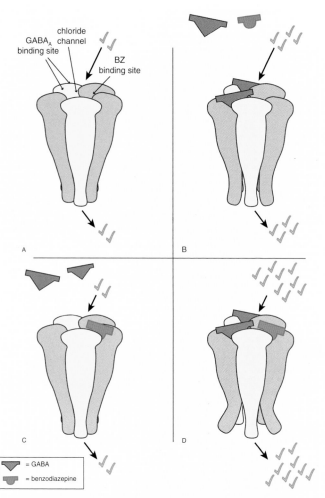

Figure 1.2 Positive allosteric modulation of GABA$_A$ receptors.
(A) Benzodiazepine (BZD)-sensitive GABA$_A$ receptors, like the one shown here, consist of five subunits with a central chloride channel, and have binding sites not only for GABA but also for positive allosteric modulators (e.g. benzodiazepines). (B) When GABA binds to its sites on the GABA$_A$ receptor, it increases the frequency of opening of the chloride channel, and thus allows more chloride ions to pass through. (C) When a positive allosteric modulator such as benzodiazepine binds to the GABA$_A$ receptor in the absence of GABA, it has no effect on the chloride channel. (D) When a positive allosteric modulator such as benzodiazepine binds to the GABA$_A$ receptor in the presence of GABA, it causes the channel to open even more frequently than when GABA alone is present. Reproduced from *Stahl's Essential Psychopharmacology*, 2021.

Highly Lipophilic	Less Lipophilic
• Enter the brain more quickly • "Turn on" the effect promptly • "Turn off" the effect more quickly and disappear quickly into fat • More intense effect	• Less lipophilic BZDs (e.g. lorazepam) produce slower effect • Provide more sustained relief, despite a shorter half-life • Less intense effect

Figure 1.3

Two-minute tutorial: benzodiazepines

- Despite the fact that trials of benzodiazepines in adults with anxiety disorders consistently demonstrate benefit (Strawn et al. 2018a; Williams et al. 2017), benzodiazepine trials in pediatric patients have produced mixed results, and double-blind placebo-controlled trials and meta-analyses do not reveal differences between benzodiazepines and placebo (Dobson et al. 2019). However, these studies were small and included very young children and high doses of short-acting benzodiazepines (e.g. alprazolam)
- In these pediatric benzodiazepine trials, the poor tolerability – particularly in younger patients, unlike the patient described in this case – may be related to age-related pharmacodynamic factors
- Importantly, the pharmacodynamics of the GABA receptor in children and adolescents differ from those in adults, with adult expression/function not being achieved until age 14–17½ years for subcortical regions and 18–22 years for cortical regions (Figure 1.4), although adult expression of GABA receptors occurs slightly earlier in girls than in boys (Chugani et al. 2001)
- Interactions are particularly important with benzodiazepines, and these interactions are often overlooked
- Clinically significant interactions for benzodiazepines include grapefruit juice (CYP3A4 inhibition), food, and antacids (Figure 1.5)
- Grapefruit juice boosts the peak benzodiazepine blood level (C_{MAX}) by almost 60%, increases the time to maximum concentration (t_{MAX}) by 80%, and significantly increases absorption by up to 50% (Figure 1.5)
- Food slows down benzodiazepine absorption, although it does not alter the total absorption (Figure 1.6)
- Antacids decrease the peak benzodiazepine blood concentrations (C_{MAX}) and the rate of absorption; medication requires longer to reach maximum concentration (t_{MAX}) (Greenblatt et al. 1980) (Figure 1.6)

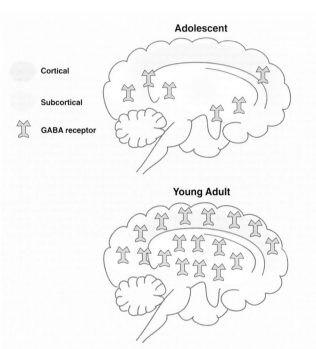

Figure 1.4 Benzodiazepine receptor expression changes significantly during development. This difference may affect the tolerability of these medications in children compared with adolescents and adults.

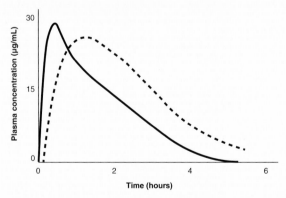

Figure 1.5 Grapefruit juice significantly alters the pharmacokinetics of several benzodiazepines. Dashed and solid lines represent diazepam with and without grapefruit juice, respectively. In this study, administration of the benzodiazepine with grapefruit juice increased absorption by 50% and altered the time to maximum concentration (t_{MAX}) by 80%. Adapted from Kupferschmidt et al. (1995).

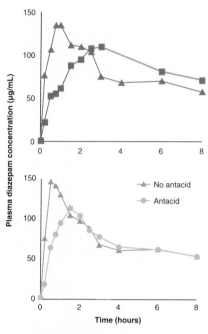

Figure 1.6 Food and antacids can significantly affect the pharmacoki-netics of benzodiazepines. Red squares and purple triangles represent diazepam administration with and without food, respectively.

Post test question

Which of the following represents an evidence-based intervention for a patient with treatment-resistant anxiety?

A. Duloxetine (Cymbalta)
B. High-dose escitalopram (Lexapro)
C. Adjunctive clonazepam (Klonopin)
D. Guanfacine (Tenex, Intuniv)
E. All of the above

Answer: C (Adjunctive clonazepam, Klonopin)

Duloxetine is approved by the U.S. Food and Drug Administration (FDA) to treat generalized anxiety disorder in adolescents (Strawn et al. 2015); however, SNRIs are less efficacious compared with SSRIs in pediatric anxiety disorders (Strawn et al. 2018b). High-dose escitalopram, in and of itself, is unlikely to help with refractory anxiety disorders, and it places pediatric patients at risk of side effects, particularly those who are CYP2C19 poor metabolizers

(Aldrich et al. 2019; Strawn et al. 2019). Guanfacine extended-release formulation has been examined in one small trial of children and adolescents with generalized, separation, and social anxiety disorders, and produced a greater response compared with placebo (Strawn et al. 2017), but it has not been studied in pediatric patients with SSRI-refractory anxiety disorders.

References

1. Aldrich, S. L., Poweleit, E. A., Prows, C. A., et al. Influence of CYP2C19 metabolizer status on escitalopram/citalopram tolerability and response in youth with anxiety and depressive disorders. *Front Pharmacol* 2019; 10: 99. https://doi.org/10.3389/fphar.2019.00099
2. Chugani, D. C., Muzik, O., Juhász, C., et al. Postnatal maturation of human GABA$_A$ receptors measured with positron emission tomography. *Ann Neurol* 2001; 49: 618–26. https://doi.org/10.1002/ana.1003
3. Compton, S. N., Peris, T. S., Almirall, D., et al. Predictors and moderators of treatment response in childhood anxiety disorders: results from the CAMS trial. *J Consult Clin Psychol* 2014; 82: 212–24. https://doi.org/10.1037/a0035458
4. Dobson, E. T., Bloch, M. H., Strawn, J. R. Efficacy and tolerability of pharmacotherapy for pediatric anxiety disorders: a network meta-analysis. *J Clin Psychiatry* 2019; 80: 17r12064. https://doi.org/10.4088/JCP.17r12064
5. Greenblatt, D. J., Allen, M. D., Harmatz, J. S., Shader, R. I. Diazepam disposition determinants. *Clin Pharmacol Ther* 1980; 27: 301–12. https://doi.org/10.1038/clpt.1980.40
6. Kupferschmidt, H. H., Ha, H. R., Ziegler, W. H., Meier, P. J., Krähenbühl, S. Interaction between grapefruit juice and midazolam in humans. *Clinical Pharmacol Ther* 1995; 58: 20–28. https://doi.org/10.1016/0009-9236(95)90068-3
7. Locher, C., Koechlin, H., Zion, S. R., et al. Efficacy and safety of selective serotonin reuptake inhibitors, serotonin–norepinephrine reuptake inhibitors, and placebo in common psychiatric disorders: a meta-analysis in children and adolescents. *JAMA Psychiatry* 2017; 74: 1011–20. https://doi.org/10.1001/jamapsychiatry.2017.2432
8. Peris, T. S., Sugar, C. A., Lindsey Bergman, R., et al. Family factors predict treatment outcome for pediatric obsessive compulsive disorder. *J Consult Clin Psychol* 2012; 80: 255–63. https://doi.org/10.1037/a0027084

9. Peris, T. S., Compton, S. N., Kendall, P. C., et al. Trajectories of change in youth anxiety during cognitive–behavior therapy. *J Consult Clin Psychol* 2015; 83: 239–52. https://doi.org/10.1037/a0038402

10. Peris, T. S., Caporino, N. E., O'Rourke, S., et al. Therapist-reported features of exposure tasks that predict differential treatment outcomes for youth with anxiety. *J Am Acad Child Adolesc Psychiatry* 2017; 56: 1043–52. https://doi.org/10.1016/j.jaac.2017.10.001

11. Stahl, S., Grady, M. M., Muntner, N. *Stahl's Essential Psychopharmacology: Neuroscientific Basis and Practical Applications*, 5th edn. Cambridge, UK: Cambridge University Press, 2021.

12. Strawn, J. R., Stimpfl, J. Practical pharmacology: optimizing benzodiazepine treatment in anxiety disorders. *Current Psychiatry* 2023; in press.

13. Strawn, J. R., Prakash, A., Zhang, Q., et al. A randomized, placebo-controlled study of duloxetine for the treatment of children and adolescents with generalized anxiety disorder. *J Am Acad Child Adolesc Psychiatry* 2015; 54: 283–93. https://doi.org/10.1016/j.jaac.2015.01.008

14. Strawn, J. R., Compton, S. N., Robertson, B., et al. Extended release guanfacine in pediatric anxiety disorders: a pilot, randomized, placebo-controlled trial. *J Child Adolesc Psychopharmacol* 2017; 27: 29–37. https://doi.org/10.1089/cap.2016.0132

15. Strawn, J. R., Geracioti, L., Rajdev, N., Clemenza, K., Levine, A. Pharmacotherapy for generalized anxiety disorder in adults and pediatric patients: an evidence-based treatment review. *Expert Opin Pharmacother* 2018a; 19: 1057–70. https://doi.org/10.1080/14656566.2018.1491966

16. Strawn, J. R., Mills, J. A., Sauley, B. A., Welge, J. A. The impact of antidepressant dose and class on treatment response in pediatric anxiety disorders: a meta-analysis. *J Am Acad Child Adolesc Psychiatry* 2018b; 57: 235–44.e2. https://doi.org/10.1016/j.jaac.2018.01.015

17. Strawn, J. R., Mills, J. A., Schroeder, H., et al. Escitalopram in adolescents with generalized anxiety disorder: a double-blind, randomized, placebo-controlled study. *J Clin Psychiatry* 2020; 81: 20m13396. https://doi.org/10.4088/JCP.20m13396

18. Strawn, J. R., Lu, L., Peris, T. S., Levine, A., Walkup, J. T. Research review: pediatric anxiety disorders – what have we learnt in the last

10 years? *J Child Psychol Psychiatry* 2021; 62: 114–39. https://doi.org/10.1111/jcpp.13262

19. Walkup, J. T., Albano, A. M., Piacentini, J., et al. Cognitive behavioral therapy, sertraline, or a combination in childhood anxiety. *N Engl J Med* 2008; 359: 2753–66. https://doi.org/10.1056/NEJMoa0804633

20. Williams, T., Hattingh, C. J., Kariuki, C. M., et al. Pharmacotherapy for social anxiety disorder (SAnD). *Cochrane Database Syst Rev* 2017; 10: CD001206. https://doi.org/10.1002/14651858.CD001206.pub3

Case 2: From anxious to activated: selective serotonin reuptake inhibitor (SSRI)-related activation

The Question: How can clinicians predict side effects associated with SSRIs in children and adolescents?

The Psychopharmacological Dilemma: Balancing side effects, side-effect management, and efficacy is challenging

Pretest self-assessment question

Which of the following represents an evidence-based intervention for a child with SSRI-related activation?

A. Immediate discontinuation of the SSRI
B. Decrease in SSRI dose
C. Initiation of adjunctive guanfacine (Tenex)
D. Initiation of an adjunctive mixed dopamine serotonin receptor antagonist
E. Cross-titration of the SSRI to a tricyclic antidepressant (TCA)

Answer: B (Decrease the SSRI dose)

Patient evaluation on intake

- A 10-year-old Asian fourth grader with separation and generalized anxiety
- The patient meets criteria for social and generalized anxiety disorders
- His anxiety persists despite psychotherapy, including the Coping Cat – an evidence-based psychotherapy for pediatric anxiety disorders

Psychiatric history

- Generalized anxiety symptoms began about 1 year ago, although this patient has been "shy" and behaviorally inhibited since toddlerhood
- His parents note that he has initial insomnia (sleep latency of 1½ hours), and they comment that this worsens on school nights
- He feels fatigued and has difficulty concentrating, but denies depressed mood and irritability
- He still enjoys playing video games online, watching short videos on the internet with his friends, and swimming
- His parents and teachers, as well as his swim coach, have been concerned about his anxiety

Social and personal history

- The patient is in 4th grade at a public elementary school, and lives with his mother and father. His mother is a teacher and his father works in IT. Neither of his parents travel for work, and his father intermittently works from home
- He does well academically, and does not have an Individualized Education Plan (IEP) or 504 Plan. He achieves A grades in most classes
- There is no history of abuse or trauma

Medical history

- The patient was delivered at 40 weeks to a 24-year-old mother and 27-year-old father
- He had normal developmental milestones, although separation anxiety persisted until age 8–9

Family history

- Mother with generalized anxiety disorder (GAD) and a history of postpartum depression
- Maternal grandmother with anxiety
- There is no family history of bipolar disorder or completed suicide

Medication history

- The patient's pediatric nurse practitioner prescribed hydroxyzine (Vistaril) 10 mg twice daily as needed to address episodes of anxiety, in addition to clonidine (Catapres) 0.1 mg every night at bedtime as a soporific
- Melatonin 3–6 mg every night at bedtime failed to improve his insomnia

Current medications

- Clonidine (Catapres) 0.1 mg every night at bedtime
- Hydroxyzine (Vistaril) 10 mg twice daily as needed

Psychotherapy history

- When his parents first noted his anxiety and heard the concerns expressed by his teachers and his friends' parents, they sought treatment with a cognitive–behavioral therapist who utilized the Coping Cat program for six sessions. These sessions included some discussion of "coping skills," and an introduction to the notion that anxious thoughts and feelings were linked to the patient's anxiety and somatic symptoms

- Most recently, he worked with a "play therapist" weekly. He has been in treatment with this therapist for approximately 6 months, and his anxiety remains minimally improved
- His anxiety has persisted despite both therapies

Further investigation

Is there anything else that you would like to know about the patient? What about additional rating scales or symptoms?

- No reports of guilt, anhedonia, or suicidal ideation
- Regarding attention and distractibility, the patient struggles to focus at school when others are around or when he is doing group work, but when working one to one with a teacher or by himself on homework he does quite well
- His score on the Screen for Child Anxiety Related Emotional Disorders (SCARED) is 40 (cut-off point for high likelihood of anxiety disorder is > 30)

What about additional physical symptoms and vital signs?

- Vital signs are within normal limits; the patient's body mass index (BMI) is in the 45th percentile for age and sex
- There is no heat or cold intolerance, or recent weight loss
- He reports occasional abdominal pain but there are no red flag symptoms (i.e. weight loss, pain that awakens him from sleep, bloody stools, chronic diarrhea)

Attending physician's mental notes: initial psychiatric evaluation

- This patient has moderate generalized and separation anxiety disorder. The SCARED was used to track symptoms, and can be helpful not only in providing an inventory of symptoms but also for clarifying symptom burdens within specific areas (e.g. separation anxiety, social anxiety, etc.). The SCARED is a child and parent self-report instrument that can be used to screen for childhood anxiety disorders, including general anxiety disorder, separation anxiety disorder, panic disorder, and social anxiety disorder. It consists of 41 items and 5 factors that parallel the *Diagnostic and Statistical Manual of Mental Disorders (DSM)* classification of anxiety disorders. The SCARED has been validated in children aged 8–18 years, and takes about 10 minutes to complete. The form can be accessed at www.pediatricbipolar.pitt.edu and is available in Arabic, Chinese, English, French, German, Italian, Portuguese, Spanish, and Thai

- The patient's anxiety symptoms are in the moderate range, and failed to improve despite cognitive behavior therapy (CBT)
- His inattentive symptoms are probably better accounted for by his anxiety disorder, given that they have fluctuated contemporaneously with his anxiety, and that he is still able to perform well when he is removed from anxiety-provoking situations and given reassurance (e.g. when working with his teacher)
- An α_2 agonist has been ineffective for sleep, although hydroxyzine provided intermittent – albeit inconsistent – relief

Question

Which of the following would be your next step?

- Begin escitalopram (Lexapro) 10 mg each morning
- Begin duloxetine (Cymbalta) 30 mg each morning
- Begin adjunctive clonazepam (Klonopin) 0.25 mg twice daily
- Begin aripiprazole (Abilify) 2 mg each evening

Case outcome: first interim follow-up (week 2)

- At the patient's last visit, escitalopram was initiated at 10 mg each morning
- Within 10 days, he noted that his thoughts were "calmer," and his mother commented that his anxiety-related abdominal pain was "actually gone"
- However, the patient and his parents reported that although his anxiety was improving, he fidgeted more and was restless
- He also had worsening insomnia and more hyperactivity

Attending physician's mental notes: first interim follow-up (week 2)

- The patient's symptoms are concerning for activation, which involves a constellation of symptoms, namely disinhibition, impulsivity, insomnia, restlessness, hyperactivity, and irritability (Figure 2.1). Importantly, these symptoms frequently co-occur
- Activation symptoms are more common in children compared with adolescents and adults. Also, activation is more common with SSRIs than with serotonin–norepinephrine reuptake inhibitors (SNRIs) (Luft et al. 2018; Mills and Strawn 2020)
- Antidepressant-related activation emerges early in treatment or following an increase in dose (Reinblatt et al. 2009), and symptoms resolve when the antidepressant dose is decreased or when the antidepressant is discontinued (Riddle et al. 1990; Wilens et al. 2003)

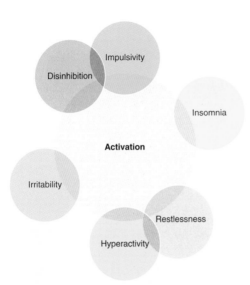

Figure 2.1 Activation syndrome symptoms. The activation syndrome represents a constellation of symptoms that emerge early in the course of treatment with SSRIs, particularly in younger patients and those with anxiety disorders.

- The emergence of activation at a relatively low dose and the relationship between the patient's escitalopram metabolism and blood levels is of concern to the attending physician. He suspects that this patient may have higher than expected escitalopram concentrations and lower clearance compared with other 10-year-olds. Both of these have been linked to activation in children and adolescents. Given this, it would be helpful to understand whether the patient is a poor CYP2C19 metabolizer (or has decreased CYP2C19 activity)

- The patient is Asian and would be expected to be more likely to be a poor CYP2C19 metabolizer compared with someone of Northern European or African ancestry (Goldstein 2001). Additionally, the attending clinician knows that for most pharmacokinetically related genes there is a spectrum of activity that affects medication exposure (Figure 2.2)

- Based on the possibility that variation in pharmacokinetic genes may affect escitalopram tolerability and plasma concentrations, the clinician ordered pharmacogenetic testing for both *CYP2C19* and *CYP2D6*

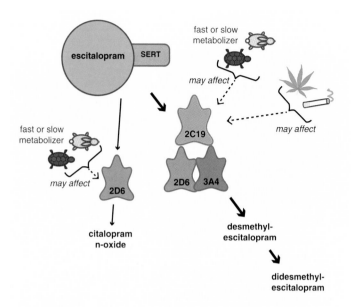

Figure 2.2 Metabolism of escitalopram. Escitalopram metabolism is predominantly driven by CYP2C19. Although numerous mutations can increase or decrease CYP2C19 activity, CYP2C19 can also be significantly inhibited by smoking and by tetrahydrocannabinol (THC) and cannabidiol (CBD).

Case outcome (continued): first interim follow-up (week 2)

- The clinician decreased escitalopram to 5 mg each morning
- Pharmacogenetic testing was ordered

Pharmacogenetic testing

```
•  CYP2D6 genotype: *1/*1  |  CYP2D6 phenotype: normal metabolizer
•  CYP2C19 genotype: *2/*2  |  CYP2C19 phenotype: poor metabolizer
•  CYP2C9 genotype: *1/*1  |  CYP2C9 phenotype: normal metabolizer
•  CYP3A4 genotype: *1/*1  |  CYP3A4 phenotype: normal
```

Case outcome: second interim follow-up (week 3)

- The patient's symptoms continued to improve while he was on escitalopram 5 mg each morning
- His SCARED score has decreased to 13; he has also been able to spend the night at a friend's house, and his mother notes that he

is no longer seeking reassurance in the evenings and is generally "back to his usual self"

- The clinician continues escitalopram 5 mg each morning

Attending physician's mental notes: second interim follow-up (week 3)

- Activation symptoms responded to a dose reduction, although should a dose titration be needed in the future, the attending physician is aware that this patient would again be at greater risk for activation (Luft et al. 2018; Wilens et al. 2003)
- Since he is a poor metabolizer for CYP2C19 – the primary enzyme that metabolizes escitalopram (and citalopram and sertraline) – this patient is at higher risk for activation (Aldrich et al. 2019; Strawn et al. 2020); however, this also suggests that he will respond to lower doses (Figure 2.3)

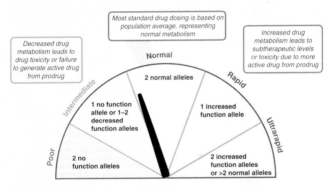

Figure 2.3 The relationship between alleles and phenotypes for pharmacokinetic genes. Reproduced from Ramsey et al. (2020).

- The reduction in escitalopram to 5 mg in a normal metabolizer produces blood concentrations that are comparable to those of a normal metabolizer treated with 10 mg (Strawn et al. 2019) (Figure 2.4)
- Also, because he is a poor CYP2C19 metabolizer, he is at greater risk for other side effects associated with escitalopram, including sedation and weight gain (Aldrich et al. 2019) (Figure 2.5)

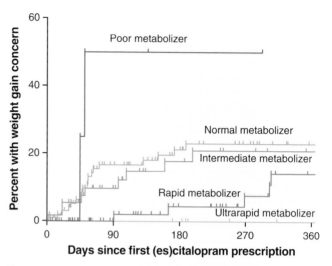

Figure 2.4 Weight gain and CYP2C19 in children and adolescents who are treated with escitalopram or citalopram. CYP2C19 status is associated with the time to first weight gain reported in the electronic medical record in a large sample of children and adolescents (p = 0.018, log-rank test for trend). Reproduced from Aldrich et al. (2019).

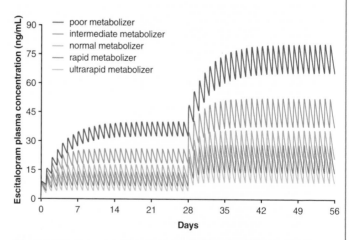

Figure 2.5 Escitalopram plasma concentrations in adolescents with different CYP2C19 phenotypes. Treatment was initiated at 10 mg daily and increased to 20 mg daily at week 4. There is considerable variation in blood concentrations of escitalopram among the CYP2C19 phenotypes, as demonstrated earlier in this series of adolescent patients. Adapted from Strawn et al. (2019).

Take-home points

- Anxiety disorders often begin in childhood and, if left untreated, can result in accumulated impairment that puts adolescents and young adults at risk for poor adaptation and maladaptive behaviors
- Anxiety symptoms can easily be monitored with measures such as the SCARED; this rating scale, which includes both parent and child versions, is sensitive to change in treatment studies, and corresponds to functional and global measures of symptom severity
- Activation is a common but manageable side effect of SSRIs and SNRIs in children and adolescents, and its risk factors include higher doses (and plasma concentrations), younger age, having an anxiety disorder, and being treated with an SSRI (compared with an SNRI). Also, slower metabolism of the SSRI increases the risk of activation
- "One size fits all" approaches with regard to SSRI dosing in children fail to take into account differences in metabolism that ultimately produce differences in plasma concentrations

Performance in practice: confessions of a psychopharmacologist

- In treating this young anxious Asian boy, it might be prudent to use an SSRI that is not metabolized through CYP2C19, or to have begun treatment at a lower dose
- Fortunately, the patient was monitored closely, and the clinician quickly recognized the patient's activation symptoms

Tips and pearls

- SSRIs and psychotherapy remain the mainstay of treating pediatric anxiety disorders (Locher et al. 2017; Strawn et al. 2018, 2021), although the SSRIs may be associated with more side effects, including activation, compared with the SNRIs (Mills and Strawn 2020)
- SSRI exposure – particularly for CYP2C19-metabolized agents – varies significantly across patients, depending on CYP2C19 phenotypes. This is particularly the case for escitalopram in adolescents wherein medication clearance varies by phenotype (Figure 2.6) and suggests differences in dosing (Figure 2.4)
- Case reports (Guile 1996; King et al. 1991), as well as a few controlled trials, suggest that activation is more likely to occur with higher doses of SSRIs as well as rapid titration of antidepressants
- Common strategies for preventing the activation syndrome, as well as other side effects, include starting SSRIs at low doses with slow

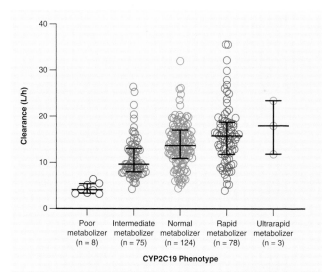

Figure 2.6 Escitalopram clearance in adolescents with different CYP2C19 phenotypes. PM, poor metabolizer; IM, intermediate metabolizer; NM, normal metabolizer; RM, rapid metabolizer; UM, ultrarapid metabolizer. *Adapted from* Poweleit et al. (2023).

planned titrations. If a patient develops activation once they begin a higher SSRI dose, decreasing the total daily dose or stopping the medication can effectively reduce this side effect (Guile 1996)

- Because activation is related to high plasma concentrations of SSRIs, switching to an extended-release form of medication (when available) may also be helpful in that the peak plasma drug concentration (i.e. C_{max}) for the medication will generally be reduced with extended-release formulations
- Another treatment strategy could be to switch to a different antidepressant, keeping in mind that patients who have experienced activation with one agent may be more likely to experience this side effect again
- Pharmacotherapy to target specific symptoms within activation syndrome, such as treating insomnia with melatonin, is another option for managing symptoms (Luft et al. 2018)

Mechanism of action moment

- The mechanism of action of SSRIs and their characteristic delayed onset of therapeutic benefit may be relevant to the pathophysiology of activation
- During the 2- to 4-week period that often precedes clinical benefit, increased synaptic serotonin (5-HT) may activate presynaptic

Mechanism of action of SSRIs: part 1. When an SSRI is administered, it immediately blocks the serotonin reuptake pump or serotonin transporter (SERT) (see icon of an SSRI blocking SERT). However, this causes 5-HT to increase initially only in the somatodendritic area of the 5-HT neuron (left) and not very much in the areas of the brain where the axons terminate (right). When 5-HT levels rise in the somatodendritic area, this stimulates nearby 5-HT$_{1A}$ auto receptors.

Mechanism of action of SSRIs: part 2. The consequence of increased serotonergic binding at somatodendritic 5-HT$_{1A}$ auto receptors is that they desensitize or downregulate (red circle).

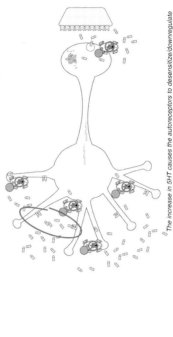

B The increase in 5HT causes the autoreceptors to desensitize/downregulate

	5HT1A autoreceptor
	5HT postsynaptic receptor
	SERT
	SSRI

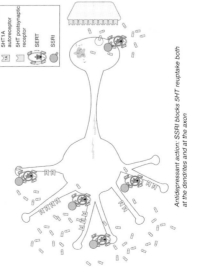

Antidepressant action: SSRI blocks 5HT reuptake both at the dendrites and at the axon

Mechanism of action of SSRIs: part 3. Once the somatodendritic 5-HT$_{1A}$ receptors downregulate, there is no longer inhibition of impulse flow in the 5-HT neuron. Thus, neuronal impulse flow is turned on. The consequence of this is release of 5-HT in the axon terminal (red circle). This increase is delayed compared with the increase in 5-HT in the somatodendritic areas of the 5-HT neuron; the delay is the result of the time it takes for somatodendritic 5-HT to downregulate the 5-HT$_{1A}$ auto receptors and turn on neuronal impulse flow in the 5-HT neuron. This delay may explain why SSRIs do not relieve depression immediately. It is also the reason why the mechanism of action of SSRIs may be linked to increasing neuronal impulse flow in 5-HT neurons, with 5-HT levels increasing at axon terminals before an SSRI can exert its therapeutic effects.

Mechanism of action of SSRIs: part 4. Finally, once the SSRIs have blocked the reuptake pump (or the SERT), increased somatodendritic 5-HT, desensitized somatodendritic 5-HT$_{1A}$ auto receptors, turned on neuronal impulse flow, and increased the release of 5-HT from axon terminals, the final step may be the desensitization of postsynaptic 5-HT receptors (red circle). This desensitization may mediate the reduction of side effects of SSRIs as tolerance develops.

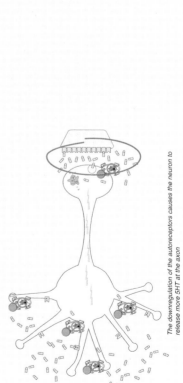

The downregulation of the autoreceptors causes the neuron to release more 5HT at the axon

The increase of 5HT at the axon causes the postsynaptic receptors to desensitize/downregulate, reducing side effects

Figure 2.7 Mechanism of action of SSRIs and the role of 5-HT$_{1A}$ auto receptors.

5-HT$_{1A}$ receptors to inhibit the release of 5-HT (Barnes and Sharp 1999). Such paradoxical decreases in serotonergic tone are associated with impulsivity similar to activation (Kruesi et al. 1990; Placidi et al. 2001) (Figure 2.6). Therefore, the early onset of activation-related adverse events may be linked to 5-HT$_{1A}$-associated depression of 5-HT release

- Interestingly, 5-HT$_{1A}$ receptor stimulation – which occurs early in the course of SSRI treatment – may underlie akathisia associated with some second-generation antipsychotics (Newman-Tancredi and Kleven 2011). Also, some studies suggest that the more rapidly maximum drug concentrations are reached, the greater the likelihood of "anxiogenic behavior" in rodent models of antidepressant-induced activation

Two-minute tutorial: activation

- Despite recognition that antidepressant-related activation is a risk factor for medication discontinuation, the activation syndrome lacks a clear definition (Reinblatt et al. 2009; Strawn et al. 2015)
- Currently, several symptoms are considered to be activation-related adverse events, namely disinhibition, impulsivity, insomnia, restlessness, hyperactivity, and irritability, and these symptoms frequently co-occur (Figure 2.1). This overlap among activation cluster symptoms complicates the assessment and measurement of activation
- Because it is related to the pharmacokinetics of the SSRI, activation emerges early in treatment or following an increase in dose (Reinblatt et al. 2009), and symptoms resolve when the antidepressant dose is decreased or when the antidepressant is discontinued (Riddle et al. 1990; Wilens et al. 2003)
- The rate of symptom resolution is related to the rate of onset of activation symptoms
- Risk factors for activation include:
  - being a child as opposed to an adolescent
  - being a slow metabolizer for the primary enzyme that metabolizes the SSRI
  - having higher concentrations of the SSRI
  - having a slower clearance of the SSRI

Two-minute tutorial: pharmacogenetics and SSRIs

- For each gene (e.g. *CYP2C19*), the patient's two alleles are represented by a /*/ followed by a number that corresponds to the specific allele. Each patient's two alleles are separated by a slash. For example, a patient who is *17/*2 has one *17 allele and one *2 allele. The two alleles (e.g. *1, *2, *17, etc.) represent the patient's genotype. This genotype corresponds to a phenotype (i.e. poor metabolizer, intermediate metabolizer, normal metabolizer, rapid metabolizer, or ultrarapid metabolizer)

- There is considerable genetic variation for CYP2C19, the primary enzyme that metabolizes escitalopram, citalopram, and sertraline
- For the patient discussed in this case, we should focus on CYP2C19. CYP2C19*2 is the most common CYP2C19 loss-of-function allele, with allele frequencies of approximately 12% in Caucasians, 15% in African Americans, and 29–35% in Asians (Hicks et al. 2015; Scott et al. 2013)
- It is also important to remember that there are alleles which increase the activity of an enzyme. For *CYP2C19,* patients may have a *17 allele which increases CYP2C19 activity. This allele is more common in Caucasians (21%) and African Americans (16%) (Hicks et al. 2015; Scott et al. 2013)
- Knowledge of the patient's CYP2C19 phenotype can be used to adjust dosing (Figure 2.5). For escitalopram, in adolescents, poor metabolizers require 10 mg daily, and ultrarapid metabolizers need 30 mg daily to achieve an exposure equivalent to 20 mg daily in a normal metabolizer. For sertraline, to achieve similar plasma levels to those in normal metabolizers who are receiving 150 mg daily, poor metabolizers require 100 mg daily. In contrast, a dose of 200 mg daily is required in rapid and ultrarapid metabolizers. For ultrarapid metabolizers, escitalopram twice daily is necessary to achieve trough levels and exposure comparable to those in normal metabolizers (Strawn et al. 2019)

Post test self-assessment question

Which of the following represents an evidence-based intervention for a child with SSRI-related activation?

A. Immediate discontinuation of the SSRI
B. Decrease in SSRI dose
C. Initiation of adjunctive guanfacine (Tenex)
D. Initiation of an adjunctive mixed dopamine serotonin receptor antagonist
E. Cross-titration of the SSRI to a tricyclic antidepressant (TCA)

Answer: B (Decrease the SSRI dose)

Discontinuing the SSRI would potentially deprive the patient of the most effective class of medication for treating pediatric anxiety disorders, namely SSRIs (Dobson et al. 2019; Strawn et al. 2018). Decreasing the dose is a pharmacokinetically informed strategy for managing activation; this strategy will lower SSRI plasma concentrations related to activation risk. Although guanfacine has been evaluated in one double-blind placebo-controlled trial in children and adolescents with anxiety disorders (Strawn et al. 2017), it is less efficacious than SSRIs. There is limited evidence for mixed dopamine serotonin receptor antagonists in pediatric anxiety disorders, and TCAs, although efficacious in some studies of young people with anxiety disorders, are not considered first- or second-line interventions for children and adolescents with anxiety disorders, and may be associated with more side effects compared with other medication classes.

References

1. Aldrich, S. L., Poweleit, E. A., Prows, C. A., et al. Influence of CYP2C19 metabolizer status on escitalopram/citalopram tolerability and response in youth with anxiety and depressive disorders. *Front Pharmacol* 2019; 10: 99. https://doi.org/10.3389/fphar.2019.00099

2. Barnes, N. M., Sharp, T. A review of central 5-HT receptors and their function. *Neuropharmacology* 1999; 38: 1083–152. https://doi.org/10.1016/s0028-3908(99)00010-6

3. Dobson, E. T., Bloch, M. H., Strawn, J. R. Efficacy and tolerability of pharmacotherapy in pediatric anxiety disorders: a network meta-analysis. *J Clin Psychiatry* 2019; 80: 17r12064. https://doi.org/10.4088/JCP.17r12064

4. Goldstein, J. A. Clinical relevance of genetic polymorphisms in the human CYP2C subfamily. *Br J Clin Pharmacol* 2001; 52: 349–55. https://doi.org/10.1046/j.0306-5251.2001.01499.x

5. Guile, J. M. Sertraline-induced behavioral activation during the treatment of an adolescent with major depression. *J Child Adolesc Psychopharmacol* 1996; 6: 281–85. https://doi.org/10.1089/cap.1996.6.281

6. Hicks, J. K., Bishop, J. R., Sangkuhl, K., et al. Clinical Pharmacogenetics Implementation Consortium (CPIC) guideline for CYP2D6 and CYP2C19 genotypes and dosing of selective serotonin reuptake inhibitors. *Clin Pharmacol Ther* 2015; 98: 127–34. https://doi.org/10.1002/cpt.147

7. King, R. A., Riddle, M. A., Chappell, P. B., et al. Emergence of self-destructive phenomena in children and adolescents during fluoxetine treatment. *J Am Acad Child Adolesc Psychiatry* 1991; 30: 179–86. https://doi.org/10.1097/00004583-199103000-00003

8. Kruesi, M. J., Rapoport, J. L., Hamburger, S., et al. Cerebrospinal fluid monoamine metabolites, aggression, and impulsivity in

disruptive behavior disorders of children and adolescents. *Arch Gen Psychiatry* 1990; 47: 419–26. https://doi.org/10.1001/archpsyc.1990.01810170019003

9. Locher, C., Koechlin, H., Zion, S. R., et al. Efficacy and safety of selective serotonin reuptake inhibitors, serotonin–norepinephrine reuptake inhibitors, and placebo in common psychiatric disorders among children and adolescents: a systematic review and meta-analysis. *JAMA Psychiatry* 2017; 74: 1011–20. https://doi.org/10.1001/jamapsychiatry.2017.2432

10. Luft, M. J., Lamy, M., DelBello, M. P., McNamara, R. K., Strawn, J. R. Antidepressant-induced activation in children and adolescents: risk, recognition and management. *Curr Probl Pediatr Adolesc Health Care* 2018; 48: 50–62. https://doi.org/10.1016/j.cppeds.2017.12.001

11. Mills, J. A., Strawn, J. R. Antidepressant tolerability in pediatric anxiety and obsessive-compulsive disorders: a Bayesian hierarchical modeling meta-analysis. *J Am Acad Child Adolesc Psychiatry* 2020; 59: 1240–51. https://doi.org/10.1016/j.jaac.2019.10.013

12. Newman-Tancredi, A., Kleven, M. S. Comparative pharmacology of antipsychotics possessing combined dopamine D2 and serotonin 5-HT1A receptor properties. *Psychopharmacology (Berl)* 2011; 216: 451–73. https://doi.org/10.1007/s00213-011-2247-y

13. Placidi, G. P. A., Oquendo, M. A., Malone, K. M., et al. Aggressivity, suicide attempts, and depression: relationship to cerebrospinal fluid monoamine metabolite levels. *Biol Psychiatry* 2001; 50: 783–91. https://doi.org/10.1016/s0006-3223(01)01170-2

14. Poweleit, E. A., Mizuno, T., Taylor, Z. L., et al. *A Population Pharmacokinetic Analysis of Escitalopram and the Effect of CYP2C19 on Clearance in Children and Adolescents. Annual Meeting of the American Society for Clinical Pharmacology & Therapeutics, Atlanta GA, March 22–24, 2023.* Alexandria, VA: American Society for Clinical Pharmacology & Therapeutics, 2023.

15. Ramsey, L. B., Brown, J. T., Vear, S. I., Bishop, J. R., Van Driest, S. L. Gene-based dose optimization in children. *Annu Rev Pharmacol Toxicol* 2020; 60: 311–31. https://doi.org/10.1146/annurev-pharmtox-010919-023459

16. Reinblatt, S. P., DosReis, S., Walkup, J. T., Riddle, M. A. Activation adverse events induced by the selective serotonin reuptake inhibitor fluvoxamine in children and adolescents. *J Child Adolesc Psychopharmacol* 2009; 19: 119–26. https://doi.org/10.1089/cap.2008.040

17. Riddle, M. A., King, R. A., Hardin, M. T., et al. Behavioral side effects of fluoxetine in children and adolescents. *J Child Adolesc*

Psychopharmacol 1990; 1: 193–8. https://doi.org/10.1089/cap.1990.1.193

18. Scott, S. A., Sangkuhl, K., Stein, C. M., et al. Clinical Pharmacogenetics Implementation Consortium guidelines for CYP2C19 genotype and clopidogrel therapy: 2013 update. *Clin Pharmacol Ther* 2013; 94: 317–23. https://doi.org/10.1038/clpt.2013.105

19. Strawn, J. R., Welge, J. A., Wehry, A. M., Keeshin, B., Rynn, M. A. Efficacy and tolerability of antidepressants in pediatric anxiety disorders: a systematic review and meta-analysis. *Depress Anxiety* 2015; 32: 149–57. https://doi.org/10.1002/da.22329

20. Strawn, J. R., Compton, S. N., Robertson, B., et al. Extended release guanfacine in pediatric anxiety disorders: a pilot, randomized, placebo-controlled trial. *J Child Adolesc Psychopharmacol* 2017; 27: 29–37. https://doi.org/10.1089/cap.2016.0132

21. Strawn, J. R., Mills, J. A., Sauley, B. A., Welge, J. A. The impact of antidepressant dose and class on treatment response in pediatric anxiety disorders: a meta-analysis. *J Am Acad Child Adolesc Psychiatry* 2018; 57: 235–44.e2. https://doi.org/10.1016/j.jaac.2018.01.015

22. Strawn, J. R., Poweleit, E. A., Ramsey, L. B. CYP2C19-guided escitalopram and sertraline dosing in pediatric patients: a pharmacokinetic modeling study. *J Child Adolesc Psychopharmacol* 2019; 29: 340–47. https://doi.org/10.1089/cap.2018.0160

23. Strawn, J. R., Mills, J. A., Schroeder, H., et al. Escitalopram in adolescents with generalized anxiety disorder: a double-blind, randomized, placebo-controlled study. *J Clin Psychiatry* 2020; 81: 20m13396. https://doi.org/10.4088/JCP.20m13396

24. Strawn, J. R., Lu, L., Peris, T. S., Levine, A., Walkup, J. T. Research review: pediatric anxiety disorders – what have we learnt in the last 10 years? *J Child Psychol Psychiatry* 2021; 62: 114–39. https://doi.org/10.1111/jcpp.13262

25. Wilens, T. E., Biederman, J., Kwon, A., et al. A systematic chart review of the nature of psychiatric adverse events in children and adolescents treated with selective serotonin reuptake inhibitors. *J Child Adolesc Psychopharmacol* 2003; 13: 143–52. https://doi.org/10.1089/104454603322163862

Case 3: The girl who couldn't sleep: posttraumatic stress disorder (PTSD) in a young girl

The Question: When should adjunctive medications be used in pediatric PTSD?

The Psychopharmacological Dilemma: First-line medications, such as selective serotonin reuptake inhibitors (SSRIs), that work in randomized clinical trials involving adults with PTSD generally fail to show benefit in children and adolescents with PTSD

Pretest self-assessment question

Which of the following represents an evidence-based intervention for a child with PTSD and prominent intrusive symptoms?

A. Paroxetine (Paxil)
B. Propranolol (Inderal)
C. Prazosin (Minipress)
D. Quetiapine (Seroquel)
E. All of the above

Answer: C (Prazosin, Minipress)

Patient evaluation on intake

- A 7-year-old girl with attention-deficit hyperactivity disorder (ADHD), combined presentation and PTSD (*Diagnostic and Statistical Manual of Mental Disorders, DSM-5* criteria)
- The patient has a relatively limited ability to relate her current symptoms to the house fire, and has difficulties articulating her current anxiety about her parents' safety

Psychiatric history

- History of ADHD, combined type
- Approximately 1 year ago the child was trapped in her upstairs bedroom during a house fire that began in the downstairs laundry room. Her parents, who had been in the basement, had difficulty reaching her, but her mother was able to get to her room and eventually they were rescued through a window by a firefighter. At the scene there were concerns about smoke inhalation. The child was taken to the local pediatric hospital, where she was observed overnight. Her parents were taken to a community hospital, where they received supportive care and monitoring. Both parents were discharged from the hospital within 24 hours
- At the time of the patient's initial evaluation, 6 months after the fire, she complained of severe initial insomnia, recurrent nightly

nightmares associated with middle insomnia, and intrusive and hyperarousal symptoms. Because her trauma had occurred in a bedroom, she always slept with the lights on and would not allow her parents to close the door to her room or to shut the window blinds
- She does well at school, although she is fearful and becomes tearful when she hears sirens
- In addition to extended-release dexmethylphenidate 5 mg each morning for her ADHD, her parents have given her low-dose melatonin 1.5 mg every night at bedtime on an as needed basis to help with her insomnia, although this has yielded minimal benefit

Social and personal history

- The patient lives with her mother and father in a single-family home, and lived briefly with her maternal aunt while the family home was being renovated and repaired following the house fire
- Her mother and father report low conflict within the home
- She has a small group of friends, both from her neighborhood and from school
- Academically, she does well and does not have an Individualized Education Plan (IEP) or 504 Plan

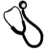

Medical history

- Delivered at 40 weeks to a 23-year-old mother and 25-year-old father
- There were some difficulties with early feeding, and also mild expressive language delays. The patient was seen in speech therapy for six sessions, and her expressive language improved
- Otherwise, her parents report normal developmental milestones

Family history

- Father with no psychiatric history
- Mother with a history of adjustment-related depressive symptoms when she moved to college. These resolved within 5 months and were associated with minimal functional impairment

Medication history

- Extended-release dexmethylphenidate (Focalin XR), 5 mg each morning

Current medications

- Extended-release dexmethylphenidate (Focalin XR), 5 mg each morning
- Melatonin 6 mg each evening as needed for insomnia

Psychotherapy history

- The patient met with a school-based therapist for four sessions approximately 2 months after posttraumatic stress symptoms began. There was no improvement in symptoms, and the sessions consisted of drawing pictures of her family and practicing relaxation strategies (e.g. deep breathing)

Further investigation

Is there anything else that you would like to know about the patient? What about details related to the emergence of her posttraumatic stress symptoms?

- Her posttraumatic stress symptoms emerged within 1–2 weeks of the trauma, and her intrusive symptoms have persisted, whereas her avoidance symptoms emerged later, beginning about 6–8 weeks after the trauma

What about additional physical symptoms and vital signs?

- No reports of depressed mood, guilt, anhedonia, or suicidal ideation
- Her vital signs are within normal limits; her body mass index (BMI) is in the 50th percentile for age and sex
- She denies cardiac symptoms, including palpitations

Attending physician's mental notes: initial psychiatric evaluation

- This patient has severe posttraumatic stress disorder and ADHD, and some features of separation anxiety disorder. However, based on her age, her separation anxiety could represent an extreme variant of normal anxiety or be related to her PTSD and trauma
- Regarding her current medication treatment, the treating clinician will need to explore her ADHD symptoms in relation both to the most recent trauma and to prior trauma
- In thinking about her co-occurring ADHD and separation anxiety it is important to bear in mind that some – but not all – comorbidity codevelops with PTSD (following trauma). Notably, the relationship between PTSD symptoms and co-occurring attentional symptoms is complex. Prospective studies suggest that some comorbidity is a "vulnerability factor" for developing PTSD (Cohen and Scheeringa 2009)
- It is noteworthy that the psychotherapy did not appear to have been trauma focused, and was more consistent with supportive psychotherapy

Question

Given the patient's prior psychotherapy and current pharmacological treatment, which of the following would be your next step?

- Discontinue her stimulant medication
- Titrate melatonin to 9 mg every night at bedtime as needed for insomnia
- Begin trauma-focused cognitive behavior therapy (TF-CBT)
- Begin interpersonal psychotherapy (IPT)

Case outcome: first interim follow-up (week 12)

- At her last visit, the patient was referred to trauma-focused psychotherapy, and she has now completed ten sessions
- Her nightmares decreased from four or five per night to twice per night, and she experiences one night per week when nightmares do not awaken her
- She continues to deny depressive symptoms, and her mother notes that she has been less fearful when she is away from her parents. She was also able to spend the night at a friend's house the week prior to the appointment
- She continues to have difficulty talking about fires and hospitals, and she struggled when the local fire department visited her elementary school for a planned educational activity

Given her prior psychotherapy and current pharmacological treatment, which of the following would be your next step?

- Discontinue her stimulant medication
- Titrate melatonin to 9 mg every night at bedtime as needed for insomnia
- Add prazosin (Minipress) 1 mg every night at bedtime to her medication regimen
- Add guanfacine (immediate release, Tenex) 1 mg every morning to her medication regimen
- Begin sertraline (Zoloft) 25 mg every morning

Attending physician's mental notes: first interim follow-up (week 12)

- TF-CBT represents the first-line treatment for children and adolescents with PTSD (Keeshin and Strawn 2012). This structured psychotherapy involves several specific components which are easily remembered with the acronym PRACTICE:
  - Psychoeducation and parenting skills
  - Relaxation

- ◦ A̲ffective expression and modulation
- ◦ C̲ognitive coping
- ◦ T̲rauma narrative processing
- ◦ I̲n vivo mastery of trauma
- ◦ C̲onjoint parent–child sessions
- ◦ E̲nhancing safety and future development
- The patient's psychiatric clinician is concerned both that she continues to experience relatively significant intrusive symptoms, and also by her parents' report that she has increased difficulty at school secondary to her daytime tiredness
- Titration of melatonin beyond 6 mg is unlikely to significantly benefit her symptoms, which are probably related to her PTSD rather than to a circadian-related sleep problem. However, attention to sleep hygiene and a discussion of sleep routines could still be helpful
- There are limited data on antidepressants in pediatric PTSD, although in general double-blind placebo-controlled studies do not suggest benefit (Keeshin and Strawn 2014). Current recommendations from the American Academy of Child and Adolescent Psychiatry (AACAP) do not support the use of SSRIs in pediatric patients with PTSD (Cohen et al. 2010). The first randomized controlled evaluation of sertraline (mean dose 150 mg daily; range 50–200 mg daily) compared with placebo occurred in the context of an adjunctive treatment trial in which children and adolescents with PTSD were receiving an evidence-based psychosocial intervention, namely TF-CBT. In this study, sertraline was associated with minimal improvement relative to placebo (Cohen et al. 2007). A subsequent 10-week study of sertraline did not observe significant differences (compared with placebo) in University of California Los Angeles (UCLA) PTSD Reaction Index scores. Finally, one additional study of children and adolescents with PTSD who were treated with fluoxetine or imipramine (compared with placebo) failed to detect differences in acute stress disorder symptoms following acute thermal burn trauma (Thombs et al. 2006). Currently, the only evidence that has suggested benefits from SSRIs in pediatric PTSD is from two open-label studies of citalopram (Seedat et al. 2002)

Case outcome: second interim follow-up (week 16)

- Since beginning a regimen of prazosin 1 mg every night at bedtime for 2 weeks, followed by titration to 2 mg every night at bedtime for an additional 2 weeks, the patient has noted fewer and fewer nightmares and commented that she is awakened by nightmares no more than once per night, on four or five nights a week

- She has a typical sleep latency and reduced hyperarousal symptoms
- However, she continues to experience avoidant symptoms
- Her blood pressure and heart rate are stable; both are in the 50th percentile for her age, sex, and height

Attending physician's mental notes: second interim follow-up (week 16)

- Prazosin has been helpful in relieving the patient's intrusive PTSD symptoms. However, her symptoms continue to interfere with functioning, and are occurring on more nights than not. Thus, titration to 3 mg is reasonable and evidence based (Keeshin et al. 2017)
- The attending physician is reassured by the patient's vital signs. However, he knows that orthostatic intolerance or orthostatic symptoms are less common in pediatric patients treated with α_1 antagonists compared with adults, given how blood pressure is differentially regulated in pediatric compared with adult patients. Also, her attending physician has considered how her blood pressure was measured. In pediatric patients, oscillometric blood pressure measurement – which measures mean arterial pressure (MAP) – uses an algorithm to determine the systolic and diastolic blood pressure, and systematically reports higher systolic and diastolic blood pressure. Therefore, auscultation-based blood pressure determination is preferred, as it directly determines the systolic and diastolic blood pressure (Flynn et al. 2014, 2017)

Case outcome: third interim follow-up (week 20)

- With titration of prazosin to 3 mg every night at bedtime and continued work in TF-CBT, the patient's sleep has normalized and her posttraumatic stress symptoms are in remission
- She is continuing her stimulant regimen and is no longer experiencing daytime tiredness. She can focus on her schoolwork and continues to be able to separate from her parents in a developmentally appropriate manner

Take-home points

- The mainstay of treatment for pediatric PTSD is TF-CBT
- Prazosin appears to be selectively effective for managing intrusive and hyperarousal symptoms in children and adolescents with PTSD. The onset of action is generally rapid, with a reduction in

the frequency and severity of nightmares; the onset of maximum efficacy occurs within 4 weeks, and the effect is usually sustained
- In children and adolescents, intrusive PTSD symptoms such as nightmares are related to noradrenergic hyperactivation (Keeshin et al. 2015; Pervanidou 2008; Pervanidou et al. 2007)

Tips and pearls

- Prazosin may effectively reduce intrusive symptoms in children and adolescents with PTSD, although the mainstay of treatment is TF-CBT
- The tolerability of prazosin may differ in younger patients, due to differences in pediatric regulation of blood pressure compared with that in adults
- Prazosin should be initiated at 1 mg 30 minutes before bedtime. It may be titrated by 1 mg every 3–4 days for the first 2 weeks, starting lower and titrating slower in younger children, and in children and adolescents who are experiencing nausea, dizziness, or other side effects
- Gradual titration of prazosin will minimize orthostatic side effects if these are present
- Additionally, although there is no clear evidence of a dose–response relationship for prazosin in pediatric patients with PTSD, the standard practice is to titrate to at least 5 mg, if this is tolerated by the patient, before concluding that the therapeutic trial has failed
- In the largest study of prazosin in children and adolescents with PTSD, patients were divided into two groups – low-dose responders and high-dose responders. In this sample, 35% of patients were treated with more than 5 mg every night at bedtime, including six patients who were treated with 10 mg or more. In general, we found that children and adolescents who were sensitive to the medication (including most patients with reported side effects) were receiving doses of 4 mg or less when the side effects were reported. In contrast, those who required higher doses were less likely to report any side effects when the medication was adjusted above 4 mg (Keeshin et al. 2017). Additionally, in this study (Figure 3.1) the response varied, with many individuals improving early and at doses of less than 5 mg daily (or less than 0.1 mg/kg)

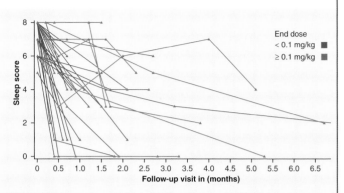

Figure 3.1 Improvement in pediatric patients with PTSD who were treated with prazosin. Adapted from Keeshin et al. (2017).

Mechanism of action moment

- Prazosin blocks noradrenergic effects, putatively at the level of the amygdala, and in doing so it decreases the generation of fear/anxiety outputs (Figure 3.2). This is particularly relevant in PTSD, where increased sympathetic activity in unmedicated traumatized adolescents is directly linked to the severity of intrusive PTSD symptoms, including nightmares (Keeshin et al. 2015)

- The α-adrenergic modulators commonly used in pediatric patients include guanfacine, clonidine, and prazosin. These agents differ in terms of their targets; however, because of differences in the distribution of these α receptors, they may vary in terms of tolerability and side effects

- α_1 receptors are located throughout the cortical and subcortical areas (Jones et al. 1985) and peripheral vasculature, although α_{1B} receptors can also be found in renal vasculature. α_2 agonists vary in their selectivity for α_2 receptors. Those that are most selective (e.g. guanfacine) appear to affect the α_{2A} receptor preferentially, and therefore may produce less sedation (Figure 3.2)

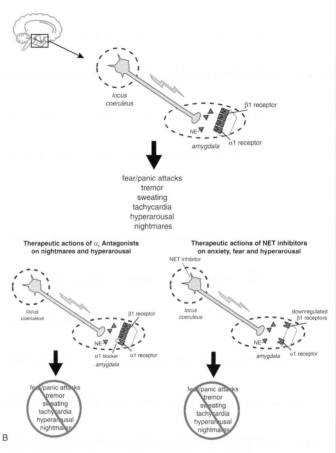

Figure 3.2 Noradrenergic hyperactivity in anxiety/fear. Norepinephrine provides input not only to the amygdala but also to many regions to which the amygdala projects; thus, it plays an important role in the fear response. Noradrenergic hyperactivation can lead to anxiety, panic attacks, tremors, sweating, tachycardia, hyperarousal, and nightmares. α_1 and β_1-adrenergic receptors may be specifically involved in these reactions. Reproduced from *Stahl's Essential Psychopharmacology*, 2021.

Two-minute tutorial

- In pediatric patients with PTSD, cortisol concentrations appear to be acutely increased (Figure 3.3) and then decrease over time. By contrast, norepinephrine concentrations continue to increase as PTSD symptoms are consolidated (Figure 3.3) (Pervanidou 2008; Pervanidou et al. 2007)

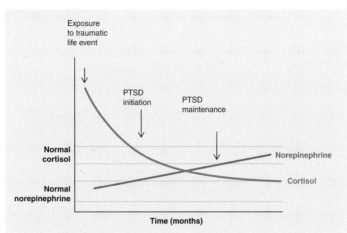

Figure 3.3 Norepinephrine and cortisol dynamics in the initiation and maintenance of PTSD in children and adolescents. In traumatized pediatric patients, trauma exposure results in significant increases in cortisol, although in patients who go on to develop PTSD, norepinephrine concentrations are generally in the "normal" range. Over time, in some pediatric patients with PTSD the cortisol concentrations decrease, but norepinephrine levels increase.

- The central role of the hypothalamic–pituitary–adrenal (HPA) axis in stress processing suggests that it would be involved in the risk and maintenance of PTSD in children and adolescents (Keeshin et al. 2014; Pervanidou 2008)
- The normal stress response involves activation of the hypothalamus and an increase in corticotropin-releasing hormone (CRH), which stimulates adrenocorticotropic hormone (ACTH) release. Cortisol binds to and stimulates receptors in the hypothalamus, pituitary, and hippocampus. In the hypothalamus, glucocorticoid binding inhibits corticotropin-releasing factor (CRF), ending the stress response, which in turn stimulates the release of ACTH from the pituitary gland. ACTH causes the release of glucocorticoid (cortisol in humans) from the adrenal gland, which binds to receptors in the hypothalamus, pituitary, and hippocampus. Glucocorticoid binding in the hypothalamus inhibits CRF release, ending the stress response. In addition, the hippocampus plays a role in inhibiting the stress response (Figure 3.4)
- In situations of chronic stress, excessive glucocorticoid release may eventually lead to atrophy of the hippocampus, thus preventing it from inhibiting the HPA axis. This could contribute to the chronic activation of the HPA axis that is seen in some patients with PTSD

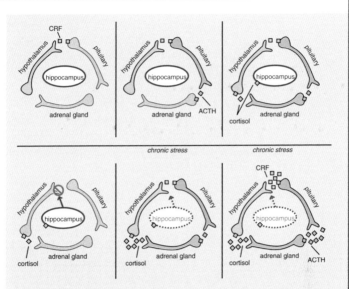

Figure 3.4 The HPA axis orchestrates the normal stress response.

Post test question

Which of the following represents an evidence-based intervention for nightmares in a child with PTSD who has been engaged in TF-CBT?

A. Paroxetine (Paxil)

B. Propranolol (Inderal)

C. Prazosin (Minipress)

D. Quetiapine (Seroquel)

E. All of the above

Answer: C (Prazosin, Minipress)

Neither paroxetine nor propranolol have been studied in pediatric patients with PTSD, although two prospective studies have evaluated the potential utility of propranolol as a means of secondary prevention in traumatized children (Famularo et al. 1988; Rosenberg et al. 2012). Melatonin is commonly used for insomnia in children and adolescents, but may lack efficacy for intrusive symptoms in pediatric PTSD, which are linked with increased sympathetic activity (Keeshin et al. 2015). Thus, prazosin is the correct answer. Prazosin appears to be effective based on moderate-sized cohort studies in pediatric patients with PTSD (Keeshin et al. 2017).

References

1. Cohen, J. A., Scheeringa, M. S. Post-traumatic stress disorder diagnosis in children: challenges and promises. *Dialogues Clin Neurosci* 2009; 11: 91–9. https://doi.org/10.31887/dcns.2009.11.1/jacohen

2. Cohen, J. A., Mannarino, A. P., Perel, J. M., Staron, V. A pilot randomized controlled trial of combined trauma-focused CBT and sertraline for childhood PTSD symptoms. *J Am Acad Child Adolesc Psychiatry* 2007; 46: 811–19. https://doi.org/10.1097/chi.0b013e3180547105

3. Cohen, J. A., Bukstein, O., Walter, H., et al. Practice parameter for the assessment and treatment of children and adolescents with posttraumatic stress disorder. *J Am Acad Child Adolesc Psychiatry* 2010; 49: 414–30. https://doi.org/10.1016/j.jaac.2009.12.020

4. Famularo, R., Kinscherff, R., Fenton, T. Propranolol treatment for childhood posttraumatic stress disorder, acute type. A pilot study. *Am J Dis Child* 1988; 142: 1244–7. http://www.ncbi.nlm.nih.gov/pubmed/3177336

5. Flynn, J. T., Daniels, S. R., Hayman, L. L., et al. Update: ambulatory blood pressure monitoring in children and adolescents: a scientific statement from the American Heart Association. *Hypertension* 2014; 63: 1116–35. https://doi.org/10.1161/HYP.0000000000000007

6. Flynn, J. T., Kaelber, D. C., Baker-Smith, C. M., et al. Clinical practice guideline for screening and management of high blood pressure in children and adolescents. *Pediatrics* 2017; 140: e20171904. https://doi.org/10.1542/peds.2017-1904

7. Jones, L. S., Gauger, L. L., Davis, J. N. Anatomy of brain alpha 1-adrenergic receptors: in vitro autoradiography with [^{125}I]-heat. *J Comp Neurol* 1985; 231: 190–208. https://doi.org/10.1002/cne.902310207

8. Keeshin, B. R., Strawn, J. R. Treatment of children and adolescents with posttraumatic stress disorder (PTSD): a review of current evidence. *Child Adolesc Psychopharmacol News* 2012; 17: 5–10. https://doi.org/10.1080/15374416.2020.1823849

9. Keeshin, B. R., Strawn, J. R. Psychological and pharmacologic treatment of youth with posttraumatic stress disorder: an evidence-based review. *Child Adolesc Psychiatr Clin N Am* 2014; 23: 399–411. https://doi.org/10.1016/j.chc.2013.12.002

10. Keeshin, B. R., Strawn, J. R., Out, D., Granger, D. A., Putnam, F. W. Cortisol awakening response in adolescents with acute sexual abuse related posttraumatic stress disorder. *Depress Anxiety* 2014; 31: 107–14. https://doi.org/10.1002/da.22154

11. Keeshin, B. R., Strawn, J. R., Out, D., Granger, D. A., Putnam, F. W. Elevated salivary alpha amylase in adolescent sexual abuse survivors with posttraumatic stress disorder symptoms. *J Child Adolesc Psychopharmacol* 2015; 25: 344–50. https://doi.org/10.1089/cap.2014.0034

12. Keeshin, B. R., Ding, Q., Presson, A. P., Berkowitz, S. J., Strawn, J.R. Use of prazosin for pediatric PTSD-associated nightmares and sleep disturbances: a retrospective chart review. *Neurol Ther* 2017; 6: 247–57. https://doi.org/10.1007/s40120-017-0078-4

13. Pervanidou, P. Biology of post-traumatic stress disorder in childhood and adolescence. *J Neuroendocrinol* 2008; 20: 632–8. https://doi.org/10.1111/j.1365-2826.2008.01701.x

14. Pervanidou, P., Kolaitis, G., Charitaki, S., et al. The natural history of neuroendocrine changes in pediatric posttraumatic stress disorder (PTSD) after motor vehicle accidents: progressive divergence of noradrenaline and cortisol concentrations over time. *Biol Psychiatry* 2007; 62: 1095–102. https://doi.org/10.1016/j.biopsych.2007.02.008

15. Rosenberg, L., Rosenberg, M., Fuchs, H., et al. Does propranolol prevent symptoms of posttraumatic stress disorder (PTSD) in children with large burns? *J Burn Care Res* 2012; 33: S119. http://onlinelibrary.wiley.com/o/cochrane/clcentral/articles/767/CN-01010767/frame.html

16. Seedat, S., Stein, D. J., Ziervogel, C., et al. Comparison of response to a selective serotonin reuptake inhibitor in children, adolescents, and adults with posttraumatic stress disorder. *J Child Adolesc Psychopharmacol* 2002; 12: 37–46. https://doi.org/10.1089/10445460252943551

17. Stahl, S., Grady, M. M., Muntner, N. *Stahl's Essential Psychopharmacology: Neuroscientific Basis and Practical Applications*, 5th edn. Cambridge, UK: Cambridge University Press, 2021.

18. Thombs, B. D., Bresnick, M. G., Magyar-Russell, G., Kim, T. J. *Pediatr Crit Care Med* 2006; 7: 498; author reply 498–9. https://doi.org/10.1089/10445460252943551

Case 4: Depressed and still depressed: major depressive disorder (MDD) in an adolescent

The Question: When should adjunctive medications be used in adolescents with treatment-resistant MDD?

The Psychopharmacological Dilemma: There is uncertainty regarding how and when to "change course" in managing treatment-resistant MDD in adolescents, and adjunctive medications may have unique tolerability concerns related to primary pharmacotherapy in this age group

Pretest self-assessment question

Which of the following represents the best and most evidence-based intervention for an adolescent with MDD who failed to respond to escitalopram (Lexapro) 20 mg daily for 4 months, and in whom escitalopram was discontinued 2 months ago?

A. Paroxetine (Paxil)

B. Venlafaxine (Effexor)

C. Fluoxetine (Prozac)

D. Duloxetine (Cymbalta)

E. All of the above

Answer: C (Fluoxetine, Prozac)

Patient evaluation on intake

- A 16-year-old boy with MDD (*The Diagnostic and Statistical Manual of Mental Disorders, DSM-5* criteria)
- Moderate to severe depressive symptoms, which are not accompanied by significant anxiety symptoms, and there is no suicidal ideation, intent, or plan currently
- The patient denies any recent stressors, although he is concerned about his academic performance, and this concern is shared by his parents

Psychiatric history

- History of some early expressive language difficulties for which the patient was seen by a speech and language pathologist. He received weekly speech therapy for 12 weeks at the age of 5, and he "graduated"
- Approximately 6 months ago he developed increasing withdrawal and anger. He has progressively stopped doing activities with his friends, including riding all-terrain vehicles. His only relationship is with his girlfriend of 8 months, and she has noted that he has been "different." They still video chat with each other most nights, but rarely go out together

- He denies tearfulness, but notes generally feeling "numb and sad"
- He experiences significant irritability, initial insomnia, and daytime tiredness, and he has had increasing difficulties at school, including in mathematics – a course which he is currently failing

Social and personal history

- The patient lives with his mother and father and attends a public school. He lives in a rural community and enjoys riding all-terrain vehicles
- As noted earlier, he is struggling to engage with his schoolwork, and in particular he struggles with mathematics
- As noted earlier, he has a girlfriend of 8 months and video chats with her most nights
- There is no history of abuse or trauma

Medical history

- Delivered at 40 weeks to a 41-year-old mother and 43-year-old father
- Some difficulties with expressive language delays, as described earlier
- Otherwise, the patient's parents report normal developmental milestones

Family history

- Father with no psychiatric history
- Mother with a history of MDD; she has done well with extended-release venlafaxine 37.5 mg daily

Medication history

- Melatonin 3 mg every night at bedtime

Current medications

- Melatonin 3 mg each evening as needed for insomnia

Psychotherapy history

- The patient met with a counselor in the community for 10 sessions and continues to attend, but comments that "it's hard to talk … it's a lot of work." He is generally limited in terms of his ability to describe the ongoing work in psychotherapy. He notes that there has been a mild improvement in depressive symptoms, and that he no longer thinks about "dying" as much since beginning therapy

Further investigation

Is there anything else that you would like to know about this patient? What about accompanying symptoms?

- The patient denies significant anxiety symptoms, although he does feel increasingly tense, overwhelmed, and on edge. However, he denies concerns related to panic attacks, agoraphobia, social anxiety, or separation anxiety

What about additional physical symptoms and vital signs?

- Vital signs are within normal limits; his body mass index (BMI) is in the 40th percentile for age and sex
- He has had a recent weight loss of approximately 2 kg over the past 6 weeks
- He denies cardiac symptoms, including palpitations

What about symptom inventories?

- Some clinicians prefer the Patient Health Questionnaire-9 (PHQ-9) for assessing depressive symptoms (see later for this patient)

PATIENT HEALTH QUESTIONNAIRE - 9 (PHQ - 9)

Over the <u>last 2 weeks</u>, how often have you been bothered by any of the following problems? (*Use "✔" to indicate your answer*)	Not at all	Several days	More than half the days	Nearly every day
1. Little interest or pleasure in doing things	0	1	2	3
2. Feeling down, depressed, or hopeless	0	1	2	3
3. Trouble falling or staying asleep, or sleeping too much	0	1	2	3
4. Feeling tired or having little energy	0	1	2	3
5. Poor appetite or overeating	0	1	2	3
6. Feeling bad about yourself — or that you are a failure or have let yourself or your family down	0	1	2	3
7. Trouble concentrating on things, such as reading the newspaper or watching television	0	1	2	3
8. Moving or speaking so slowly that other people could have noticed? Or the opposite — being so fidgety or restless that you have been moving around a lot more than usual	0	1	2	3
9. Thoughts that you would be better off dead or of hurting yourself in some way	0	1	2	3

FOR OFFICE CODING _____ + _____ + _____ + _____

= Total Score: _____

- However, the Quick Inventory of Depressive Symptomatology – Self-Report (QIDS-SR) probes more dimensions and can be helpful in determining the directionality of symptoms (e.g. assessing decreased appetite or increased appetite as opposed to a change in appetite). Given that specific types of sleep disturbance, appetite disturbance, and weight change vary and may predict differential responses, we prefer this inventory. The QIDS-SR for this patient is shown here:

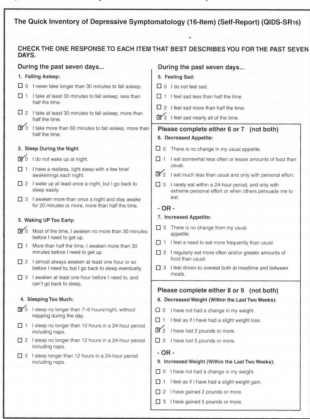

The Quick Inventory of Depressive Symptomatology (16-Item) (Self-Report) (QIDS-SR16)

CHECK THE ONE RESPONSE TO EACH ITEM THAT BEST DESCRIBES YOU FOR THE PAST SEVEN DAYS.

During the past seven days...

1. Falling Asleep:
- ☐ 0 I never take longer than 30 minutes to fall asleep.
- ☐ 1 I take at least 30 minutes to fall asleep, less than half the time.
- ☐ 2 I take at least 30 minutes to fall asleep, more than half the time.
- ☑ 3 I take more than 60 minutes to fall asleep, more than half the time.

2. Sleep During the Night:
- ☑ 0 I do not wake up at night.
- ☐ 1 I have a restless, light sleep with a few brief awakenings each night.
- ☐ 2 I wake up at least once a night, but I go back to sleep easily.
- ☐ 3 I awaken more than once a night and stay awake for 20 minutes or more, more than half the time.

3. Waking UP Too Early:
- ☑ 0 Most of the time, I awaken no more than 30 minutes before I need to get up.
- ☐ 1 More than half the time, I awaken more than 30 minutes before I need to get up.
- ☐ 2 I almost always awaken at least one hour or so before I need to, but I go back to sleep eventually.
- ☐ 3 I awaken at least one hour before I need to, and can't go back to sleep.

4. Sleeping Too Much:
- ☑ 0 I sleep no longer than 7–8 hours/night, without napping during the day.
- ☐ 1 I sleep no longer than 10 hours in a 24-hour period including naps.
- ☐ 2 I sleep no longer than 12 hours in a 24-hour period including naps.
- ☐ 3 I sleep longer than 12 hours in a 24-hour period including naps.

During the past seven days...

5. Feeling Sad:
- ☐ 0 I do not feel sad.
- ☐ 1 I feel sad less than half the time.
- ☐ 2 I feel sad more than half the time.
- ☑ 3 I feel sad nearly all of the time.

Please complete either 6 or 7 (not both)

6. Decreased Appetite:
- ☐ 0 There is no change in my usual appetite.
- ☐ 1 I eat somewhat less often or lesser amounts of food than usual.
- ☑ 2 I eat much less than usual and only with personal effort.
- ☐ 3 I rarely eat within a 24-hour period, and only with extreme personal effort or when others persuade me to eat.

- OR -

7. Increased Appetite:
- ☐ 0 There is no change from my usual appetite.
- ☐ 1 I feel a need to eat more frequently than usual.
- ☐ 2 I regularly eat more often and/or greater amounts of food than usual.
- ☐ 3 I feel driven to overeat both at mealtime and between meals.

Please complete either 8 or 9 (not both)

8. Decreased Weight (Within the Last Two Weeks):
- ☐ 0 I have not had a change in my weight.
- ☐ 1 I feel as if I have had a slight weight loss.
- ☑ 2 I have lost 2 pounds or more.
- ☐ 3 I have lost 5 pounds or more.

- OR -

9. Increased Weight (Within the Last Two Weeks):
- ☐ 0 I have not had a change in my weight.
- ☐ 1 I feel as if I have had a slight weight gain.
- ☐ 2 I have gained 2 pounds or more.
- ☐ 3 I have gained 5 pounds or more.

- Both the QIDS-SR and the PHQ-9 are freely available

What about psychological testing?

- The Personality Assessment Inventory for Adolescents (PAI-A) was administered, and revealed the following:
  - At times, the patient describes being socially isolated and having few interpersonal relationships that could be described as close and warm
  - In terms of his self-concept, there appears to be a generally negative self-evaluation that may vary from states of harsh self-criticism and self-doubt to periods of relative self-confidence and intact self-esteem. This fluctuation is

The Quick Inventory of Depressive Symptomatology (16-Item) (Self-Report) (QIDS-SR16)

During the past seven days...

10. Concentration / Decision Making:

- ☐ 0 There is no change in my usual capacity to concentrate or make decisions.
- ☐ 1 I occasionally feel indecisive or find that my attention wanders.
- ☑ 2 Most of the time, I struggle to focus my attention or to make decisions.
- ☐ 3 I cannot concentrate well enough to read or cannot make even minor decisions.

11. View of Myself:

- ☐ 0 I see myself as equally worthwhile and deserving as other people.
- ☐ 1 I am more self-blaming than usual.
- ☑ 2 I largely believe that I cause problems for others.
- ☐ 3 I think almost constantly about major and minor defects in myself.

12. Thoughts of Death or Suicide:

- ☐ 0 I do not think of suicide or death.
- ☑ 1 I feel that life is empty or wonder if it's worth living.
- ☐ 2 I think of suicide or death several times a week for several minutes.
- ☐ 3 I think of suicide or death several times a day in some detail, or I have made specific plans for suicide or have actually tried to take my life.

13. General Interest:

- ☐ 0 There is no change from usual in how interested I am in other people or activities.
- ☐ 1 I notice that I am less interested in people or activities.
- ☑ 2 I find I have interest in only one or two of my formerly pursued activities.
- ☐ 3 I have virtually no interest in formerly pursued activities.

During the past seven days...

14. Energy Level:

- ☐ 0 There is no change in my usual level of energy.
- ☐ 1 I get tired more easily than usual.
- ☑ 2 I have to make a big effort to start or finish my usual daily activities (for example, shopping, homework, cooking, or going to work).
- ☐ 3 I really cannot carry out most of my usual daily activities because I just don't have the energy.

15. Feeling Slowed Down:

- ☐ 0 I think, speak, and move at my usual rate of speed.
- ☐ 1 I find that my thinking is slowed down or my voice sounds dull or flat.
- ☑ 2 It takes me several seconds to respond to most questions and I'm sure my thinking is slowed.
- ☐ 3 I am often unable to respond to questions without extreme effort.

16. Feeling Restless:

- ☑ 0 I do not feel restless.
- ☐ 1 I'm often fidgety, wringing my hands, or need to shift how I am sitting.
- ☐ 2 I have impulses to move about and am quite restless.
- ☐ 3 At times, I am unable to stay seated and need to pace around.

- likely to vary as a function of his current circumstances
- During stressful times, he is prone to be self-critical and pessimistic, dwelling on past failures and lost opportunities, with considerable uncertainty and indecision about his plans and goals for the future. Given this self-doubt, he tends to blame himself for setbacks, and he sees any prospects for future success as dependent upon the actions of others
- His interpersonal style is characterized as withdrawn and introverted. He is likely to be rather passive and distant in those relationships that are maintained
- With respect to anger management, he describes himself as a very meek and unassertive person who has difficulty standing up for himself, even when assertiveness is warranted

PATIENT FILE

Attending physician's mental notes: initial psychiatric evaluation

- This patient has MDD, moderate to severe, with anxious distress
- Regarding psychotherapy, it is noteworthy that, even with significant questioning, he is unable to describe many aspects of the psychotherapeutic process. There are concerns that this may be supportive rather than interpersonally focused or cognitively focused

Question

Given this patient's prior psychotherapy, which of the following would be your next step?

- Begin fluoxetine 10 mg daily with titration to 20 mg daily in 1 week
- Begin extended-release venlafaxine 37.5 mg each morning
- Begin interpersonal psychotherapy for adolescents (IPT-A)
- Titrate melatonin to 9 mg every night at bedtime as needed for insomnia

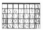

Case outcome: first interim follow-up (week 4)

- At the patient's initial visit, he began fluoxetine which was titrated to 20 mg daily. At a telehealth visit 2 weeks after beginning fluoxetine, he denied any side effects and commented that he feels he is "a little bit less sad"
- He continues to struggle in school, and his mother notes that he has been eating dinner with the family more often, and that he is more engaged with the family overall
- His sleep remains problematic, and he frequently naps (for 1–2 hours) on school days

Question

Given this patient's current psychotherapy and current pharmacological treatment (fluoxetine 20 mg daily for 26 days), which of the following would be your next step?

- Continue fluoxetine (Prozac) at 20 mg daily
- Titrate fluoxetine (Prozac) to 40 mg daily
- Add trazodone (Desaryl) (50 mg every night at bedtime) to assist with his initial insomnia
- Obtain pharmacogenetic testing

Attending physician's mental notes: first interim follow-up (week 4)

- The patient's depressive symptoms are partially improving while he is continuing supportive psychotherapy. Additionally, now that the patient is more able to engage with others, the clinician has reached out to his therapist to gauge whether there has been a contemporaneous improvement in his ability to work in therapy
- His psychiatric clinician is concerned that he continues to experience relatively significant depressive symptoms
- Given the mild improvement in depressive symptoms, evidence suggests titration of fluoxetine to 40 mg early in the course of treatment rather than waiting an additional 4 weeks (Gunlicks-Stoessel et al. 2019)
- Trazodone should be avoided in adolescents with MDD who are treated with fluoxetine, given findings from the Treatment of Resistant Depression in Adolescents (TORDIA) study and concerns that this may decrease the antidepressant response (Shamseddeen et al. 2012)
- Pharmacogenetic testing is unlikely to be beneficial in this situation, given that the patient is tolerating fluoxetine well and demonstrating an early – albeit modest – improvement in depressive symptoms. Currently, the strongest support for pharmacogenetic testing related to selective serotonin reuptake inhibitors (SSRIs) is for escitalopram and sertraline dosing (Bousman et al. 2023), and there is no clear evidence that it may be used for medication selection in adolescents with MDD

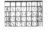

Case outcome: second interim follow-up (week 12)

- Since titration of fluoxetine (Prozac) to 40 mg and then to 60 mg daily at a telehealth visit during week 8 of treatment, the patient has noted a significant improvement in depressive symptoms, although the gains reported by his parents are more modest
- His score on the QIDS-SR has decreased from 16 to 15, but this is still consistent with moderate depressive symptoms
- He continues to struggle with initial insomnia, and withdrawal from friends, although since his last visit he has gone to his girlfriend's house twice, and he went out to dinner with her family

CHECK THE ONE RESPONSE TO EACH ITEM THAT BEST DESCRIBES YOU FOR THE PAST SEVEN DAYS.

During the past seven days...

1. Falling Asleep:

☑ 0   I never take longer than 30 minutes to fall asleep.

☐ 1   I take at least 30 minutes to fall asleep, less than half the time.

☐ 2   I take at least 30 minutes to fall asleep, more than half the time.

☐ 3   I take more than 60 minutes to fall asleep, more than half the time.

2. Sleep During the Night

☐ 0   I do not wake up at night.

☑ 1   I have a restless, light sleep with a few brief awakenings each night.

☐ 2   I wake up at least once a night, but I go back to sleep easily.

☐ 3   I awaken more than once a night and stay awake for 20 minutes or more, more than half the time.

3. Waking Up Too Early:

☑ 0   Most of the time, I awaken no more than 30 minutes before I need to get up.

☐ 1   More than half the time, I awaken more than 30 minutes before I need to get up.

☐ 2   I almost always awaken at least one hour or so before I need to, but I go back to sleep eventually.

☐ 3   I awaken at least one hour before I need to, and can't go back to sleep.

4. Sleeping Too Much:

☐ 0   I sleep no longer than 7–8 hours/night, without napping during the day.

☑ 1   I sleep no longer than 10 hours in a 24-hour period including naps.

☐ 2   I sleep no longer than 12 hours in a 24-hour period including naps.

☐ 3   I sleep longer than 12 hours in a 24-hour period including naps.

During the past seven days...

5. Feeling Sad:

☐ 0   I do not feel sad.

☐ 1   I feel sad less than half the time.

☑ 2   I feel sad more than half the time.

☐ 3   I feel sad nearly all of the time.

Please complete either 6 or 7   (not both)

6. Decreased Appetite:

☐ 0   There is no change in my usual appetite.

☐ 1   I eat somewhat less often or lesser amounts of food than usual.

☐ 2   I eat much less than usual and only with personal effort.

☐ 3   I rarely eat within a 24-hour period, and only with extreme personal effort or when others persuade me to eat.

- OR -

7. Increased Appetite:

☐ 0   There is no change from my usual appetite.

☑ 1   I feel a need to eat more frequently than usual.

☐ 2   I regularly eat more often and/or greater amounts of food than usual.

☐ 3   I feel driven to overeat both at mealtime and between meals.

Please complete either 8 or 9   (not both)

8. Decreased Weight (Within the Last Two Weeks):

☑ 0   I have not had a change in my weight.

☐ 1   I feel as if I have had a slight weight loss.

☐ 2   I have lost 2 pounds or more.

☐ 3   I have lost 5 pounds or more.

- OR -

9. Increased Weight (Within the Last Two Weeks):

☐ 0   I have not had a change in my weight.

☐ 1   I feel as if I have had a slight weight gain.

☐ 2   I have gained 2 pounds or more.

☐ 3   I have gained 5 pounds or more.

During the past seven days...

10. Concentration / Decision Making:

☐ 0   There is no change in my usual capacity to concentrate or make decisions.

☐ 1   I occasionally feel indecisive or find that my attention wanders.

☑ 2   Most of the time, I struggle to focus my attention or to make decisions.

☐ 3   I cannot concentrate well enough to read or cannot make even minor decisions.

11. View of Myself:

☐ 0   I see myself as equally worthwhile and deserving as other people.

☐ 1   I am more self-blaming than usual.

☑ 2   I largely believe that I cause problems for others.

☐ 3   I think almost constantly about major and minor defects in myself.

12. Thoughts of Death or Suicide:

☐ 0   I do not think of suicide or death.

☑ 1   I feel that life is empty or wonder if it's worth living.

☐ 2   I think of suicide or death several times a week for several minutes.

☐ 3   I think of suicide or death several times a day in some detail, or I have made specific plans for suicide or have actually tried to take my life.

13. General Interest:

☐ 0   There is no change from usual in how interested I am in other people or activities.

☐ 1   I notice that I am less interested in people or activites.

☑ 2   I find I have interest in only one or two of my formerly pursued activities.

☐ 3   I have virtually no interest in formerly pursued activities.

During the past seven days...

14. Energy Level:

☐ 0   There is no change in my usual level of energy.

☐ 1   I get tired more easily than usual.

☑ 2   I have to make a big effort to start or finish my usual daily activities (for example, shopping, homework, cooking, or going to work).

☐ 3   I really cannot carry out most of my usual daily activities because I just don't have the energy.

15. Feeling Slowed Down:

☐ 0   I think, speak, and move at my usual rate of speed.

☐ 1   I find that my thinking is slowed down or my voice sounds dull or flat .

☑ 2   It takes me several seconds to respond to most questions and I'm sure my thinking is slowed.

☐ 3   I am often unable to respond to questions without extreme effort.

16. Feeling Restless:

☑ 0   I do not feel restless.

☐ 1   I'm often fidgety, wringing my hands, or need to shift how I am sitting.

☐ 2   I have impulses to move about and am quite restless.

☐ 3   At times, I am unable to stay seated and need to pace around.

Question

Given the patient's current psychotherapy and current pharmacological treatment (fluoxetine 60 mg daily for nearly 8 weeks), which of the following would be your next step?

- Continue fluoxetine (Prozac) at 60 mg daily
- Add aripiprazole (Abilify) 5 mg every night at bedtime
- Discontinue fluoxetine (Prozac) and begin escitalopram (Lexapro)

Attending physician's mental notes: second interim follow-up (week 12)

- Titration of fluoxetine has been helpful, and the patient's therapist reports more engagement and has begun working with behavioral activation strategies; however, the therapist also feels that "things have somewhat stalled" in terms of his improvement

- The attending physician has discussed adherence and substance use, and there are no concerns. The patient has missed only one dose in the last month, and did not report any withdrawal symptoms associated with this

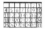

Case outcome: third interim follow-up (week 14)

- With the addition of aripiprazole 5 mg to his regimen, the patient notes that his sleep has normalized, but despite this he feels increasingly tired and notes more restlessness and feeling "agitated … like I have to just get up and walk or do something"
- He continues to work in psychotherapy and feels that this has been more helpful over the past 2 weeks
- He has not noted any weight gain

Attending physician's mental notes: third interim follow-up (week 14)

- The psychopharmacologist was concerned about akathisia following the addition of aripiprazole. She was even more concerned when she considered the strong likelihood of phenoconversion (Shah and Smith 2015) related to cytochrome P4502D6
- Fluoxetine is a potent inhibitor of CYP2D6 (mechanism-based inhibition), and this resulted in the patient – through phenoconversion – being a slower metabolizer (likely poor metabolizer) with regard to CYP2D6
- According to the recommended dosing of aripiprazole, in patients who are CYP2D6 poor metabolizers, aripiprazole should be started at half of the typical dose
- The dose of aripiprazole was decreased to 2.5 mg, and at a telehealth visit the following week the patient commented that "it's definitely working, I feel so much better." Additionally, his akathisia had resolved, and he continued to deny any weight gain

Take-home points

- The first-line psychopharmacological treatment for depression in adolescents is an SSRI, and the SSRIs are generally well tolerated
- For fluoxetine, which is approved for the treatment of MDD in children and adolescents, pharmacogenetic testing may not be helpful in determining dose, except in patients who are already poor or intermediate metabolizers of CYP2D6
- Concomitant medications affect CYP2D6 activity, and these include strong inhibitors such as fluoxetine. This is important when considering adjunctive medications such as aripiprazole, which is metabolized by CYP2D6

PATIENT FILE

Tips and pearls

- Regarding when to change medications or increase dose, there is evidence from adaptive trials that titration should occur early in the course of treatment, rather than waiting for 6–8 weeks
- Phenoconversion represents an important concept in pediatric and adult psychopharmacology, and may explain side effects that emerge at unusually low doses or contrast with what might be expected based on pharmacogenetic testing (Figure 4.1)

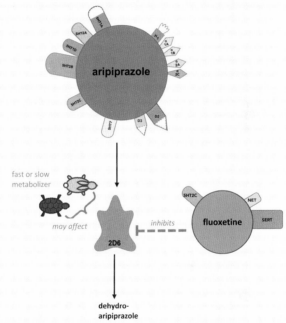

Figure 4.1 Aripiprazole is metabolized by CYP2D6. Fluoxetine is a potent inhibitor of CYP2D6, which results in higher than expected concentrations of aripiprazole and increases the likelihood of concentration-related adverse effects.

- When considering the differences in aripiprazole exposure based on CYP2D6, it is important to recall that CYP2D6 activity varies substantially across individuals (Figure 4.2)
- Studies in adults reveal that poor metabolizers have significantly increased maximum concentrations (C_{MAX}) and total exposure (area under curve, AUC) compared with normal metabolizers (Figure 4.3)

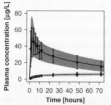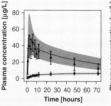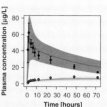

Figure 4.2 Plasma concentration–time curves (mean and standard deviation) of aripiprazole (filled circles) and its metabolite dehydro-aripiprazole (open circles) after the administration of a single 10-mg dose of aripiprazole in healthy adults according to their cytochrome CYP2D6 phenotype. Solid colored lines indicate the mean, and the colored area indicates the ± standard deviation of the physiologically based pharmacokinetic model. Circles indicate observed plasma concentrations. Normal metabolizers are shown on the left, intermediate metabolizers are shown in the middle, and poor metabolizers are shown on the right. Adapted from Kneller et al. (2021).

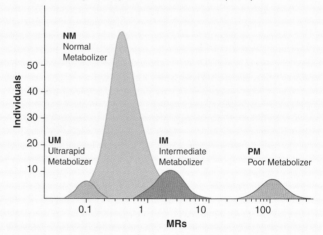

Figure 4.3 Frequency of various CYP2D6 phenotypes in a northern European cohort. Metabolic ratios (MRs) are shown on the x-axis. Adapted from Zanger and Schwab (2013).

Post test self-assessment question

Which of the following represents an evidence-based intervention for an adolescent with MDD?

A. Paroxetine (Paxil)

B. Venlafaxine (Effexor)

C. Fluoxetine (Prozac)

D. Duloxetine (Cymbalta)

E. All of the above

Answer: C (Fluoxetine, Prozac)

Paroxetine has been studied in adolescents with MDD, and there is some evidence for efficacy; however, it has been associated with poorer tolerability relative to other SSRIs and is not approved by the U.S. Food and Drug Administration (FDA) for any condition in children and adolescents. Duloxetine is approved by the FDA to treat generalized anxiety disorder in adolescents (Strawn et al. 2015); however, studies of duloxetine in adolescents with MDD have failed to demonstrate benefit (Emslie et al. 2014). Venlafaxine has not demonstrated efficacy relative to placebo in adolescents with MDD, although it was evaluated in the treatment of SSRI-resistant depression in adolescents (Asarnow et al. 2009). More recent analyses of these data also suggest that venlafaxine is about 10% less effective than an SSRI in adolescents with SSRI-resistant depression (Suresh et al. 2020). Fluoxetine is associated with a substantial evidence base in children and adolescents with MDD, and is FDA-approved for this condition.

References

1. Asarnow, J. R., Emslie, G., Clarke, G., et al. Treatment of selective serotonin reuptake inhibitor-resistant depression in adolescents: predictors and moderators of treatment response. *J Am Acad Child Adolesc Psychiatry* 2009; 48: 330–39. https://doi.org/10.1097/chi.0b013e3181977476

2. Bousman, C. A., Stevenson, J. M., Ramsey, L. B., et al. Clinical Pharmacogenetics Implementation Consortium (CPIC) guideline for CYP2D6, CYP2C19, CYP2B6, SLC6A4, and HTR2A genotypes and serotonin reuptake inhibitor antidepressants. *Clin Pharmacol Ther* 2023; 114: 51–68. https://doi.org/10.1002/cpt.2903

3. Compton, S. N., Peris, T. S., Almirall, D., et al. Predictors and moderators of treatment response in childhood anxiety disorders: results from the CAMS trial. *J Consult Clin Psychol* 2014; 82: 212–24. https://doi.org/10.1037/a0035458

4. Dobson, E. T., Bloch, M. H., Strawn, J. R. Efficacy and tolerability of pharmacotherapy in pediatric anxiety disorders: a network meta-analysis. *J Clin Psychiatry* 2019; 80: 17r12064. https://doi.org/10.4088/JCP.17r12064

5. Emslie, G. J., Prakash, A., Zhang, Q., et al. A double-blind efficacy and safety study of duloxetine fixed doses in children and adolescents with major depressive disorder. *J Child Adolesc Psychopharmacol* 2014; 24: 170–79. https://doi.org/10.1089/cap.2013.0096

6. Greenblatt, D. J., Divoll Allen, M., Harmatz, J. S., Shader, R. I. Diazepam disposition determinants. *Clin Pharmacol Ther* 1980; 27: 301–12. https://doi.org/10.1038/clpt.1980.40

7. Gunlicks-Stoessel, M., Mufson, L., Bernstein, G., et al. Critical decision points for augmenting interpersonal psychotherapy for depressed adolescents: a pilot sequential multiple assignment randomized trial. *J Am Acad Child Adolesc Psychiatry* 2019; 58: 80–91. https://doi.org/10.1016/j.jaac.2018.06.032

8. Kneller, L. A., Zubiaur, P., Koller, D., Abad-Santos, F., Hempel, G. Influence of CYP2D6 phenotypes on the pharmacokinetics of aripiprazole and dehydro-aripiprazole using a physiologically based pharmacokinetic approach. *Clin Pharmacokinet* 2021; 60: 1569–82. https://doi.org/10.1007/s40262-021-01041-x

9. Locher, C., Koechlin, H., Zion, S. R., et al. Efficacy and safety of selective serotonin reuptake inhibitors, serotonin–norepinephrine reuptake inhibitors, and placebo in common psychiatric disorders: a meta-analysis in children and adolescents. *JAMA Psychiatry* 2017; 74: 1011–20. https://doi.org/10.1001/jamapsychiatry.2017.2432

10. Shah, R. R., Smith, R. L. Addressing phenoconversion: the Achilles' heel of personalized medicine. *Br J Clin Pharmacol* 2015; 79: 222–40. https://doi.org/10.1111/bcp.12441

11. Shamseddeen, W., Clarke, G., Keller, M. B., et al. Adjunctive sleep medications and depression outcome in the treatment of serotonin-selective reuptake inhibitor resistant depression in adolescents study. *J Child Adolesc Psychopharmacol* 2012; 22: 29–36. https://doi.org/10.1089/cap.2011.0027

12. Strawn, J. R., Prakash, A., Zhang, Q., et al. A randomized, placebo-controlled study of duloxetine for the treatment of children and adolescents with generalized anxiety disorder. *J Am Acad Child Adolesc Psychiatry* 2015; 54: 283–93. https://doi.org/10.1016/j.jaac.2015.01.008

13. Strawn, J. R., Geracioti, L., Rajdev, N., Clemenza, K., Levine, A. Pharmacotherapy for generalized anxiety disorder in adult and pediatric patients: an evidence-based treatment review. *Expert Opin Pharmacother* 2018a; 19: 1057–70. https://doi.org/10.1080/14656566.2018.1491966

14. Strawn, J. R., Mills, J. A., Sauley, B. A., Welge, J. A. The impact of antidepressant dose and class on treatment response in pediatric anxiety disorders: a meta-analysis. *J Am Acad Child Adolesc Psychiatry* 2018b; 57: 235–44.e2. https://doi.org/10.1016/j.jaac.2018.01.015

15. Strawn, J. R., Lu, L., Peris, T. S., Levine, A., Walkup, J. T. Research review: pediatric anxiety disorders – what have we learnt in the last 10 years? *J Child Psychol Psychiatry* 2021; 62: 114–39. https://doi.org/10.1111/jcpp.13262

16. Suresh, V., Mills, J. A., Croarkin, P. E., Strawn, J. R. What next? A Bayesian hierarchical modeling re-examination of treatments for adolescents with selective serotonin reuptake inhibitor-resistant depression. *Depress Anxiety* 2020; 37: 926–34. https://doi.org/10.1002/da.23064

17. Walkup, J. T., Albano, A. M., Piacentini, J., et al. Cognitive behavioral therapy, sertraline, or a combination in childhood anxiety. *N Engl J Med* 2008; 359: 2753–66. https://doi.org/10.1056/NEJMoa0804633

18. Williams, T., Hattingh, C. J., Kariuki, C. M., et al. Pharmacotherapy for social anxiety disorder (SAnD). *Cochrane Database Syst Rev* 2017; 10: CD001206. https://doi.org/10.1002/14651858.CD001206.pub3

19. Zanger, U. M., Schwab, M. Cytochrome P450 enzymes in drug metabolism: regulation of gene expression, enzyme activities, and impact of genetic variation. *Pharmacol Ther* 2013; 138: 103–41. https://doi.org/10.1016/j.pharmthera.2012.12.007

Case 5: A 13-year-old adolescent who feels "amazing": selective serotonin reuptake inhibitor (SSRI)-induced mania in an adolescent

The Questions: What medications should be used in an adolescent who develops mania when treated with an SSRI? Does SSRI-related mania represent bipolar disorder?

The Psychopharmacological Dilemma: How to treat patients who are at "high risk" for developing bipolar disorder but are experiencing depressive and/or anxiety symptoms presents a challenge for many clinicians, particularly as SSRIs are the first-line pharmacotherapy for adolescents with depressive and anxiety disorders

Pretest self-assessment question

Which of the following is approved by the U.S. Food and Drug Administration (FDA) for the treatment of bipolar mania in adolescents?

A. Divalproex (Depakote)
B. Carbamazepine (Tegretol)
C. Asenapine (Saphris)
D. Clozapine (Clozaril)
E. All of the above

Answer: C (Asenapine, Saphris)

Patient evaluation on intake

- A 13-year-old adolescent who developed depressive symptoms over a period of 6 months
- She feels disengaged at school and with friends, and when at home she spends most of her time in her room
- She wishes to not be alive several days per week, and when this wish is present she is thinking about it for several hours at a time, although she denies having thought about specific ways in which she might end her life
- She sleeps up to 12 hours per day, chronically feels tired, and feels unmotivated
- She was treated with interpersonal psychotherapy for adolescents (IPT-A) for 4 months, but continued to experience significant depressive symptoms
- Significant depressive symptoms and ongoing heavy neurovegetative burden
- No significant anxiety symptoms
- No history of attention-deficit hyperactivity disorder (ADHD)

Psychiatric history

- The onset of depressive symptoms was at age 11 years 5 months

Social and personal history

- The patient lives with her mother and father
- She achieved As and Bs in middle school (prior to the onset of her mood symptoms), and has always had a small group of friends
- Active in a local archery club, and gets on well with friends
- No history of abuse or trauma, and no legal history

Medical history

- Delivered at 39 weeks to a 30-year-old mother and 31-year-old father
- Her mother was treated with quetiapine for an affective disorder during the last 8 weeks of her pregnancy
- Normal developmental milestones

Family history

- Mother with bipolar I disorder, who is currently being treated with quetiapine (extended-release formulation) 200 mg daily with adjunctive metformin 1000 mg twice daily for second-generation antipsychotic (SGA)-associated weight gain
- There is no family history of substance use disorders or endocrinopathy

Medication history

- No pharmacotherapy currently

Current medications

- Fexofenadine 180 mg daily

Psychotherapy history

- IPT-A has been ongoing for 4 months, and occurs weekly

Further investigation

Is there anything else that you would like to know about the patient? What about possible manic or hypomanic symptoms?

- When asked about her decreased need for sleep, the patient comments that she once stayed up while spending the night with

a friend, but "crashed" the next day and was "so exhausted that I couldn't function"
- She denies hypersexuality, grandiosity, pressured speech, flight of ideas, or other manic symptoms

Attending physician's mental notes: initial psychiatric evaluation

- This patient has a moderate major depressive episode and a maternal family history of bipolar I disorder
- Her symptoms have persisted despite IPT-A, and there is no evidence of prior mania
- In considering the evidence for pharmacotherapy in adolescents with a family history of bipolar I disorder the guidelines are unclear, and current recommendations are for a trial of an SSRI prior to careful observation. Trials of divalproex plus SSRIs have not suggested substantial benefit (Findling et al. 2008). However, some studies – without comparison groups – suggest that antidepressants may not be as well tolerated in children and adolescents with a family history of bipolar disorder (Strawn et al. 2014)

Question

Given the patient's current symptoms, what would be your next step?

- Begin fluoxetine 10 mg daily
- Omega-3 fatty acid supplementation
- Quetiapine 100 mg every night at bedtime
- A trial of high-frequency transcranial magnetic stimulation (TMS) of the left dorsolateral prefrontal cortex for 6 weeks

Case outcome: first interim follow-up (week 2)

- The patient began fluoxetine 10 mg every morning while continuing psychotherapy
- One week after beginning fluoxetine, she commented that she felt "amazing," and showed a rapid and significant improvement in depressive symptoms
- She was no longer sleeping for 12 hours per day, was no longer napping, had improved energy and motivation, and her parents mentioned that she was more engaged with friends, and was spending less time in her room
- The patient had complete resolution of her previously reported Columbia–Suicide Severity Rating Scale (CSSRS) 1-2 suicidal ideation (Posner et al. 2011)

Attending physician's mental notes: first interim follow-up (week 2)

- Given the patient's significant response, the attending physician is concerned. However, a thorough interview with the patient and her parents (including both conjoint and separate time) reveals no hypomanic or manic symptoms

Question

This patient has had a robust and early response to fluoxetine within 2 weeks, and almost complete resolution of her symptoms. Which of the following would be your next step?

- Discontinue fluoxetine (Prozac)
- Re-evaluate symptoms in 1 week
- Begin quetiapine (Seroquel) 50 mg every night at bedtime

Case outcome: second interim follow-up (week 3)

- The patient is re-evaluated in 1 week
- She reports feeling "better than ever," although her parents noted that there were times when she would still cry and would be particularly irritable with family members, friends, and teachers
- Her parents were concerned by several recent events, including the patient having stolen her mother's credit card, spent $1,300 on underwear, talked to several older men online, and used sexually explicit language during these conversations
- The patient was only sleeping for 4–5 hours per night, was struggling with attention at school, and was experiencing deteriorating academic performance. She was at times more irritable in her interactions with her family members, but continued to do well in terms of her peer interactions
- She noted that her "thinking speed was about 80 miles per hour," and on examination was found to have tangential thought processes and pressured speech
- Fluoxetine was discontinued, and asenapine was initiated at 2.5 mg twice daily. After 2 weeks it was titrated to 5 mg twice daily. Then, 2 weeks later, it was titrated to 10 mg twice daily

Attending physician's mental notes: second interim follow-up (week 3)

- The patient has clear symptoms of mania and significant functional impact
- Given the severity of her symptoms, inpatient hospitalization was considered. Compared with adults, the decision to admit pediatric patients to a psychiatric unit is based on developmental factors. In considering this, suicidality is of particular importance. When children and adolescents consider suicide, the time between consideration of suicide and a suicide attempt is significantly shorter than in adults, narrowing the window for intervention. In part, this shortened window for intervention relates to neuromaturational factors and underdevelopment of the prefrontal cortex, which is also delayed in boys compared with girls
- In considering psychiatric admission for this adolescent, clinicians may use the Child and Adolescent Service Intensity Instrument (CASII). This was developed by the American Academy of Child & Adolescent Psychiatry in 2007 (www.aacap.org/aacap/Member_Resources/Practice_Information/CASII.aspx) and evaluates several important domains:

  Dimension I: Risk of harm
  Dimension II: Functional status
  Dimension III: Co-occurring conditions (developmental, medical, substance use related)
  Dimension IV: Recovery environment – environmental stress
  Dimension IV: Recovery environment – environmental support
  Dimension V: Resilience and/or response to services

The first two dimensions for this patient are shown here.

- The clinician was also very concerned about the kinetics of fluoxetine. Given that the mania-producing effects of the fluoxetine would persist for weeks, an antidepressant with a shorter half-life would have been cleared much more quickly
- Additionally, the clinician is concerned about the presence of mixed features, which are more common in pediatric patients with bipolar I disorder than in adults, and considers this particularly with regard to the patient's increased risk of suicide. The clinician is also conceptualizing her symptoms with regard to the affective spectrum (Figure 5.1)
- The clinician chose asenapine based on the evidence for its efficacy in the pediatric population (Findling et al. 2015a, 2015b, 2018). Also, given the severity of the patient's current symptoms, he hopes that some of the initial sedation might be helpful in addressing

her sleep and psychomotor agitation. However, he knows that asenapine may be more sedating than other medications within this class, including other SGAs that are approved for pediatric patients with mania (e.g. lurasidone, aripiprazole). He is also concerned about the risk of weight gain (Dogterom et al. 2018; Findling et al. 2015a), and will monitor this carefully, although prior to prescribing asenapine he considered the patient's baseline body mass index (BMI) percentile and reviewed recent labs from her pediatrician, including her HbA1C and her last fasting lipids (Figure 5.2)

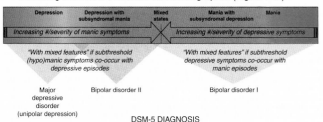

Depression	Depression with subsyndromal mania	Mixed states	Mania with subsyndromal depression	Mania

Increasing #/severity of manic symptoms | Increasing #/severity of depressive symptoms

"With mixed features" if subthreshold (hypo)manic symptoms co-occur with depressive episodes

"With mixed features" if subthreshold depressive symptoms co-occur with manic episodes

Major depressive disorder (unipolar depression)

Bipolar disorder II

Bipolar disorder I

DSM-5 DIAGNOSIS

Figure 5.1 Mixed features and the mood disorders continuum.

Child and Adolescent Service Intensity Instrument (CASII)

Dimension I. Risk of Harm (*Circle the number below that best represents the child's or adolescent's current potential to be harmed by others or cause significant harm to self or others*)

Low Risk of Harm (1)	Some Risk of Harm (2)	Significant Risk of Harm (3)	Serious Risk of Harm (4)*	Extreme Risk of Harm (5)**
a. No indication of current suicidal or homicidal thoughts or impulses, with no significant distress, and no history of suicidal or homicidal ideation. b. No indication or report of physically or sexually aggressive impulses. c. Developmentally appropriate ability to maintain physical safety and/or use environment for safety. d. Low risk for victimization, abuse, or neglect e. Other:	a. Past history of fleeting suicidal or homicidal thoughts with no current ideation, plan, or intention and no significant distress. b. Mild suicidal ideation with no intent or conscious plan and with no past history. c. Indication or report of occasional impulsivity, and/or some physically or sexually aggressive impulses with minimal consequences for self or others. d. Substance use without significant endangerment of self or others. e. Infrequent, brief lapses in the ability to care for self and/or use environment for safety. f. Some risk for victimization, abuse, or neglect. g. Other:	a. Significant current suicidal or homicidal ideation with some intent and plan, with the ability of the child or adolescent and his/her family to contract for safety and carry out a safety plan. Child or adolescent expresses some aversion to carrying out such behavior. b. No active suicidal/ homicidal ideation, but extreme distress and/or a history of suicidal/ homicidal behavior. c. Indication or report of episodic impulsivity, or physically or sexually aggressive impulses that are moderately endangering to self or others (e.g. status offenses, impulsive acts while intoxicated; self – mutilation; running away from home or facility with voluntary return; fire setting; violence toward animals; affiliation with dangerous peer group). d. Binge or excessive use of alcohol or other drugs resulting in potentially harmful behaviors. e. Episodic inability to care for self and/or maintain physical safety in developmentally appropriate ways. f. Serious or extreme risk for victimization, abuse, or neglect. g. Other:	a. Current suicidal or homicidal ideation with either clear expressed intentions and/or past history of carrying out such behavior. Child or adolescent has expressed ambivalence about carrying out the safety plan and/or his/her family's ability to carry out the safety plan is compromised. b. Indication or report of significant impulsivity and/or physical or sexual aggression, with poor judgment and insight, that is/are significantly endangering to self or others (property destruction; repetitive fire setting or violence toward animals). c. Indication of consistent deficits in ability to care for self and/or use environment for safety. d. Recent pattern of excessive substance use resulting in clearly harmful behaviors with no demonstrated ability of child/adolescent or family to restrict use. e. Clear and persistent inability, given developmental abilities, to maintain physical safety and/or use environment for safety. f. Other:	a. Current suicidal or homicidal behavior or such intentions with a plan and available means to carry out this behavior; without expressed ambivalence or significant barriers to doing so, or with a history of serious past attempts that are not of a chronic, impulsive, or consistent nature, or in presence of command hallucinations or delusions that threaten to override usual impulse control. b. Indication or report of repeated behavior, including physical or sexual aggression, that is clearly injurious to self or others (e.g. fire setting with intent of serious property destruction or harm to others or self, planned violence and/or group violence with other perpetrators) with history, plan or intent, and no insight and judgment (forcible and violent, repetitive sexual acts against others), c. Relentless engaging in acutely self endangering behaviors. d. A pattern of nearly constant and uncontrolled use of alcohol or other drugs, resulting in behavior that is clearly endangering. e. Other:

* Requires level 5 independent of other dimensions
** Requires level 6, independent of other dimensions

Child and Adolescent Service Intensity Instrument (CASII)

Dimension II. Functional Status (*Circle the number below that best represents the child's or adolescent's current level of functioning*)

Minimal Impairment (1)	Mild Impairment (2)	Moderate Impairment (3)	Serious Impairment (4)*	Severe Impairment (5)**
a. Consistent functioning appropriate to age and developmental level in school behavior and/or academic achievement, relationships with peers, adults, and family, and self care/hygiene/control of bodily functions. b. No more than transient impairment in functioning following exposure to an identifiable stressor with consistent and normative vegetative status. c. Other:	a. Evidence of minor deterioration, or episodic failure to achieve expected levels of functioning, in relationships with peers, adults, and/or family (e.g. defiance, provocative behavior, lying/cheating/not sharing, or avoidance/lack of follow through); school behavior and/or academic achievement (difficulty turning in homework, occasional attendance problems), or biologic functions (feeding or elimination problems) but with adequate functioning in at least some areas and/or ability to respond to redirection/intervention. b. Sporadic episodes during which some aspects of self-care/hygiene/control of bodily functions are compromised. c. Demonstrates significant improvement in function following a period of deterioration. d. Other:	a. Conflicted, withdrawn, or otherwise troubled in relationships with peers, adults, and/or family, but without episodes of physical aggression. b. Self-care/hygiene deteriorates below usual or expected standards on a frequent basis. c. Significant disturbances in vegetative activities, (such as sleeping, eating habits, activity level, or sexual interest), that do not pose a serious threat to health. d. School behavior has deteriorated to the point that in-school suspension has occurred and the child is at risk for placement in an alternative school or expulsion due to their disruptive behavior. Absenteeism may be frequent. The child is at risk for repeating their grade. e. Chronic and/or variably severe deficits in interpersonal relationships, ability to engage in socially constructive activities, and responsibilities. f. Recent gains and/or stabilization in functioning have been achieved while participating in treatment in a structured, protected, and/or enriched setting. g. Other:	a. Serious deterioration of interpersonal interactions with consistently conflictual or otherwise disrupted relations with others, which may include impulsive or abusive behaviors. b. Significant withdrawal and avoidance of almost all social interaction. c. Consistent failure to achieve self-care/hygiene at levels appropriate to age and/or developmental level. d. Serious disturbances in vegetative status such as weight change, disrupted sleep or fatigue, and feeding or elimination, which threaten physical functioning. e. Inability to perform adequately even in a specialized school setting due to disruptive or aggressive behavior. School attendance may be sporadic. The child or adolescent has multiple academic failures. f. Other:	a. Extreme deterioration in interactions with peers, adults, and/or family that may include chaotic communication or assaultive behaviors. with little or no provocation, minimal control over impulses that may result in abusive behaviors. b. Complete withdrawal from all social interactions c. Complete neglect of, and inability to attend to self-care/hygiene/control of biological functions with associated impairment in physical status. d. Extreme disruption in vegetative function causing serious compromise of health and well being. e. Nearly complete inability to maintain any appropriate school behavior and/or academic achievement given age and developmental level. f. Other:

* Requires level 5 independent of other dimensions
** Requires level 6, independent of other dimensions

Weight Gain

unusual   not unusual   common   problematic

- Occurs in a significant minority
- May be less than for some antipsychotics, more then for others

Sedation

unusual   not unusual   common   problematic

Figure 5.2 Weight gain and sedation associated with asenapine.

Case outcome: third interim follow-up (week 5)

- As an outpatient, after titration of asenapine to 10 mg twice daily she felt better and was free of depressive and manic symptoms. Asenapine titration followed the current recommendations: initially 5 mg daily in two divided doses; after 3 days it can be increased to 10 mg daily in two divided doses; after 3 more days it can be increased to 20 mg daily in two divided doses

- Her mixed features had resolved
- She was doing better in terms of family functioning, although she experienced some anxiety related to the amount of school that she had missed as a result of her manic episode
- Additionally, she was doing well in terms of appetite, although she had gained 0.5 kg over the past 10 days

Attending physician's mental notes: third interim follow-up (week 5)

- The attending physician is very encouraged by the patient's early improvement with asenapine; however, he is concerned about her weight gain and will monitor this closely, in addition to recommended metabolic parameters
- Increasingly, in the pediatric setting, there is evidence for beginning metformin early, particularly in those patients who have a BMI above the 85th percentile and who have experienced early SGA-related weight gain. Metformin is initiated at 500 mg twice daily, and can be titrated to 1000 mg twice daily over several weeks (DelBello et al. 2017; Strawn and DelBello 2018)
- The attending physician will discuss communication with the school system so that accommodations might be considered for the patient's missed assignments and additional missed instruction secondary to her symptoms. Such coordination with school systems and school counselors is common in child and adolescent psychiatry. Additionally, depending on persistent impairment or effects of symptoms on school functioning, the clinician may work with the school to evaluate the patient for specific accommodations, including those provided by 504 Plans and Individualized Education Plans (IEPs)

Take-home points

- Mixed symptoms are common in pediatric patients with bipolar disorder, and evidence suggests that antidepressants are poorly tolerated in pediatric patients with a family history of bipolar disorder. However, randomized prospective trials of this population have only recently been completed, and the results are expected soon
- Low omega-3 fatty acid concentrations have been observed in adolescents with major depressive disorder (MDD) and in those with depressive symptoms who have a parent with bipolar disorder (McNamara and Strawn 2013; McNamara et al. 2014). Additionally, several prospective studies have shown that, in patients with mild to moderate depressive symptoms and a family history of bipolar disorder, omega-3 fatty acid supplementation is helpful and

may affect functional activity in brain areas that are implicated in pediatric bipolar disorder. However, the dose and source of fatty acids are particularly important, and the recommended dose is at least 3 grams of eicosatetraenoic acid (EPA) plus docosahexaenoic acid (DHA) per day (McNamara and Strawn 2013). In general, omega-3 fatty acids are well tolerated

Tips and pearls

- Asenapine is poorly absorbed after swallowing (less than 2% bioavailability orally) and thus must be administered sublingually (35% bioavailability), as swallowing would render the medication inactive. However, peak concentrations generally occur within 1 hour in pediatric patients (Figure 5.3)

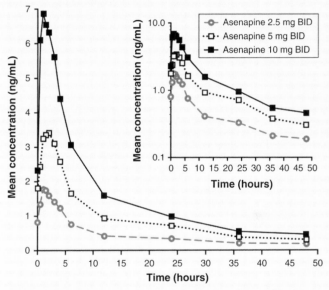

Figure 5.3 Mean asenapine plasma concentration–time profiles in children and adolescents aged 10–17. BID, twice daily. Reproduced from Dogterom et al. (2018).

- Also, daily use seems to be theoretically possible because the half-life of asenapine is 13–39 hours, but this has not been extensively studied, and may be complicated by the need to expose the sublingual surface area to a limited amount of sublingual drug dosage
- Peak concentrations tend to be about 30% higher in younger patients (age 10–11) compared with older adolescents (Dogterom et al. 2018)
- Pediatric patients should be instructed to place the tablet under the tongue and allow it to dissolve completely, which will occur in seconds; the tablet should not be divided, crushed, chewed, or swallowed

- Patients should not eat or drink for 10 minutes following sublingual administration, so that the drug in the oral cavity can be absorbed locally and is not washed into the stomach (where it would not be absorbed)

Mechanism of action moment

- Asenapine, like other SGAs, or mixed dopamine/serotonin receptor antagonists, antagonizes D_2 and 5-HT_{2A} receptors; however, asenapine has a complex binding profile and potent binding at multiple serotonergic and dopaminergic receptors. In addition, it binds at α_1 and α_2 receptors. However, the effects of α_1 antagonism on blood pressure tend to be less pronounced in pediatric patients, given that blood pressure in younger patients is primarily regulated by heart rate and stroke volume rather than by peripheral vascular resistance. That said, adolescent females may be more sensitive to these orthostatic effects
- Asenapine has activity at 5-HT_{2C} receptors (Figure 5.4), which potentially – in combination with its H_1 histamine-receptor antagonism – contributes to weight gain

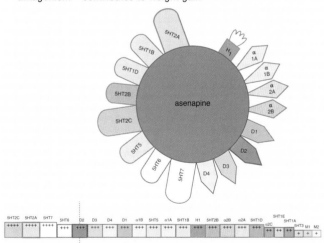

Figure 5.4 Pharmacological and binding profile of asenapine. This figure portrays a qualitative consensus of current thinking about the binding properties of asenapine. It has a complex binding profile, with potent binding at multiple serotonergic and dopaminergic receptors, α_1 and α_2 receptors, and H_1 histamine receptors. In particular, 5-HT_{2C} antagonist properties may contribute to its efficacy for mood and cognitive symptoms, whereas 5-HT_7 antagonist properties may contribute to its efficacy for mood, cognitive, and sleep symptoms. As with all of the agents discussed in this case, binding properties vary greatly depending on technique and from one laboratory to another; they are constantly being revised and updated. Adapted from Stahl et al. (2021).

Post test self-assessment question

Which of the following is approved by the FDA for the treatment of bipolar mania in adolescents?

A. Divalproex (Depakote)
B. Carbamazepine (Tegretol)
C. Asenapine (Saphris)
D. Clozapine (Clozaril)
E. All of the above

Answer: C (Asenapine, Saphris)

Asenapine has been studied in multiple double-blind placebo-controlled trials of children and adolescents with bipolar disorder, including those with mixed episodes. It is approved by the FDA for this indication. Divalproex has demonstrated poor tolerability in adolescents with mania, and in adolescent females there are specific concerns related to the risk of polycystic ovarian syndrome and also the teratogenic effects should a divalproex-treated adolescent become pregnant. Finally, clozapine should not be used as a first-line treatment for mania in adolescents.

References

1. DelBello, M. P., Strawn, J. R., Duran, L. P. Recognition and management of second-generation antipsychotic-associated adverse effects. *J Am Acad Child Adolesc Psychiatry* 2017; 56: S135. https://doi.org/10.1016/j.jaac.2017.07.509
2. Dogterom, P., Riesenberg, R., de Greef, R., et al. Asenapine pharmacokinetics and tolerability in a pediatric population. *Drug Design Dev Ther* 2018; 12: 2677–93. https://doi.org/10.2147/DDDT.S171475
3. Findling, R. L., Lingler, J., Rowles, B. M., et al. A pilot pharmacotherapy trial for depressed youths at high genetic risk for bipolarity. *J Child Adolesc Psychopharmacol* 2008; 18: 615–21. https://doi.org/10.1089/cap.2008.018
4. Findling, R. L., Landbloom, R. P., Mackle, M., et al. Safety and efficacy from an 8 week double-blind trial and a 26 week open-label extension of asenapine in adolescents with schizophrenia. *J Child Adolesc Psychopharmacol* 2015a; 25: 384–96. https://doi.org/10.1089/cap.2015.0027
5. Findling, R. L., Landbloom, R. L., Szegedi, A., et al. Asenapine for the acute treatment of pediatric manic or mixed episode of bipolar I disorder. *J Am Acad Child Adolesc Psychiatry* 2015b; 54: 1032–41. https://doi.org/10.1016/j.jaac.2015.09.007

6. Findling, R. L., Earley, W., Suppes, T., et al. Post hoc analyses of asenapine treatment in pediatric patients with bipolar I disorder: efficacy related to mixed or manic episode, stage of illness, and body weight. *Neuropsychiatr Dis Treat* 2018; 14: 1941–52. https://doi.org/10.2147/NDT.S165743

7. McNamara, R. K., Strawn, J. R. Role of long-chain omega-3 fatty acids in psychiatric practice. *PharmaNutrition* 2013; 1: 41–9. https://doi.org/10.1016/j.phanu.2012.10.004

8. McNamara, R. K., Strimpfel, J., Jandacek, R. et al. Detection and treatment of long-chain omega-3 fatty acid deficiency in adolescents with SSRI-resistant major depressive disorder. *PharmaNutrition* 2014; 2: 38–46. https://doi.org/10.1016/j.phanu.2014.02.002

9. Posner, K., Brown, G. K., Stanley, B., et al. The Columbia–Suicide Severity Rating Scale: initial validity and internal consistency findings from three multisite studies with adolescents and adults. *Am J Psychiatry* 2011; 168: 1266–77. https://doi.org/10.1176/appi.ajp.2011.10111704

10. Stahl, S., Grady, M. M., Muntner, N. *Stahl's Essential Psychopharmacology: Neuroscientific Basis and Practical Applications*, 5th edn. Cambridge, UK: Cambridge University Press, 2021.

11. Strawn, J. R., DelBello, M. P. Recognizing and managing side effects of second-generation antipsychotics. *J Am Acad Child Adolesc Psychiatry* 2018; 57: S85. PMID: 16001096.

12. Strawn, J. R., Adler, C. M., McNamara, R. K., et al. Antidepressant tolerability in anxious and depressed youth at high risk for bipolar disorder: a prospective naturalistic treatment study. *Bipolar Disord* 2014; 16: 523–30. https://doi.org/10.1111/bdi.12113

Case 6: Counting on a cure: obsessive compulsive disorder (OCD) in an adolescent

The Question: When should medications other than selective serotonin reuptake inhibitors (SSRIs) be used, and how should clomipramine be dosed and monitored in pediatric OCD?

The Psychopharmacological Dilemma: The decision to move beyond SSRIs in treating adolescents with OCD is difficult for many clinicians. In addition, some clinicians experience trepidation about initiating clomipramine and using therapeutic drug-monitoring strategies

Pretest self-assessment question

Which of the following represents the best and most evidence-based intervention for an adolescent with OCD who has failed three SSRIs and cognitive behavior therapy (CBT)?

A. Duloxetine (Cymbalta)
B. Venlafaxine (Effexor)
C. Aripiprazole (Abilify)
D. Clomipramine (Anafranil)
E. Imipramine (Tofranil)

Answer: D (Clomipramine, Anafranil)

Patient evaluation on intake

- A 16-year-old girl who developed obsessive compulsive symptoms at age 10 and was treated with exposure-based CBT
- She has multiple obsessions, including thoughts that she might accidentally hurt someone. These thoughts are very ego-dystonic, and she feels intense guilt related to them, which she recognizes as "not right, since I'd never hurt anyone"
- She worries about being contaminated by germs or dirt and has several safety rituals
- She repeatedly washes her hands, even while at home, she needs to turn off her lights four times, and she must have the audio volume settings on even numbers; she has several additional repeating and ordering/arranging rituals
- She spends 3–5 hours daily attending to her obsessions and performing her compulsive behaviors, and her parents have attempted to limit her evening showering rituals to less than 90 minutes
- When she was queried regarding her ritualistic behavior, she noted that she must touch and tap things in a certain way and repeatedly asked her mother and father about the correctness of her behavior. She frequently feels as though she has to tell on herself

- She denies both trichotillomania and repeatedly having to say the same words, prayers, or sentences over and over, or eating or drinking in a special order
- She denies depressive symptoms, although she notes some concentration-related difficulties, commenting "when my OCD is bad or I'm under a lot of stress, I can't concentrate"
- She denies suicidal thoughts and self-injurious behavior
- She reports constant obsessions and functionally limiting compulsions, worrying, and difficulty concentrating
- No reports of depressed mood, anhedonia, or suicidal ideation
- No manic or psychotic symptoms
- There are no reports of heat or cold intolerance, recent weight loss, or dysmenorrhea
- The patient denies cardiac symptoms, including palpitations
- There is no suicidal ideation, intent, or plan currently
- She denies any recent stressors

Psychiatric history

- The patient was seen in individual psychotherapy as described earlier, and recently began work with a new psychotherapist
- At times when she has experienced increased symptoms she has seen the school counselor once weekly for 3–4 weeks at a time, but this was stopped "because the coping strategies didn't help"

Social and personal history

- The patient lives with her mother and father and her 6-year-old brother
- She relates that she has a good relationship with her parents, although she is closer to her mother
- She denies use of alcohol, or the use of marijuana or other illicit substances. She does not vape or use other tobacco-containing products
- She is not currently in a relationship
- She denies any history of abuse or significant trauma

Medical history

- Delivered at 36 weeks to a 27-year-old mother and 26-year-old father
- Her parents report normal developmental milestones

Family history

- Mother with a history of generalized anxiety disorder
- Father with a history of OCD
- There is no family history of substance use disorders or endocrinopathy

Medication history

- At age 12, while continuing psychotherapy, the patient began fluoxetine, which was titrated to 40 mg daily over 8 months. She continued to experience significant OCD symptoms; fluoxetine was discontinued, and sertraline was initiated at 25 mg and titrated to 150 mg daily with minimal benefit
- At age 15, she began fluvoxamine (extended-release formulation), which was titrated to 300 mg every night at bedtime
- She is tolerating fluvoxamine 300 mg daily with minimal improvement, and has experienced some weight gain

Current medications

- Fluvoxamine (extended-release formulation) 300 mg every night at bedtime
- Psychotherapy began at age 10 in early adolescence, and consisted of exposure-response prevention
- At age 12 the patient began psychotherapy with a new therapist, who met regularly with her parents, and she describes being given weekly homework by her therapist
- During her prior work in psychotherapy, her therapist worked with her parents to reduce blame for her symptoms

Further investigation

What about additional physical symptoms and vital signs?

- Vital signs are within normal limits; the patient's body mass index (BMI) is in the 78th percentile for age and sex
- There has been no recent weight loss
- She denies cardiac symptoms, including palpitations

What about structured rating scales?

The Children's Yale-Brown Obsessive-Compulsive Scale (CY-BOCS) is an evidence-based scale for evaluating the frequency and severity of obsessions and compulsions (Scahill et al. 1997). It is freely available and has been incorporated into several electronic medical record systems. This patient's CY-BOCS score is shown here:

Rating scales

Children's Yale-Brown Obsessive Compulsive Scale

Administering the CY-BOCS Symptom Checklist and CY-BOCS Severity Ratings

1. Establish the diagnosis of obsessive compulsive disorder.
2. Using the CY-BOCS Symptom Checklist (other form), ascertain current and past symptoms.
3. Next, administer the 10-item severity ratings (below) to assess the severity of the OCD during the last week.
4. Readminister the CY-BOCS Severity Rating Scale to monitor progress.

Obsession Rating Scale (circle appropriate score)

Note: Scores should reflect the composite effect of all the patient's obsessive compulsive symptoms.
Rate the average occurrence of each item during the prior week up to and including the time of interview.

QUESTIONS ON OBSESSIONS (ITEMS 1–5) *"I AM NOW GOING TO ASK YOU QUESTIONS ABOUT THE THOUGHTS YOU CANNOT STOP THINKING ABOUT."* (Review for the informant(s) the Target Symptoms and refer to them while asking questions 1–5).

1. Time Occupied by Obsessive Thoughts
[Be sure to exclude ruminations and preoccupations which, unlike obsessions, are ego-syntonic and rational (but exaggerated)]

	None	Mild	Moderate	Severe	Extreme
		less than 1 hr/day or occasional intrusion	1 to 3 hrs/day or frequent intrusion	greater than 3 and up to 8 hrs/day or very frequent intrusion	greater than 8 hrs/day or near constant intrusion
Score	0	1	2	(3)	4

2. Interference Due to Obsessive Thoughts
* How much do these thoughts get in the way of school or doing things with friends?
* Is there anything that you don't do because of them? (If currently not in school, determine how much performance would be affected if patient were in school)

	None	Mild	Moderate	Severe	Extreme
		slight interference with social or school activities, but overall performance not impaired	definite interference with social or school performance, but still manageable	causes substantial impairment in social or school performance	incapacitating
Score	0	1	2	(3)	4

3. Distress Associated with Obsessive Thoughts

	None	Mild	Moderate	Severe	Extreme
		infrequent, and not too disturbing	frequent, and disturbing, but still manageable	very frequent, and very disturbing	near constant, and disabling distress/frustration
Score	0	1	(2)	3	4

4. Resistance Against Obsessions
* How hard do you try to stop the thoughts or ignore them? (Only rate effort made to resist, not success or failure in actually controlling the obsessions. If the obsessions are minimal, the patient may not feel the need to resist them, in such cases, a rating of "0" should be given.)

	None	Mild	Moderate	Severe	Extreme
	makes an effort to always resist, or symptoms so minimal doesn't need to actively resist	tries to resist most of the time	makes some effort to resist	yields to all obsessions without attempting to control them, but does so with some reluctance	completely and willingly yields to all obsessions
Score	0	1	2	(3)	4

5. Degree of Control Over Obsessive Thoughts

	Complete Control	Much Control	Moderate Control	Little Control	No Control
		usually able to stop or divert obsessions with some effort and concentration	sometimes able to stop or divert obsessions	rarely successful in stopping obsessions, can only divert attention with difficulty	experienced as completely involuntary, rarely able to even momentarily divert thinking
Score	0	1	(2)	3	4

Obsession subtotal (add items 1–5) _____ 13

<u>QUESTIONS ON COMPULSIONS (ITEMS 6–10)</u> *"I AM NOW GOING TO ASK YOU QUESTIONS ABOUT THE HABITS YOU CAN'T STOP"* (Review for the informant(s) the Target Symptoms and refer to them while asking questions 6–10).

6. Time Spent Performing Compulsive Behaviors

	None	Mild less than 1 hr/day	Moderate 1 to 3 hrs/day	Severe greater than 3 & up to 8 hrs/day	Extreme greater than 8 hrs/day
Score	0	1	2	(3)	4

7. Interference Due to Compulsive Behaviors
- How much do these habits get in the way of school or doing things with friends?
- Is there anything that you don't do because of them? (If currently not in school, determine how much performance would be affected if patient were in school.)

	None	Mild slight interference with social or school activities, but overall performance not impaired	Moderate definite interference with social or school performance, but still manageable	Severe causes substantial impairment in social or school performance	Extreme incapacitating
Score	0	1	(2)	3	4

8. Distress Associated with Compulsive Behavior
- How would you feel if prevented from carrying out your habits? How upset would you become?

	None	Mild only slightly anxious if compulsions prevented	Moderate anxiety would mount but remain manageable if compulsions prevented	Severe prominent and very disturbing increase in anxiety if compulsions interrupted	Extreme incapacitating anxiety from any intervention aimed at modifying activity
Score	0	1	(2)	3	4

9. Resistance Against Compulsions
- How much do you try to fight the habits? (Only rate effort made to resist, not success or failure in actually controlling the compulsions.)

	None makes an effort to always resist, or symptoms so minimal doesn't need to actively resist	Mild tries to resist most of the time	Moderate makes some effort to resist	Severe yields to all obsessions without attempting to control them, but does so with some reluctance	Extreme completely and willingly yields to all obsessions
Score	0	1	(2)	3	4

10. Degree of Control Over Compulsive Thoughts
- How strong is the feeling that you have to carry out the habit(s)?
- When you try to fight them, what happens?

	Complete Control	Much Control experiences pressure to perform the behavior, but usually able to exercise voluntary control over it	Moderate Control moderate control, strong pressure to perform behavior, can control it only with difficulty	Little Control little control, very strong drive to perform behavior, must be carried to completion, can only delay with difficulty	Extreme no control, drive to perform behavior experienced as completely involuntary and overpowering, rarely able to delay activity [even momentarily]
Score	0	1	(2)	3	4

Compulsion subtotal (add items 6–10)	11
CY-BOCS total (add items 1–10)	24

Total CY-BOCS score: range of severity for patients who have both obsessions and compulsions

0–7	Subclinical	24–31	Severe
8–15	Mild	32–40	Extreme
16–23	Moderate		

Attending physician's mental notes: initial psychiatric evaluation

- This patient has severe OCD that is refractory to multiple SSRIs and traditional psychotherapies
- Her CY-BOCS score is 24, and is consistent with severe OCD
- Several family factors predict poor response to psychotherapy in pediatric patients with OCD, including high family conflict, explicit blame for the child's symptoms, and poor family cohesion (Bloch and Storch 2015; Peris et al. 2012). These factors have a synergistic effect, and the attending physician notes that blame was a form of treatment in prior psychotherapy. In the largest trial of psychotherapy and pharmacotherapy for adolescents with OCD, 80% of patients with none of these risk factors responded (Figure 6.1). However, barely 1 in 10 patients with all three risk factors responded (Peris et al. 2012)

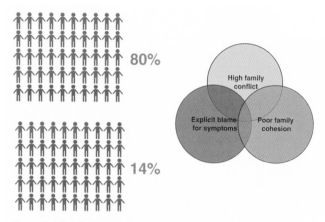

Figure 6.1 Family factors associated with response in pediatric patients with OCD. Only 14% of patients with all three of these characteristics responded to treatment. Adapted from Peris et al. (2012).

- The attending physician also considered several factors in the patient's history that may have predicted (or explained) her poor outcome with prior treatments (Figure 6.2)

Symptoms
- Greater symptom severity
- Greater OCD-related functional impairment
- Higher comorbid externalizing symptoms

Psychological factors
- Lower willingness to experience unpleasant thoughts
- Greater resistance to change
- Less insight

Family characteristics
- High family conflict
- Poor cohesion
- Explicit blame for symptoms
- Greater family accommodation

Other characteristics
- Family history of OCD → sixfold decrease in CBT monotherapy response
- Poor treatment adherence

Figure 6.2 Predictors of poor outcomes in pediatric OCD.

Question

Given the patient's current treatment, which of the following would be your next step?

- Laboratory screening for hyperthyroidism
- Pharmacogenetic testing for pharmacokinetic genes
- Augmentation of her fluvoxamine (Luvox) with risperidone (Risperdal) 0.5 mg every night at bedtime
- Discontinuation of fluvoxamine (Luvox) and a trial of clomipramine (Anafranil)

Given the patient's age, normal vital signs, lack of family history, and lack of clinical symptoms of hyperthyroidism, as well as the lack of medications known to impact thyroid function, laboratory screening for hyperthyroidism may be of limited utility (Luft et al. 2019).

She has had trials of several SSRIs, including medications that are metabolized through both CYP2C19 and CYP2D6 as well as CYP3A4 and CYP1A2. She has tolerated these, even at high doses, without side effects and much response. As such, pharmacogenetic testing is unlikely to be useful in this patient.

Augmentation of fluvoxamine with risperidone is unlikely to produce significant benefit in adolescents, and may be particularly problematic in adolescent females secondary to the risk of hyperprolactinemia (higher in adolescents compared with adults), which produces secondary amenorrhea and affects bone mineralization during this developmental period.

Case outcome: first interim follow-up (week 2)

- Before beginning clomipramine, an electrocardiogram (EKG) was obtained and was remarkable only for sinus arrhythmia (common in athletic individuals and adolescents)
- Clomipramine was initiated, was titrated to 25 mg every morning and 50 mg every night at bedtime, and is well tolerated
- The patient and her parents have noted an improvement in her anxiety, specifically in terms of her intrusive thoughts
- Her mother reports that her "rituals" consume significantly less time during the day and interfere less with family activities
- There continues to be high family cohesion and low family conflict
- The patient is sleeping better and reports having more "restful" sleep

Testing: laboratory results, imaging, EKGs

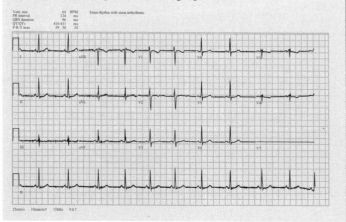

Attending physician's mental notes: first interim follow-up (week 2)

- The attending physician is encouraged by the lack of significant side effects, and there has been a 25% reduction in the patient's CY-BOCS score, even during the second week of treatment
- Based on this, the physician titrates clomipramine to 50 mg twice daily, then 50 mg every morning and 75 mg every night at bedtime, and then 75 mg twice daily over 4 weeks
- The attending physician is also aware that the response to clomipramine in pediatric patients with OCD may be not only greater than for SSRIs, but also faster (Figure 6.3)

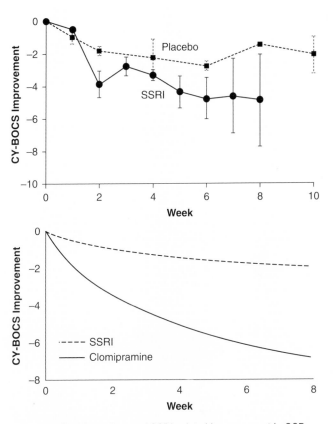

Figure 6.3. Clomipramine- and SSRI-related improvement in OCD symptoms. Reproduced from Varigonda et al. (2016).

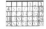 ### Case outcome: second interim follow-up (week 6)

- After approximately 6 weeks on clomipramine 150 mg daily, the patient is doing well and has very infrequent obsessions and almost complete resolution of her compulsions. Her CY-BOCS score has decreased to 6
- However, she developed some constipation, fatigue, and dry mouth in addition to feeling "like I'm slowing down," and she fell asleep twice during the past week while working on a music project

 ### Question

Given this patient's current pharmacological treatment, which of the following would be your next step?

- Re-check the EKG to evaluate for bradyarrhythmia

- Discontinue clomipramine
- Obtain a 12-hour trough level of clomipramine and norclomipramine (desmethylclomipramine) and re-evaluate her clomipramine dose, which may need to be reduced (even if the 12-hour concentrations are in the reference range)
- Prescribe armodafinil, docusate, and Biotene

Testing: laboratory results, imaging, EKGs

Therapeutic drug monitoring

	Value	Reference range
Norclomipramine + clomipramine	510	230-450

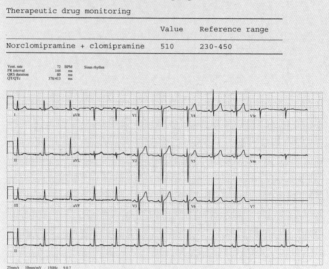

Attending physician's mental notes: second interim follow-up (week 6)

- There is concern that the patient's symptoms are related to the anticholinergic effects of clomipramine
- Her EKG may be unlikely to reveal a bradyarrhythmia unless it was obtained at the time when she was symptomatic. Additionally, cardiac etiology would be unlikely to account for her anticholinergic symptoms
- Clomipramine has been effective in reducing her symptoms and, given her prior treatment failure, it would not be advisable to discontinue an efficacious agent after such a short trial, especially in view of her significant improvement

Case outcome: third interim follow-up (week 8)

- The patient's 12-hour norclomipramine + clomipramine concentration was 510 ng/mL (reference range: 230–450 ng/mL), and this level was obtained after the patient had been on 75 mg twice daily for 3 weeks
- Given that her symptoms were significantly improved and based on her anticholinergic symptoms, the clomipramine dose was decreased to 50 mg each morning and 75 mg every night at bedtime. This asymmetric dosing was used so that the C_{MAX} would occur in the evening at a time when she was already asleep or in the process of falling asleep
- In general, asymmetric dosing for some sedating medications may decrease peak-related (i.e. C_{MAX}-associated) side effects
- Approximately 6 weeks after the dose decrease, her constipation resolved, and she again felt more alert. However, her dry mouth persisted
- Her OCD symptoms remained largely in remission

Attending physician's mental notes: third interim follow-up (week 8)

- The attending physician is encouraged by the patient's progress and will perform therapeutic drug monitoring regularly
- He will also monitor for anticholinergic symptoms, particularly if other medications are added which could affect the metabolism of clomipramine. Adding medications, using marijuana, cannabidiol (CBD), or smoking may affect specific cytochrome P450 enzymes, which could in turn affect not only her total clomipramine + norclomipramine level, but also the ratio of clomipramine to norclomipramine (Figure 6.4)
- Regarding dry mouth, tricyclic antidepressants (TCAs) are notorious for their propensity to produce this symptom. In one study of antidepressant-treated adults, TCAs reduced salivary flow by nearly 60%, whereas SSRIs reduced salivary flow by approximately 30% (Hunter and Wilson 1995). Proposed treatments for dry mouth, regardless of pharmacological etiology, include lozenges, sprays, mouth rinses, gels, oils, and chewing gum, which broadly fall into two categories – saliva stimulants and saliva substitutes. Recent systematic reviews of treatments for xerostomia have failed to identify any topical therapies that are effective for symptomatic relief. However, oxygenated glycerol triester (OGT) saliva substitute spray is more effective than an aqueous electrolyte spray. Chewing gums appear to increase saliva production in individuals with

residual secretory capacity, and may be preferred by patients; there is no evidence that gum is better or worse than saliva substitutes (Furness et al. 2011). Certainly, saliva substitutes have been used in pediatric patients with multiple disorders and are a reasonable first-line intervention

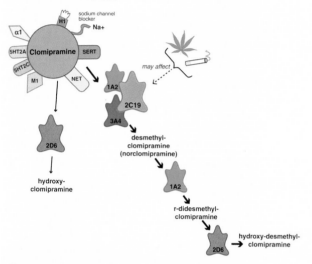

Figure 6.4 Metabolism of clomipramine.

Take-home points

- Treatment of OCD in children and adolescents generally involves SSRIs (Geller et al. 2003, 2001; Pediatric OCD Treatment Study (POTS) Team 2004), CBT (Pediatric OCD Treatment Study (POTS) Team 2004), or a combination of the two (Pediatric OCD Treatment Study (POTS) Team 2004; Storch et al. 2013) (Figure 6.5)
- Multiple SSRIs, including sertraline (Pediatric OCD Treatment Study (POTS) Team 2004), fluvoxamine, fluoxetine (Geller et al. 2001), and sertraline (Pediatric OCD Treatment Study (POTS) Team 2004; Storch et al. 2013), have demonstrated efficacy in prospective randomized controlled trials. Similarly, CBT has generally been superior to waitlist control conditions in children and adolescents. However, treatment response varies substantially in children and adolescents with OCD regardless of whether they are treated with SSRIs, other medication classes (e.g. TCAs) (Varigonda et al. 2016), or a combination of CBT plus SSRIs
- Using symptom ratings and tracking forms can be helpful in assessing progress, and the CY-BOCS is an evidence-based

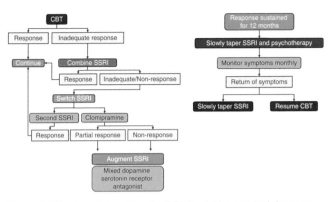

Figure 6.5 Treatment algorithm for OCD in children and adolescents. Adapted from Stein et al. (2019).

instrument that is sensitive to change with both pharmacotherapy and psychotherapy in children and adolescents
- Clomipramine, although not the first-line treatment for OCD in pediatric patients, is approved by the U.S. Food and Drug Administration (FDA) and may be associated with greater improvement compared with SSRIs (Varigonda et al. 2016)
- It should remain in the armamentarium for the treatment of patients with OCD. In adolescents, checking an EKG at baseline and following dose titration is important, and is recommended practice
- Clomipramine is well absorbed and undergoes first-pass metabolism to desmethyl-clomipramine (norclomipramine), its pharmacologically active metabolite

Mechanism of action moment

- All TCAs block reuptake of norepinephrine and are antagonists at histamine-1 (H_1), α_1-adrenergic, and muscarinic cholinergic receptors; they also block voltage-sensitive sodium channels. Some TCAs are also potent inhibitors of the serotonin reuptake pump, and some may additionally be antagonists at two serotonin receptors – 5-HT_{2A} and 5-HT_{2C}. However, they vary considerably in their anticholinergic properties and in their selectivity for norepinephrine or serotonin
- The major limitation of the TCAs has never been their efficacy – these are quite effective agents. The problem with this class of medications is the fact that all of them share at least four other unwanted pharmacological actions, namely blockade of muscarinic cholinergic receptors, H_1 histamine receptors, α_1-adrenergic receptors, and voltage-sensitive sodium channels

- Clomipramine represents one of the most serotonergic of the TCAs, and has effects at 5-HT$_{2C}$ and 5-HT$_{2A}$ receptors. Like the other TCAs, it has antihistaminic effects, anti-muscarinic effects, and α_1 antagonism (Figure 6.6)

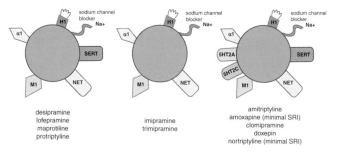

Figure 6.6 Receptor pharmacology of TCAs. Reproduced from *Stahl's Essential Psychopharmacology*, 2021.

Tips and pearls

- TCAs, and specifically clomipramine, should be considered in pediatric patients who have failed multiple SSRIs and evidence-based psychotherapy
- For clomipramine, the time to steady state for active moieties is approximately 3 weeks
- When ordering therapeutic drug monitoring, clinicians should keep several points in mind:
  - Include the active metabolite in testing
  - The ratio of parent compound to metabolite may help to evaluate metabolic state or adherence
  - A higher clomipramine/norclomipramine ratio in adults is associated with a better OCD response
  - The OCD response is correlated with clomipramine levels in adults (Mavissakalian et al. 1990)
  - Most side effects are anticholinergic (rather than serotonergic) and may not always be reflected by therapeutic drug monitoring, given that the concentration can fluctuate considerably and may be affected by several patient-specific and pharmacodynamic factors
- In general, meta-analyses suggest that there are dose–response relationships for SSRIs in pediatric patients with OCD – higher doses are associated with a greater response (Figure 6.7)

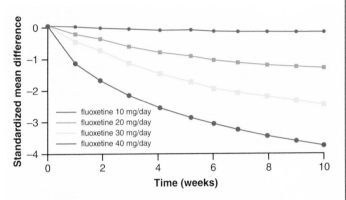

Figure 6.7 SSRI response in a meta-analysis of children and adolescents with OCD. *Reproduced from* Varigonda et al. (2016).

Post test self-assessment question

Which of the following represents the best and most evidence-based intervention for an adolescent with OCD who has failed three SSRIs and CBT?

A. Duloxetine (Cymbalta)
B. Venlafaxine (Effexor)
C. Aripiprazole (Abilify)
D. Clomipramine (Anafranil)
E. Imipramine (Tofranil)

Answer: D (Clomipramine, Anafranil)

Clomipramine is FDA-approved for the treatment of OCD in children and adolescents, and may be associated with a greater treatment response compared with SSRIs. Duloxetine, venlafaxine, and aripiprazole have not demonstrated efficacy compared with placebo in pediatric patients with OCD. Finally, imipramine is associated with less response compared with clomipramine in children and adolescents.

References

1. Bloch, M. H., Storch, E. A. Assessment and management of treatment-refractory obsessive-compulsive disorder in children. *J Am Acad Child Adolesc Psychiatry* 2015; 54: 251–62. https://doi .org/10.1016/j.jaac.2015.01.011
2. Furness, S., Worthington, H. V., Bryan, G., Birchenough, S., McMillan, R. Interventions for the management of dry mouth: topical therapies. *Cochrane Database Syst Rev* 2011; 12: CD008934. https://doi.org/10.1002/14651858.CD008934.pub2

3. Geller, D. A., Hoog, S. L., Heiligenstein, J. H., et al. Fluoxetine treatment for obsessive-compulsive disorder in children and adolescents: a placebo-controlled clinical trial. *J Am Acad Child Adolesc Psychiatry* 2001; 40: 773–9. https://doi.org/10.1097/00004583-200107000-00011

4. Geller, D. A., Biederman, J., Stewart, S. E., et al. Which SSRI? A meta-analysis of pharmacotherapy trials in pediatric obsessive-compulsive disorder. *Am J Psychiatry* 2003; 160: 1919–28. https://doi.org/10.1176/appi.ajp.160.11.1919

5. Hunter, K. D., Wilson, W. S. The effects of antidepressant drugs on salivary flow and content of sodium and potassium ions in human parotid saliva. *Arch Oral Biol* 1995; 40: 983–9. https://doi.org/10.1016/0003-9969(95)00079-5

6. Luft, M. J., Aldrich, S.L., Poweleit, E., et al. Thyroid function screening in children and adolescents with mood and anxiety disorders. *J Clin Psychiatry* 2019; 80: 18m12626. https://doi.org/10.4088/JCP.18m12626

7. Mavissakalian, M. R., Jones, B., Olson, S., Perel, J. M. Clomipramine in obsessive-compulsive disorder: clinical response and plasma levels. *J Clin Psychopharmacol* 1990; 10: 261–8. PMID: 2286699.

8. Pediatric OCD Treatment Study (POTS) Team. Cognitive-behavior therapy, sertraline, and their combination for children and adolescents with obsessive-compulsive disorder: the Pediatric OCD Treatment Study (POTS) randomized controlled trial. *JAMA* 2004; 292: 1969–76. https://doi.org/10.1001/jama.292.16.1969

9. Peris, T. S., Sugar, C. A., Lindsey Bergman, R., et al. Family factors predict treatment outcome for pediatric obsessive compulsive disorder. *J Consult Clin Psychol* 2012; 80: 255–63. https://doi.org/10.1037/a0027084

10. Scahill, L., Riddle, M. A., McSwiggin-Hardin, M., et al. Children's Yale-Brown Obsessive Compulsive Scale: reliability and validity. *J Am Acad Child Adolesc Psychiatry* 1997; 36: 844–52. https://doi.org/10.1097/00004583-199706000-00023

11. Stahl, S., Grady, M. M., Muntner, N. *Stahl's Essential Psychopharmacology: Neuroscientific Basis and Practical Applications*, 5th edn. Cambridge, UK: Cambridge University Press, 2021.

12. Stein, D. J., Costa, D. L. C., Lochner, C., et al. Obsessive-compulsive disorder. *Nat Rev Dis Primers* 2019; 5: 52. https://doi.org/10.1038/s41572-019-0102-3

13. Storch, E. A., Bussing, R., Small, B. J., et al. Randomized, placebo-controlled trial of cognitive-behavioral therapy alone or combined

with sertraline in the treatment of pediatric obsessive-compulsive disorder. *Behav Res Ther* 2013; 51: 823–9. https://doi.org/10.1016/j.brat.2013.09.007

14. Storch, E. A., Peris, T. S., de Nadai, A., et al. Little doubt that CBT works for pediatric OCD. *J Am Acad Child Adolesc Psychiatry* 2020; 59: 785–7. https://doi.org/10.1016/j.jaac.2020.01.026

15. Varigonda, A. L., Jakubovski, E., Bloch, M. H. Systematic review and meta-analysis: early treatment responses of selective serotonin reuptake inhibitors and clomipramine in pediatric obsessive-compulsive disorder. *J Am Acad Child Adolesc Psychiatry* 2016; 55: 851–9.e2. https://doi.org/10.1016/j.jaac.2016.07.768

Case 7: Struggles in the second grade: attention-deficit hyperactivity disorder (ADHD) in a child

The Question: When should nonstimulant medications be used in pediatric patients with ADHD?

The Psychopharmacological Dilemma: When to add nonstimulants to stimulant medications in children with ADHD is unclear for many clinicians. Furthermore, how to choose a nonstimulant, based on the mechanism of action, is a source of uncertainty

Pretest self-assessment question

How does an α_{2A} receptor agonist improve attention?

A. It lowers brainstem noradrenergic output, similar to its antihypertensive effects
B. It promotes dopaminergic activity in the dorsolateral prefrontal cortex (DLPFC) secondarily
C. It lowers γ-aminobutyric acid (GABA) activity, which allows greater glutamate activity in the thalamus
D. It allows fine-tuning of cortical pyramidal glutamate neurons to improve signal-to-noise ratios in frontocortical information processing

Answer: D (It allows fine-tuning of cortical pyramidal glutamate neurons to improve signal-to-noise ratios in frontocortical information processing)

Patient evaluation on intake

- An 8½ -year-old girl with inattention and distractibility at school and difficulties with impulse control
- She denies suicidal thoughts and self-injurious behavior
- During the evaluation, she would forget rules as the child and adolescent psychiatrist played with her
- She was somewhat impulsive, restless, and wiggly. She appeared to tire easily when a puzzle was attempted. The child psychiatrist noted that moving the pace along of the activities appeared to help her
- She was very interested in her performance and was down on herself at times, if she felt that she had upset the psychiatrist as the two played
- She often perceived that she had made errors or was displaying weak performance as the psychiatrist asked questions and did some simple assessments of working memory
- She was very talkative, off-task, and required frequent redirections
- No reports of depressed mood, anhedonia, or suicidal ideation

- No manic or psychotic symptoms
- Vital signs are within normal limits, and there are no reports of heat or cold intolerance, recent weight loss, or dysmenorrhea
- She denies cardiac symptoms, including palpitations
- There is no suicidal ideation, intent, or plan currently
- She denies any recent stressors

Psychiatric history

- She has a history of difficulties with sustained attention, distractibility, and hyperactivity
- Her pediatrician began methylphenidate long-acting (Ritalin LA) 10 mg each morning 8 weeks ago
- Her pediatrician referred her to a logical psychologist for testing to "diagnose ADHD." During the course of this evaluation, the psychologist administered the Wechsler Intelligence Scale for Children: Fifth Edition, the Tower of London-DX: Second Edition, the Test of Variables of Attention, and a STROOP Color-Word Test, and obtained a Vanderbilt ADHD Assessment from the parent and one of her teachers at school

Social and personal history

- She lives with her mother and father and struggles with rule-following at home, and the family has tried numerous behavioral charting approaches and parenting approaches. Her behavior has contributed to occasional parental disagreements
- There is no history of trauma or abuse
- She attended preschool for 2 years and then attended kindergarten and first grade
- She has no history of an Individualized Education Plan (IEP) or 504 Plan
- Her first-grade teacher noted some concerns related to inattention and task persistence. However, these have been more difficult to assess during her first-grade year as she is in nontraditional instruction secondary to the COVID-19 pandemic
- Her mother notes that she may require instructions to be repeated multiple times and that she requires frequent breaks, often only completing 20–30% of a short assignment at a time
- A review of her progress report from her second-grade teacher revealed "developing skills" in math, and "independence" in reading, writing, science, and social studies

Medical history

- The prenatal course was remarkable for a twin pregnancy with in-utero growth restriction (IUGR) of her twin sister, and she was delivered via cesarian section at 36 weeks, 1 day, with a birth weight of 2,500 g
- She was breastfed until the age of 3–4 months
- Her mother's pregnancy was further remarkable for cholestasis
- Developmental milestones within normal ranges
- Peanut allergy, which has resolved, and seasonal allergies for which she takes loratadine 10 mg daily during allergy season

Family history

- ADHD in her father, maternal grandmother, and maternal aunt
- Anxiety in her mother and paternal grandmother
- Obsessive compulsive disorder (OCD), panic disorder, and depressive disorder in her maternal aunt
- There is no family history of substance-use disorders or endocrinopathy

Medication history

- Methylphenidate long-acting (Ritalin LA) 10 mg each morning

Current medications

- Methylphenidate long-acting (Ritalin LA) 10 mg each morning

Psychotherapy history

- None

Further investigation

What about the results of the intelligence testing?

Composite		Composite score	Percentile rank	95% confidence interval	Qualitative description	SEM
Verbal comprehension	VCI	118	88	109–124	High average	4.24
Visual-spatial	VSI	117	87	108–123	High average	4.24
Fluid reasoning	FRI	121	92	112–127	Very high	3.67
Working memory	WMI	107	68	99–114	Average	4.50
Processing speed	PSI	98	45	89–107	Average	5.20
General ability	FSIQ	123	94	116–128	Very high	3.00

Domain	Subtest name		Scaled score	Percentile rank	SEM
Verbal comprehension	Similarities	SI	13	84	1.08
	Vocabulary	VC	14	91	1.12
	(Information)	IN	—	—	—
	(Comprehension)	CO	—	—	—
Visual-spatial	Block design	BD	13	84	1.12
	Visual puzzles	VP	13	84	0.95
Fluid reasoning	Matrix reasoning	MR	14	91	1.04
	Figure weights	FW	13	84	0.73
	(Picture concepts)	PC	—	—	—
	(Arithmetic)	AR	—	—	—
Working memory	Digit span	DS	10	50	0.85
	Picture span	PS	12	75	1.27
	(Letter–number seq.)	LN	—	—	—
Processing speed	Coding*	CD	9	37	1.41
	Symbol search*	SS	10	50	1.24
	(Cancellation)	CA	—	—	—

On the Wechsler Intelligence Scale for Children 5 (WISC-5), the General Ability Index (GAI) is used as an ancillary index score to estimate general intelligence that is less impacted by working memory and processing speed, relative to the Full-scale Intelligence Quotient (FSIQ). This is important for patients with ADHD, in whom processing speed and working memory are significantly affected. The GAI consists of subtests from the verbal comprehension, visual-spatial, and fluid reasoning domains. Overall, this index score was very advanced for the patient's age (GAI = 123). High GAI scores indicate well-developed abstract, conceptual, visual-perceptual, and spatial reasoning, as well as verbal problem-solving. The patient's GAI score was significantly higher than her FSIQ score (GAI > FSIQ by 10%). The significant difference between her GAI and FSIQ scores indicates that the effects of cognitive proficiency, as measured by working memory and processing speed, may have led to a lower overall FSIQ score. This estimate of her overall intellectual ability was lowered by including working memory and processing speed subtests. This result supports that her working memory and processing speed skills are areas of specific weakness.

Verbal Comprehension: The Verbal Comprehension Index (VCI) assesses her ability to access and apply acquired word knowledge. Specifically, this score reflects her ability to verbalize meaningful concepts, think about verbal information, and express herself using words.

Visual-Spatial: The Visual-Spatial Index (VSI) measures the patient's ability to evaluate visual details and understand visual-spatial relationships to construct geometric designs from a model. Her performance in this area was particularly strong. The VSI is derived from two subtests, Block Design (BD) and Visual Puzzles (VP).

Fluid Reasoning: The Fluid Reasoning Index (FRI) measures her ability to detect the underlying conceptual relationship among visual objects and use reasoning to identify and apply rules. She can solve complex problems despite having difficulty with other tasks.

Working Memory: The Working Memory Index (WMI) measures the patient's ability to register, maintain, and manipulate visual and auditory information in conscious awareness, which requires attention and concentration, as well as visual and auditory discrimination. Unlike many other scales, she was in the average range for working memory. Her performance on these tasks was a relative weakness compared to her performance on logical reasoning tasks (WMI < FRI by 20%).

Processing Speed: The Processing Speed Index (PSI) measures the patient's speed and accuracy in visual identification, decision-making, and implementation. The performance here is related to visual scanning, visual discrimination, short-term visual memory, visuomotor coordination, and concentration. This index assesses her ability to rapidly identify, register, and implement decisions about visual stimuli. Her overall processing speed performance was average for her age (PSI = 98). Importantly, for this patient, this is not a weakness compared to peers, but it was an area of personal weakness for the patient compared to her overall level of ability.

Additionally, the results of the Test of Variables of Attention and the Stroop Color Word Test also support attentional problems.

What about structured rating scales?

The Vanderbilt ADHD Rating Scale is a common instrument for evaluating the frequency of multiple ADHD symptoms. Though originally published by the American Academy of Pediatrics, it has been incorporated into several electronic medical record systems and is available online. This patient's Vanderbilt Scale while treated with methylphenidate long-acting (Ritalin LA) 10 mg daily is shown below.

Rating scales

Directions: Each rating should be considered in the context of what is appropriate for the age of your child. When completing this form, please think about your child's behaviors in the past <u>6 months</u>.

Is this evaluation based on a time when the child   ☐ was on medication   ☐ was not on medication   ☐ not sure?

Symptoms	Never	Occasionally	Often	Very Often
1. Does not pay attention to details or makes careless mistakes with, for example, homework	0	1	2	③
2. Has difficulty keeping attention to what needs to be done	0	1	2	③
3. Does not seem to listen when spoken to directly	0	1	2	③
4. Does not follow through when given directions and fails to finish activities (not due to refusal or failure to understand)	0	1	②	3
5. Has difficulty organizing tasks and activities	0	1	2	③
6. Avoids, dislikes, or does not want to start tasks that require ongoing mental effort	0	1	2	③
7. Loses things necessary for tasks or activities (toys, assignments, pencils, or books)	0	1	2	③
8. Is easily distracted by noises or other stimuli	0	1	2	③
9. Is forgetful in daily activities	0	1	2	③
10. Fidgets with hands or feet or squirms in seat	0	1	2	③
11. Leaves seat when remaining seated is expected	0	1	②	3
12. Runs about or climbs too much when remaining seated is expected	0	1	②	3
13. Has difficulty playing or beginning quiet play activities	0	1	2	③
14. Is "on the go" or often acts as if "driven by a motor"	0	1	2	③
15. Talks too much	0	1	②	3
16. Blurts out answers before questions have been completed	0	①	2	3
17. Has difficulty waiting his or her turn	0	1	②	3
18. Interrupts or intrudes in on others' conversations and/or activities	0	1	2	3
19. Argues with adults	0	①	2	3
20. Loses temper	0	①	2	3
21. Actively defies or refuses to go along with adults' requests or rules	⓪	1	2	3
22. Deliberately annoys people	⓪	1	2	3
23. Blames others for his or her mistakes or misbehaviors	⓪	1	2	3
24. Is touchy or easily annoyed by others	0	1	②	3
25. Is angry or resentful	⓪	1	2	3
26. Is spiteful and wants to get even	⓪	1	2	3
27. Bullies, threatens, or intimidates others	⓪	1	2	3
28. Starts physical fights	⓪	1	2	3
29. Lies to get out of trouble or to avoid obligations (ie, "cons" others)	⓪	1	2	3
30. Is truant from school (skips school) without permission	⓪	1	2	3
31. Is physically cruel to people	⓪	1	2	3
32. Has stolen things that have value	⓪	1	2	3

Symptoms (continued)	Never	Occasionally	Often	Very Often
33. Deliberately destroys others' property	(0)	1	2	3
34. Has used a weapon that can cause serious harm (bat, knife, brick, gun)				
35. Is physically cruel to animals	(0)	1	2	3
36. Has deliberately set fires to cause damage	(0)	1	2	3
37. Has broken into someone else's home, business, or car	(0)	1	2	3
38. Has stayed out at night without permission	(0)	1	2	3
39. Has run away from home overnight	(0)	1	2	3
40. Has forced someone into sexual activity	(0)	1	2	3
41. Is fearful, anxious, or worried	0	1	(2)	3
42. Is afraid to try new things for fear of making mistakes	0	1	2	(3)
43. Feels worthless or inferior	0	1	(2)	3
44. Blames self for problems, feels guilty	(0)	1	2	3
45. Feels lonely, unwanted, or unloved; complains that "no one loves him or her"	(0)	1	2	3
46. Is sad, unhappy, or depressed	(0)	1	2	3
47. Is self-conscious or easily embarrassed	0	1	2	3

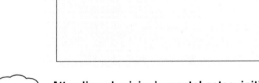

Performance	Excellent	Above Average	Average	Somewhat of a Problem	Problematic
48. Overall school performance	(1)	2	3	4	5
49. Reading	(1)	2	3	4	5
50. Writing	(1)	2	3	4	5
51. Mathematics	(1)	2	3	4	5
52. Relationship with parents	(1)	2	3	4	5
53. Relationship with siblings	1	2	(3)	4	5
54. Relationship with peers	1	2	3	4	5
55. Participation in organized activities (eg, teams)	1	2	3	4	5

Comments:

Attending physician's mental notes: initial psychiatric evaluation

- This patient has severe ADHD, despite treatment with methylphenidate long-acting (Ritalin LA) 10 mg each morning
- Her parents report some improvement associated with methylphenidate, but not by the time she is picked up from school, "It's like she never had the medication"
- Her teachers report some improvement in her symptoms with methylphenidate, but she still has to be redirected and will get out of her seat occasionally
- At recess, she has had some difficulty regulating frustration and has thrown balls at several peers' heads while playing gaga ball on the playground. She has been banned from the gaga ball pit by the recess monitor
- The attending physician also considered her partial response to methylphenidate osmotic controlled-release oral delivery system (OROS) and reviewed her vital signs, including her heart rate of 100, her blood pressure of 94/50 mmHg, and that she weighs 27.3 kg.

Question

Given her current treatment, which of the following would be your next step?

- Pharmacogenetic testing for pharmacokinetic genes
- Augmentation with extended-release guanfacine 1 mg
- Hold stimulant medication until an electrocardiogram (EKG) is obtained
- Titrate methylphenidate long-acting (Ritalin LA) 10 mg to 20 mg every morning

Attending physician's additional mental notes

Given the patient's age, normal vital signs, lack of family history, and lack of clinical symptoms, an EKG is not required (Hammerness et al. 2011), although an EKG was obtained and was unremarkable.

Pharmacogenetic testing would not be helpful in terms of predicting methylphenidate response based on pharmacokinetic genes. However, if the clinician were considering atomoxetine, which is metabolized through CYP2D6, different starting doses and titrations are recommended for patients who are poor metabolizers.

Given her very low dose of methylphenidate, it would be preferred to titrate methylphenidate, particularly given strong evidence of dose–response relationships for methylphenidate (Barkley et al. 1991; Newcorn et al. 2010; Stein et al. 2003).

Her clinician titrated methylphenidate to 20 mg. In general, titration of methylphenidate should be to a goal of 0.8–1 mg/kg in pediatric patients. Approaches for optimizing methylphenidate (MPH) dosing are shown in Table 7.1, and medication selection should include consideration of the duration of action and the proportion of the medication that is released immediately vs. that which is extended over the remainder of the day.

Table 7.1

Medication	Starting Dose	Maximum Dose*	Duration
Ritalin IR	5 mg QD/BID	2 mg/kg/day	4 hr/BID
Focalin	2.5 mg QD/BID	1 mg/kg/day	4–5 hr/BID–TID
Focalin XR	5 mg QD	1 mg/kg/day	10–12 hr QD
Daytrana	10 mg		6–16 hr
Concerta®	18 mg QD	2 mg/kg/day	12 hr/once
MetadateCD	20 mg QD		8 hr/once
Ritalin LA	20 mg QD		8 hr/once
Quillivant	<10 mg QD		12 hr/once
Quillichew	<10 mg QD		8 hr/once

Medication	Starting Dose	Maximum Dose*	Duration
Contempla XR (Dissolve tab)	8.6 mg QD	51.8 mg	12 hr/once
Aptensio XR	10 mg QD	2 mg/kg/day	12 hr/once
Adhansia XR	25 mg QD		To 16 hr/once
Jornay (Delayed release)	20 mg QD	100 mg	12 hr/once
Azstarys (SerdexMPH, MPH)	26/5 mg QD	52/10 mg	12 hr/once

*This may be higher than the FDA-labeled maximum dose

Testing: laboratory results, imaging, EKGs

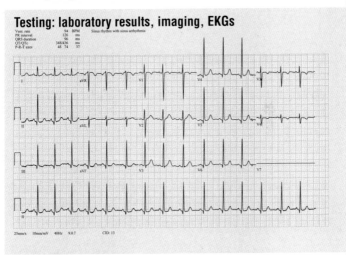

Vent. rate	94	BPM	Sinus rhythm with sinus arrhythmia
PR interval	126	ms	
QRS duration	96	ms	
QT/QTc	348/436	ms	
P-R-T axes	46 74	37	

25mm/s 10mm/mV 40Hz 9.0.7 CID: 13

Case outcome: follow-up (week 8)

- After titration of methylphenidate to 20 mg every morning, she is much better at school and parents report that she is also more focused during the early after-school period
- A repeat Vanderbilt scale completed by the parents reveals very few inattentive symptoms, although a significant number of impulsivity symptoms remain
- She is doing better academically, although she will still get in trouble for getting out of her chair at school and will still be impulsive at school and at home with her twin sister and with the family dog
- She is sleeping well but has had some difficulties with appetite
- Over the past several months, her mother notes that she has not been eating most of her lunch at school, although she generally eats a normal dinner
- Her blood pressure and heart rate remain within normal ranges for her sex, age, and height, and her growth chart is shown

PATIENT FILE

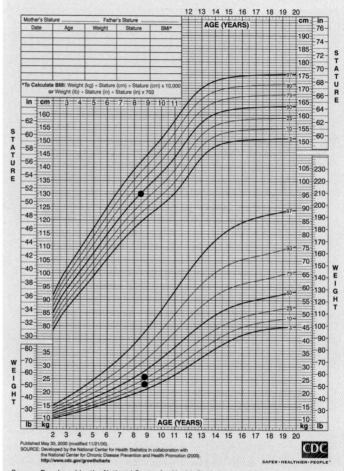

Testing: Laboratory Results, Imaging, EKGs

Source: Developed by the National Center for Health Statistics in collaboration with the National Center for Chronic Disease Prevention and Health Promotion (2000), http://www.cdc.gov/growthcharts

Attending physician's mental notes: follow-up (week 8)

- The attending physician is encouraged by the lack of significant side effects, although they are concerned about the patient's decreased appetite
- They have reviewed the growth chart and note that the patient's weight percentile has decreased from the 25th percentile to the 10th percentile. Her height has remained at the 50th percentile

- Based on this, the clinician is concerned about titration beyond 20 mg daily, particularly given that appetite suppression with methylphenidate is dose-related (Cortese et al. 2013)
- Given the appetite concerns and weight loss, the clinician reviews her eating habits pre- and post-treatment initiation and recommends giving the medication after breakfast. The clinician also encourages high-caloric snacks and late afternoon eating. The clinician will also consider dose reduction, change of stimulant (particularly to an isomeric formulation) and combination therapy, as well as medication holidays and referral to a nutritionist

Case outcome: follow-up (week 14)

- The patient's weight loss is no longer evident, and the family met with a dietitian and has begun introducing more calorically dense foods. Also, the patient was previously only eating two packages of fruit snacks and toast in the morning. Now she is eating microwavable pancakes and sausage, and the family has returned to whole milk with meals. She also eats yogurt and crackers with soy butter each evening
- Her impulsivity symptoms persist, and the family and teachers remain frustrated, despite reasonable control of her inattentive symptoms

Question

Given her current pharmacologic treatment, which of the following would be your next step?

- Discontinue methylphenidate and begin an extended-release mixed amphetamine salt
- Begin duloxetine (Cymbalta) 30 mg every morning
- Obtain a 12-hour trough methylphenidate level
- Add guanfacine extended-release formulation 1 mg every morning

Attending physician's mental notes: follow-up (week 14)

- There has been significant benefit associated with methylphenidate and there are currently no tolerability concerns. Therefore, changing to an alternative agent may not be helpful. Additionally, the risk of side effects, in general, is higher with mixed amphetamine salts compared to methylphenidate-based compounds (Cortese et al. 2018; Farhat et al. 2022; Stuckelman et al. 2017)
- Duloxetine may be helpful for pediatric anxiety disorders and is approved for generalized anxiety disorder (GAD) in the patient's age

range (Strawn et al. 2015). However, it is unlikely to have significant benefits for her ADHD

- Therapeutic drug monitoring for stimulants is not particularly helpful in terms of dose adjustment
- An α_2 agonist, such as guanfacine extended-release formulation, which is approved for the treatment of ADHD in this age range, may be helpful in addressing her impulsivity symptoms (Sallee et al. 2012) and may be effective as monotherapy or when combined with stimulant medications (Sallee et al. 2009, 2012; Wilens et al. 2012, 2015). The starting dose is 1 mg and the greatest efficacy is achieved at doses between 0.08 and 0.12 mg/kg (Martin et al. 2014; Sallee et al. 2009). However, if because of the need to split or crush tablets, an immediate-release formulation is needed, clinicians should be careful not to exchange extended-release guanfacine for immediate-release guanfacine 1:1. As shown in Figure 7.1, peak concentrations and total absorption are greater for immediate-release guanfacine compared to extended-release guanfacine at the same doses

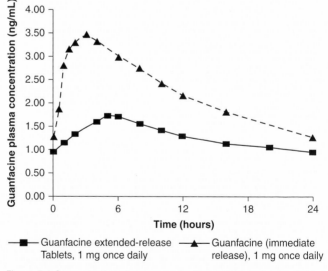

Figure 7.1 Concentration–time curves for immediate- and extended-release guanfacine in pediatric patients. Reproduced from Guanfacine extended-release formulation package insert.

Case outcome: third follow-up (week 24)

- Impulsivity symptoms are moderately improved and inattentive symptoms have improved significantly
- The patient's vital signs are within normal limits, although her heart rate is now 84 beats per minute
- There are no side effects

Attending physician's mental notes: follow-up (week 24)

- The attending physician will check vitals at each visit given treatment with a stimulant and an α_2 agonist (Hammerness et al. 2011). However, it is noteworthy that in some studies, the rates of side effects are actually lower with a simulant + α_2 agonist than with either monotherapy (Sayer et al. 2016). Mild bradycardia can be caused by α_2 agonists in some pediatric trials (Strawn et al. 2017)
- Given her current symptoms and improvement, the attending physician will titrate guanfacine to 2 mg daily. Of note, there is strong evidence for dose–response relationships with guanfacine extended-release formulation and improvement and the best outcomes are generally achieved at doses >0.08 mg/kg (Sallee et al. 2009)

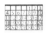

Take-home points

- ADHD is among the first disorders to emerge
- Methylphenidate is the first-line treatment for pediatric patients with ADHD and long-acting formulations are preferred
- Consider the component of the medication that is released immediately vs. the amount released later in the day
- EKGs are not required or recommended in stimulant-treated pediatric patients unless there are specific concerns (Hammerness et al. 2011)
- Regarding cardiac symptoms, controlled trials show short-term increases in pulse and blood pressure, which persist but are not deemed clinically meaningful. Multiple large studies have failed to show a relationship between drugs and severe cardiovascular events over population rates. Occasional palpitations do not cause concern (Cortese et al. 2013)
- Combining α_2 agonists and stimulants can help with impulsivity and hyperactivity symptoms in addition to ADHD symptoms and may differentially engage neurocircuitry
- Clonidine and guanfacine, both adrenergic α_2 agonists, have been used for treating childhood ADHD, off-label, for many years. Extended-release preparations of clonidine and guanfacine are approved for childhood ADHD (Kapvay and Intuniv) (Ming et al. 2011; Sallee et al. 2009, 2012)

- Using symptom ratings and tracking forms can be helpful in assessing progress, and the Vanderbilt ADHD Rating Scale is an evidence-based instrument that is sensitive to change with both pharmacotherapies

Two-minute tutorial: developmental neurophysiology of ADHD

- ADHD is among the first disorders to emerge in children and adolescents (Figure 7.2)

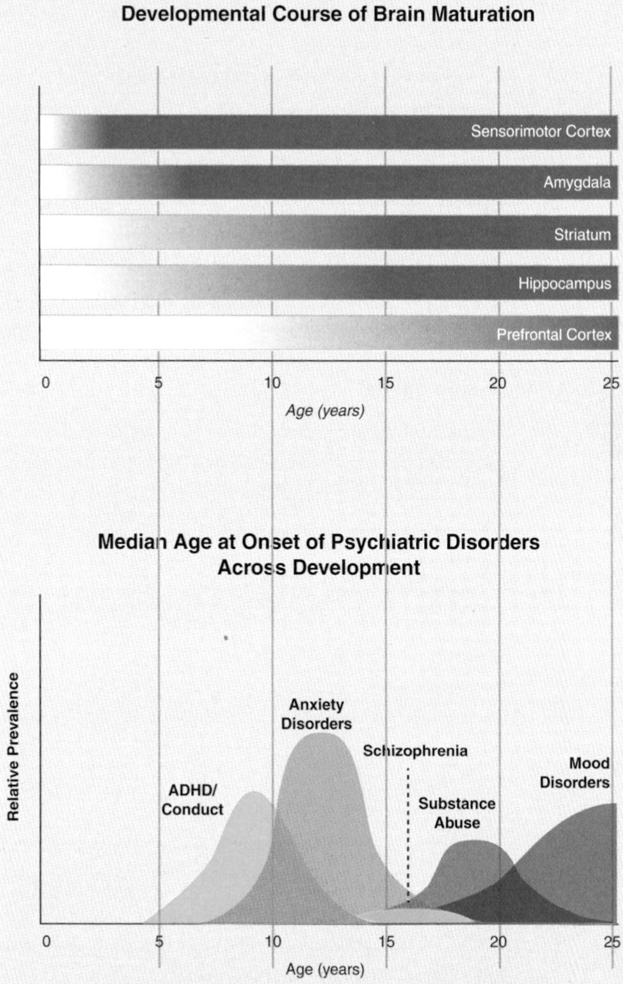

Developmental Course of Brain Maturation

Median Age at Onset of Psychiatric Disorders Across Development

Figure 7.2 Developmental course of brain maturation and onset of psychiatric disorders. The sensorimotor cortex and limbic brain regions are among the earliest to develop, followed by the prefrontal cortex. However, in patients with ADHD, cortical development is delayed.

- The developmental course of brain development is such that the sensorimotor cortex and limbic brain regions develop first, and the prefrontal cortex develops later. In ADHD, this same pattern is observed; however, cortical development is delayed. This may account for the childhood onset of ADHD and why, although ADHD may continue into adulthood, its onset does not occur in adulthood. In contrast, other disorders can also begin in childhood but are typically diagnosed later than ADHD, with onset continuing into adulthood
- The neurocircuitry of ADHD is complex, but specific symptoms can be thought of in terms of their neuroanatomic and neurofunctional basis (Figure 7.3)

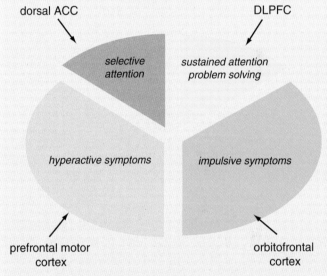

dorsal ACC

DLPFC

selective attention

sustained attention problem solving

hyperactive symptoms

impulsive symptoms

prefrontal motor cortex

orbitofrontal cortex

Figure 7.3 Matching ADHD symptoms to circuits. Problems with selective attention are believed to be linked to inefficient information processing in the dorsal anterior cingulate cortex (dACC), while problems with sustained attention are linked to inefficient information processing in the dorsolateral prefrontal cortex (DLPFC). Hyperactivity may be modulated by the prefrontal motor cortex and impulsivity by the orbital frontal cortex.

- A unifying formulation of ADHD is that it is caused by delayed maturation of prefrontal cortex circuitry that manifests in ADHD symptoms at least by age 12. Synapses rapidly increase in the prefrontal cortex by age 6, and then up to half of them are rapidly eliminated by adolescence. The timing of the onset of ADHD suggests that the formation of synapses and, perhaps more importantly, the selection of synapses for removal in the prefrontal cortex during childhood may contribute to the onset and lifelong pathophysiology of this condition. Those who are able to compensate for these prefrontal cortical abnormalities by new synapse formation after age 12 and into early adulthood may be the ones who "grow out of their ADHD" and why the prevalence of ADHD in adults is only half that in children and adolescents

Mechanism of action moment

Methylphenidate blocks the reuptake of dopamine into the terminal by binding at an allosteric site (i.e. different than the dopamine binding site) (Figure 7.4).

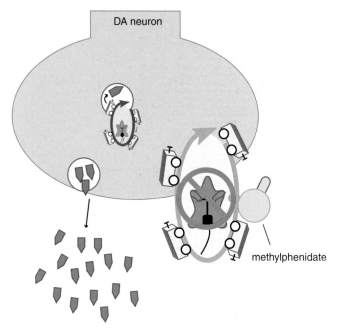

Figure 7.4 Mechanism of action of methylphenidate at dopamine and norepiphenephrine neurons. Methylphenidate blocks the reuptake of dopamine (DA) into the terminal by binding at an allosteric site (i.e. different than the DA binding site). Methylphenidate basically stops the transporter, preventing DA reuptake and thus leading to increased synaptic availability of DA. Methylphenidate blocks the reuptake of norepinephrine (NE) into the terminal by binding at an allosteric site (i.e. different than the NE binding site). Methylphenidate basically stops the transporter, preventing NE reuptake and thus leading to increased synaptic availability of NE.

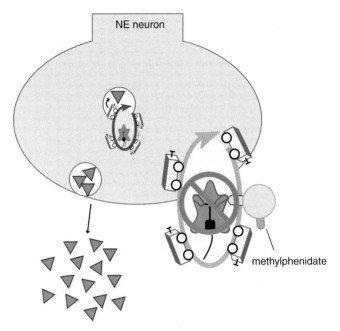

Figure 7.4 Continued

Methylphenidate basically stops the transporter, preventing dopamine reuptake and thus leading to increased synaptic availability of dopamine.

Methylphenidate blocks the reuptake of norepinephrine (NE) into the terminal by binding at an allosteric site (i.e. different than the NE binding site). Methylphenidate stops the transporter, preventing NE reuptake and thus leading to increased synaptic availability of NE.

Two-minute tutorial: neuropharmacology of ADHD

Why does adrenergic α_2 receptor agonism treat ADHD symptoms?

- Stimulating presynaptic α_{2A} receptors in the locus coeruleus, with the use of approved antihypertensive medications within this pharmacological family of medicines (e.g. guanfacine [Tenex] and clonidine [Catapres]), dampens adrenergic tone by reducing norepinephrine release, and thus causes a lowering of blood pressure
- Dampening of peripheral sympathetic noradrenergic tone makes sense from an anxiolytic point of view in that palpitations,

diaphoresis, and tremulousness is driven by the sympathetic nervous system and diminished by certain antihypertensives

- However, this mechanism may not explain how these drugs treat ADHD, where good cortical noradrenergic tone is needed to treat ADHD symptoms
- The slow-release preparations of these medications are now approved for childhood ADHD (e.g. guanfacine extended-release formulation [Intuniv] and clonidine extended-release formulation [Kapvay])
  - When prescribed for ADHD, they hypothetically stimulate postsynaptic α_2 receptors on cortical glutamate pyramidal neurons instead of those located presynaptically in brainstem regulatory centers that control blood pressure
  - When converting immediate release to extended release, clinicians should consider differences in pharmacokinetics and note that the absorption will be greater for immediate release and that peak concentrations will be increased with immediate release, which could produce peak-related side effects (e.g. sedation). For example, in Figure 7.4, see the concentration–time curves for immediate and extended-release guanfacine in pediatric patients
  - Centrally in the DLPFC, these noradrenergic agonist drugs hypothetically affect postsynaptic cortical heteroreceptors in that they bind to α_2 NE heteroreceptors located upon glutamate neurons
- α_2 Adrenergic receptors
  - Are present throughout the central nervous system (CNS), including the prefrontal cortex, but do not have high concentrations in the nucleus accumbens
  - Are believed to mediate the inattentive, hyperactive, and impulsive symptoms of ADHD, while other α_2 adrenergic receptors may have other functions
  - Clonidine is an α_2 adrenergic receptor agonist that is nonselective, and binds to α_{2A}, α_{2B}, and α_{2C} receptors
  - It also binds to imidazoline receptors, which contribute to its more sedating and hypotensive effects as well (Bousquet et al. 2020)
  - Although clonidine's actions at α_{2A} receptors make it a therapeutic option for ADHD, its actions at other receptors may increase side effects

- ◦ The slower-release preparation of clonidine (Kapvay) is approved for ADHD (Ming et al. 2011), keeping drug plasma levels lower and helping mitigate these side effects
  - Guanfacine extended-release formulation (Intuniv) is a more selective α_{2A} receptor agonist and thus has therapeutic efficacy with a reduced side-effect profile as it does not stimulate the α_{2B}, and α_{2C} receptors as much as clonidine
  - Situated on this neuron's spine is an α_{2A} adrenergic heteroreceptor and a D_1 dopaminergic receptor
  - These are both connected via cyclic adenosine monophosphate (cAMP) to cation channels called hyperpolarization-activated cyclic nucleotide-gated (HCN) channels
  - If DA and NE act in concert and are in balance, binding their respective receptors, then the HCN channels are opened to the appropriate size allowing the pyramidal glutamate neuron to fire efficiently – not too much and not too little
  - If millions of these cortical neurons fire efficiently and in synchrony, adequate attention and concentration theoretically occur
  - In ADHD, patients may have an imbalance in this cortical system, which allows inefficient processing with subsequent inattention
  - In situations such as those with inattention due to ADHD, or even anxiety, these HCN channels may be out of balance
  - In Figures 7.5 and 7.6, endogenous NE may bind to an α_{2A} heteroreceptor, and this will, in turn close down its associated HCN channel
    - This allows the glutamate pyramidal neuron to retain some of its internal electrical signal (it maintains or improves its signal-to-noise ratio) and to become focused on its own firing
    - If this occurs, in millions of these neurons, the DLPFC may become more efficient and allow for better focus and concentration symptomatically
  - It is at these α_{2A} receptor sites where ADHD medications such as clonidine extended-release formulation and guanfacine extended-release formulation may exert their anti-ADHD mechanism of action

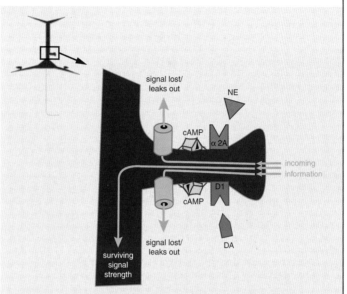

Figure 7.5 Signal distribution in a dendritic spine. The location of α_{2A} and D_1 receptors on dendritic spines of cortical pyramidal neurons in the prefrontal cortex allows them to gate incoming signals. Both α_{2A} and D_1 receptors are linked to the molecule cyclic adenosine monophosphate (cAMP). The effects on cAMP from norepinephrine (NE) and dopamine (DA) binding at their respective receptors are opposite (inhibitory in the case of NE and excitatory in the case of DA). In either case, the cAMP molecule links the receptors to the hyperpolarization-activated cyclic nucleotide-gated (HCN) cation channels. When HCN channels are open, incoming signals leak out before they can be passed along. However, when these channels are closed, the incoming signal survives and can be directed down the neuron.

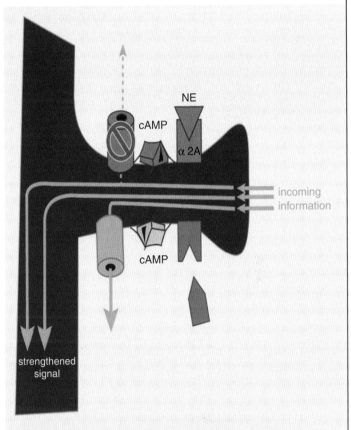

Figure 7.6 Norepinephrine actions at α_{2A} receptors strengthen the incoming signal. An inhibitor G protein (Gi) links α_{2A} receptors to cyclic adenosine monophosphate (cAMP). When NE occupies these α_{2A} receptors, the activated Gi-linked system inhibits cAMP, and the hyperpolarization-activated cyclic nucleotide-gated (HCN) channel is closed, preventing loss of the incoming signal.

Post test question

How does an α_{2A} receptor agonist really improve attention?

A. It lowers NE output similar to its antihypertensive effects

B. It promotes DA activity in the DLPFC secondarily

C. It lowers GABA activity, which allows greater glutamate activity in the thalamus

D. It allows fine-tuning of cortical pyramidal glutamate neurons to improve signal-to-noise ratios in cortical information processing

Answer: D (It allows fine-tuning of cortical pyramidal glutamate neurons to improve signal-to-noise ratios in cortical information processing)

As depicted in the figures in this case, specifically for inattention symptoms, these antihypertensive, α_2 noradrenergic receptor agonists act upon heteroreceptors. They modulate glutamate pyramidal neurons originating in the frontal cortex. In synchrony with other pyramidal neurons, α_2 receptor agonists improve signal-to-noise ratios and fine-tune neuronal firing, thus improving attention and concentration.

This is a separate mechanism of action: α_2 agonists do not promote DA activity; instead, they act in concert with endogenous dopamine activity, which occurs at the D_1 receptor also situated on glutamate neurons.

The α_2 agonists do not manipulate GABA to modulate glutamate neurons.

References

1. Barkley, R. A., DuPaul, G. J., McMurray, M. B. Attention deficit disorder with and without hyperactivity: clinical response to three dose levels of methylphenidate. *Pediatrics* 1991; 87(4): 519–31. https://doi.org/10.1542/peds.87.4.519

2. Bousquet, P., Hudson, A., García-Sevilla, J. A., Li, J. X. Imidazoline receptor system: the past, the present, and the future. *Pharmacol Rev* 2020; 72(1): 50–79. https://doi.org/10.1124/pr.118.016311

3. Cortese, S., Adamo, N., Del Giovane, C., et al. Comparative efficacy and tolerability of medications for attention-deficit hyperactivity disorder in children, adolescents, and adults: a systematic review and network meta-analysis. *The Lancet Psychiatry* 2018; 5(9): 519–31. https://doi.org/10.1016/S2215-0366(18)30269-4

4. Cortese, S., Holtmann, M., Banaschewski, T., et al. Practitioner review: current best practice in the management of adverse events during treatment with ADHD medications in children and adolescents. *J Child Psychol Psychiatry Allied Discip* 2013; 54(3): 227–46. https://doi.org/10.1111/jcpp.12036

5. Farhat, L. C., Flores, J. M., Behling, E., et al. The effects of stimulant dose and dosing strategy on treatment outcomes in attention-deficit/hyperactivity disorder in children and adolescents: a meta-analysis. *Molec Psychiatry* 2022: 27(3): 1562–72. https://doi.org/10.1038/s41380-021-01391-9

6. Hammerness, P. G., Perrin, J. M., Shelley-Abrahamson, R., Wilens, T. E. Cardiovascular risk of stimulant treatment in

pediatric attention-deficit/hyperactivity disorder: update and clinical recommendations. *J Am Acad Child Adolesc Psychiatry* 2011; 50(10): 978–90. https://doi.org/10.1016/j.jaac.2011.07.018

7. Martin, P., Satin, L., Vince, B. D., et al. Pharmacokinetics and pharmacodynamics of guanfacine extended release in adolescents aged 13–17 years with attention-deficit/hyperactivity disorder. *Clin Pharmacol Drug Devel* 2014; 3(4): 252–61. https://doi.org/10.1002/cpdd.124

8. Ming, X., Mulvey, M., Mohanty, S., Patel, V. Safety and efficacy of clonidine and clonidine extended-release in the treatment of children and adolescents with attention deficit and hyperactivity disorders. *Adolesc Health Med Ther* 2011; 2: 105–12. https://doi.org/10.2147/AHMT.S15672

9. Newcorn, J. H., Stein, M. A., Cooper, K. M. Dose-response characteristics in adolescents with attention-deficit/hyperactivity disorder treated with OROS methylphenidate in a 4-week, open-label, dose-titration study. *J Child Adolesc Psychopharmacol* 2010; 20(3): 187–96. https://doi.org/10.1089/cap.2009.0102

10. Sallee, F. R., Kollins, S. H., Wigal, T. L. Efficacy of guanfacine extended release in the treatment of combined and inattentive only subtypes of attention-deficit/hyperactivity disorder. *J Child Adolesc Psychopharmacol* 2012; 22(3): 206–14. https://doi.org/10.1089/cap.2010.0135

11. Sallee, F. R., McGough, J., Wigal, T., et al. Guanfacine extended release in children and adolescents with attention-deficit/hyperactivity disorder: a placebo-controlled trial. *J Am Acad Child Adolesc Psychiatry* 2009; 48(2): 155–65. https://doi.org/10.1097/CHI.0b013e318191769e

12. Sayer, G. R., McGough, J. J., Levitt, J., et al. Acute and long-term cardiovascular effects of stimulant, guanfacine, and combination therapy for attention-deficit/hyperactivity disorder. *J Child Adolesc Psychopharmacol* 2016; 26(10): 882–88. https://doi.org/10.1089/cap.2015.0264

13. Stein, M. A., Sarampote, C. S., Waldman, I. D., et al. A dose-response study of OROS methylphenidate in children with attention-deficit/hyperactivity disorder. *Pediatrics* 2003; 112(5): e404. https://doi.org/10.1542/peds.112.5.e404

14. Strawn, J. R., Compton, S. N., Robertson, B., et al. Extended release guanfacine in pediatric anxiety disorders: a pilot, randomized, placebo-controlled trial. *J Child Adolesc Psychopharmacol* 2017; 27 (1): 29–37. https://doi.org/10.1089/cap.2016.0132

15. Strawn, J. R., Prakash, A., Zhang, Q., et al. A randomized, placebo-controlled study of duloxetine for the treatment of children and adolescents with generalized anxiety disorder. *J Am Acad Child Adolesc Psychiatry* 2015; 54(4): 283–93. https://doi.org/10.1016/j.jaac.2015.01.008

16. Stuckelman, Z. D., Mulqueen, J. M., Ferracioli-Oda, E., et al. Risk of irritability with psychostimulant treatment in children with ADHD: a meta-analysis. *J Clin Psychiatry* 2017; 78(6): e648–55. https://doi.org/10.4088/JCP.15r10601

17. Wilens, T. E., Bukstein, O., Brams, M., et al. A controlled trial of extended-release guanfacine and psychostimulants for attention-deficit/hyperactivity disorder. *J Am Acad Child Adolesc Psychiatry* 2012; 51(1): 74–85. https://doi.org/10.1016/j.jaac.2011.10.012

18. Wilens, T. E., Robertson, B., Sikirica, V., et al. A randomized, placebo-controlled trial of guanfacine extended release in adolescents with attention-deficit/hyperactivity disorder. *J Am Acad Child Adolesc Psychiatry* 2015; 54(11): 916–25. https://doi.org/10.1016/j.jaac.2015.08.016

Case 8: From prodrome to psychosis: early-onset schizophrenia

The Question: What constitutes an evidence-based work-up for children and adolescents who have prodromal psychotic symptoms or are experiencing a first psychotic episode?

The Psychopharmacological Dilemma: The approach to the young patient with a possible psychotic disorder is unclear for many clinicians, and varies considerably in practice. How specific factors should be considered and what interventions should be used are common questions for clinicians

Pretest self-assessment question

Which of the following is U.S. Food and Drug Administration (FDA)-approved for the treatment of schizophrenia in adolescents?

A. Haloperidol (Haldol)
B. Molindone (Moban)
C. Paliperidone (Invega)
D. Clozapine (Clozaril)
E. All of the above

Answer: C (Paliperidone, Invega)

Patient evaluation on intake

- A 16-year-old adolescent had a history of depressive symptoms early in adolescence and was treated with fluoxetine (Prozac) for approximately 12 months
- More recently, he has had intermittent depressive symptoms and withdrawal and has "been hearing static in his brain" and occasionally hearing a single male voice which he recognizes as coming from "outside my head"
- The family is very supportive, and the patient appears to have good insight
- The patient shares that he is concerned about some of his recent academic difficulties (primary concern), although his parents are more concerned by this. He was previously a B student and has primarily earned Cs and Ds over the past four trimesters
- He notes that it has been challenging to focus and reports that he frequently hears "static in my brain" and has intermittently heard a male voice commenting on his school performance, his parents, and what he is saying. He denies any thought insertion or command hallucinations
- He also notes some fears related to his principal at school, whom he has felt is "against me," and when he is seen alone, he shares

that he is concerned that his principal is not his principal but has been replaced by a "fake." He is quite guarded about this, but describes that several of his teachers know that an imposter has assumed the principal's body
- He denies anhedonia, guilt, anergia, suicidal ideation, intent, or plan
- He denies manic symptoms
- He reports non-specific anxiety and an uneasy sense but denies symptoms consistent with generalized, separation, or social anxiety disorders
- No history of attention-deficit hyperactivity disorder (ADHD)

Psychiatric history

- The onset of depressive symptoms was at age 13, and he was treated with fluoxetine 20 mg daily for 12 months. He also worked in interpersonal psychotherapy for adolescents (IPT-A) for 6 months. When fluoxetine was discontinued, it was decreased to 10 mg and then stopped over 3 months

Social and personal history

- The patient lives with his parents and younger brother, aged 12
- His mother works as a clinical laboratory technologist and works the third shift at the local community hospital. His father is a project manager at a local hospital who describes recent increases in stress at work
- He is a junior in high school and does not have an Individualized Education Plan (IEP) or 504 Plan, although he has had some difficulties in math and has made use of peer tutoring
- He has limited involvement in extracurricular activities and describes few close relationships with peers, although he plays video games online with two friends who live in other states
- There is no history of abuse or neglect

Medical history

- He was delivered by cesarian section at 35 weeks to a 36-year-old mother and 39-year-old father. The prenatal course was complicated by preterm labor at 31 weeks and intrauterine growth restriction. Birth weight was 2500 g, and APGARS were 5 and 7. He was in the neonatal intensive care unit (NICU) for 3 weeks. He had hyperbilirubinemia requiring phototherapy, but otherwise, his NICU course was remarkable for a brief supplemental oxygen requirement during the first 4 days of life and supplementation of breast milk

- His mother had prenatal care throughout the pregnancy and took a multivitamin
- Developmental milestones were remarkable for expressive language delays, and he received speech therapy

Family history

- The patient's father experienced a brief period of anxiety in adolescence and again during his first year of college. He was treated with supportive psychotherapy
- The patient's paternal grandmother and paternal uncle have both been diagnosed with schizophrenia. His paternal grandmother is deceased (suicide) and had a history of coronary artery disease, type II diabetes, and obesity
- His uncle has had multiple psychiatric hospitalizations and has been treated with multiple dopamine receptor antagonists as well as serotonin-dopamine receptor antagonists, and is currently treated with clozapine 600 mg daily, aripiprazole 10 mg daily, metformin 1000 mg twice daily, atorvastatin 40 mg daily, and takes omega-3 fatty acids for hypertriglyceridemia
- There is no family history of substance-use disorders

Medication history

- No pharmacotherapy currently

Current medications

- None

Psychotherapy history

- IPT-A was successful in reducing depression and maintaining remission at 13 years of age.

Further investigation

Is there anything else that you would like to know about the patient? What about possible safety concerns?

- When asked about his principal, he denies any thoughts that he would hurt his principal or the teachers he believes to know about the "scheme"
- The family owns four handguns and three rifles. These are locked except for a handgun which is kept in a bedside table in his parents' bedroom. His parents are willing to obtain a separate gun safe for the handgun, which is kept at the parents' bedside

- The patient denies suicidal ideation, intent, and plan and is future-oriented with regard to "getting my grades fixed" and "doing better at school"
- There have been no recent exposures to suicide attempts or completed suicides, although a senior at his high school died by suicide last year. The patient knew this student superficially

Attending physician's mental notes: initial psychiatric evaluation

- This patient has a concerning family history of schizophrenia
- His deteriorating academic performance over 18 months with nonspecific anxiety and – initially vague – perceptual disturbances are concerning for a prodromal phase that has now emerged as a first psychotic episode
- From a safety standpoint, given the delusions described, the clinician has carefully evaluated homicidality, access to weapons, and risk factors for suicide. Also, in adolescents, contagion is an important factor to consider when assessing suicidality. The clinician has attended to this as he asked about recent suicides and prior suicides at the school
- In considering the management of prodromal symptoms, whether to begin a mixed serotonin–dopamine receptor antagonist vs. careful monitoring is unclear. Some advocate using N-acetylcysteine or omega-3 fatty acids if prodromal symptoms are present in a patient at high risk for developing schizophrenia (Bosnjak Kuharic et al. 2019) and they may have an adjunctive role in patients with schizophrenia (Xu et al. 2022). That said, this patient is already experiencing intermittent hallucinations and delusions, which have been present for nearly 7 months

Question

Given his current symptoms and presentation, what would be your next step?

- Obtain an electroencephalogram (EEG)
- Obtain magnetic resonance imaging (MRI), B_{12}, folic acid, thyroid-stimulating hormone (TSH)/free thyroxine (T_4), human immunodeficiency virus (HIV), complete blood count (CBC), comprehensive metabolic panel, a comprehensive drug screen, and an encephalitis panel in addition to a complete physical and neurologic examination
- Administer a Positive and Negative Symptoms of Schizophrenia (PANSS) scale
- Referral for psychological testing

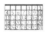

Case outcome: first interim follow-up (Day 3)

- An EEG was not obtained, and the PANSS was not obtained, given that neither would be of significant value in ruling out a nonpsychiatric etiology of his psychosis. The neurologic examination and physical examination were unremarkable

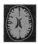

Testing: laboratory results, imaging, EKGs

The MRI was obtained, and representative T2 images are shown in Figure 8.1.

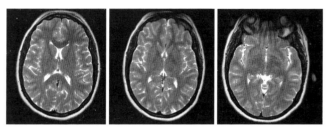

Figure 8.1

Radiologist Report: Significant susceptibility artifact related to orthodontics/dental hardware that results in suboptimal visualization of the anterior intracranial contents on many series and the posterior fossa on others. The ventricles and extra-axial spaces are within normal limits in size and shape. There are faint areas of ill-defined hyperintense T2/FLAIR signal abnormality in the bilateral periatrial white matter. There was no mass lesion or evidence of intracranial hemorrhage, and parenchymal signal and morphology are otherwise normal. There is no evidence of cortical dysplasia. The hippocampal formations are typical in appearance. There are normal flow voids in the intracranial vessels. There are no regions of restricted diffusion. The intensities are felt to reflect "subtle probable gliosis in the bilateral periatrial white matter." Otherwise, this was a normal exam, with the above-mentioned reservations regarding susceptibility artifact.

		CODE	0=None 1=Minimal, may be extreme normal 2=Mild 3=Moderate 4=Severe

	MOVEMENT RATINGS: Rate highest severity observed. Rate movements that occur upon activation one less than those observed spontaneously. Circle movement as well as code number that applies.	RATER Date	RATER Date	RATER Date
Facial and Oral Movements	**1. Muscles of Facial Expression** e.g. movements of forehead, eyebrows, periorbital area, cheeks, including frowning, blinking, smiling, grimacing	⓪1 2 3 4	0 1 2 3 4	0 1 2 3 4
	2. Lips and Perioral Area e.g. puckering, pouting, smacking	⓪1 2 3 4	0 1 2 3 4	0 1 2 3 4
	3. Jaw e.g. biting, clenching, chewing, mouth opening, lateral movement	⓪1 2 3 4	0 1 2 3 4	0 1 2 3 4
	4. Tongue Rate only increases in movement both in and out of mouth. NOT inability to sustain movement. Darting in and out of mouth.	⓪1 2 3 4	0 1 2 3 4	0 1 2 3 4
Extremity Movements	**5. Upper (arms, wrists,, hands, fingers)** Include choreic movements (i.e. rapid, objectively purposeless, irregular, spontaneous) athetoid movements (i.e. slow, irregular, complex, serpentine). DO NOT INCLUDE TREMOR (i.e. repetitive, regular, rhythmic)	⓪1 2 3 4	0 1 2 3 4	0 1 2 3 4
	6. Lower (legs, knees, ankles, toes) e.g. lateral knee movement, foot tapping, heel dropping, foot squirming, inversion and eversion of foot.	⓪1 2 3 4	0 1 2 3 4	0 1 2 3 4
Trunk Movements	**7. Neck, shoulders, hips** e.g. rocking, twisting, squirming, pelvic gyrations	⓪1 2 3 4	0 1 2 3 4	0 1 2 3 4
Global Judgments	**8. Severity of abnormal movements overall**	⓪1 2 3 4	0 1 2 3 4	0 1 2 3 4
	9. Incapacitation due to abnormal movements	⓪1 2 3 4	0 1 2 3 4	0 1 2 3 4
	10. Patient's awareness of abnormal movements Rate only patient's report No awareness 0 Aware, no distress 1 Aware, mild distress 2 Aware, moderate distress 3 Aware, severe distress 4	⓪ 1 2 3 4	0 1 2 3 4	0 1 2 3 4
Dental Status	**11. Current problems with teeth and/or dentures?**	Ⓝⓞ Yes	No Yes	No Yes
	12. Are dentures usually worn?	Ⓝⓞ Yes	No Yes	No Yes
	13. Edentia?	Ⓝⓞ Yes	No Yes	No Yes
	14. Do movements disappear in sleep?	No Yes	No Yes	No Yes

The results of the laboratory studies (Table 8.1) reveal no specific reversible causes of psychosis, and the encephalitis panel (Table 8.2) is unremarkable

Table 8.1

Hemoglobin A1C		
	Value	Ref Range
Hemoglobin A1C	5.0	

Lipid Profile W/ HDL		
	Value	Ref Range
HDL CHOLESTEROL	40	>=40 mg/dL
CHOLESTEROL LEVEL	129	<=199 mg/dL
TRIGLYCERIDES	125	<=129 mg/dL
LDL CHOLESTEROL	75	<=129 mg/dL

Insulin		
	Value	Ref Range
INSULIN	7.4	2.6 - 24.9 mIU/mL

CBC with Differential		
	Value	Ref Range
WBC	8.8	4.5 - 13.0 K/mcL
RBC	5.09	4.50 - 5.30 M/mcL

HGB	15.8	13.0 - 16.0 gm/dL
HCT	44.7	37.0 - 49.0 %
MCV	87.8	78.0 - 94.0 fL
MCH	30.9	25.0 - 35.0 pg
MCHC	35.2	31.0 - 37.0 gm/dL
RDW	11.5	$\leq$14.6 %
PLATELET	204	135 - 466 K/mcL

Comp Metabolic Panel

	Value	Ref Range
SODIUM	141	136 - 145 mmol/L
POTASSIUM	4.1	3.3 - 4.7 mmol/L
CHLORIDE	105	100 - 112 mmol/L
CO2	26	17 - 31 mmol/L
ANION GAP	10	4 - 15 mmol/L
BUN	12	6 - 21 mg/dL
CREATININE	0.96	0.46 - 1.00 mg/dL
B/C RATIO	12	$\leq$25
GLUCOSE	93	65 - 106 mg/dL
CALCIUM	9.4	8.3 - 10.6 mg/dL
ALBUMIN	4.6	3.3 - 4.8 gm/dL
TOTAL PROTEIN	7.6	6.2 - 8.1 gm/dL
ALKALINE PHOS	130	48 - 138 unit/L
ALT	34	<=49 unit/L
AST	39 (H)	10 - 36 unit/L
BILIRUBIN	1.8 (H)	0.1-1.2 mg/dL
GLOBULIN	3.0	gm/dL
A/G RATIO	2	1 - 2

GGT

	Value	Ref Range
GGT	17	9 - 49 unit/L

TSH with Reflex to T4 Free, Rapid

	Value	Ref Range
TSH WITH REFLEX TO T4 FREE, RAPID	1.861	0.430 - 4.000 mcIU/mL

TOXICOLOGY - MASS SPEC

	Value	Ref Range
AMPHETAMINES	Not Detected	Not Applicable
BARBITURATES	Not Detected	Not Applicable
BENZODIAZEPINES	Not Detected	Not Applicable
CANNABINOIDS	Not Detected	Not Applicable
COCAINE	Not Detected	Not Applicable
OPIOID	Not Detected	Not Applicable
METHADONE INTERP	Not Detected	Not Applicable
BUPRENORPHINE INTERP	Not Detected	Not Applicable
MUSCLE RELAXANTS INTERP	Not Detected	Not Applicable
PHENCYCLIDINE	Not Detected	Not Applicable
NICOTINE INTERP	Not Detected	Not Applicable

Table 8.2

AUTOIMMUNE ENCEPHALITIS PANEL	Ref Range	Value
AChR Ganglionic Neuronal Ab	≤0.02 nmol/L	0
AMPA-R Ab CBA	Negative	Negative
Amphiphysin Ab, S	<1:240 titer	Negative
AGNA-1, S	<1:240 titer	Negative
ANNA-1, S	<1:240 titer	Negative
Reflex Added		None.
ANNA-2, S	<1:240 titer	Negative
ANNA-3, S	<1:240 titer	Negative
CASPR2-IgG CBA, S	Negative	Negative
CRMP-5-IgG, S	<1:240 titer	Negative
DPPX Ab IFA	Negative	Negative
GABA-B-R Ab CBA	Negative	Negative
GAD65 Ab, S	≤0.02 nmol/L	0
GFAP IFA	Negative	Negative
IgLON5 IFA	Negative	Negative
LGI1-IgG CBA, S	Negative	Negative
mGluR1 Ab IFA	Negative	Negative
NIF IFA	Negative	Negative
NMDA-R Ab CBA	Negative	Negative
Calcium Channel Bind Ab, N-Type	≤0.03 nmol/L	0
Calcium Channel Bind Ab, P/Q Type	≤0.02 nmol/L	0
PCA-1, S	<1:240 titer	Negative
PCA-2, S	<1:240 titer	Negative
PCA-Tr, S	<1:240 titer	Negative

Question

Given his current symptoms and the results of the work-up, what would be your next step?

- Begin perphenazine 4 mg twice daily
- Begin paliperidone to 3 mg every night at bedtime
- Begin *Ashwaganda* and omega-3 fatty acids (3 g daily)
- Begin low-dose, escitalopram 5 mg daily

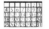

Case outcome: second interim visit (week 1)

- Paliperidone was initiated at 3 mg every night at bedtime, and he "feels better"
- He has been more talkative with his family
- He thinks more clearly and has only intermittently heard the previously described voice over the past week
- He minimizes his prior concerns related to the school staff and denies depressive and manic symptoms. His anxiety is minimal, and he can concentrate more easily at school

- He describes excellent adherence, and his parents have helped him to monitor his medication adherence
- An Abnormal Involuntary Rating Scale (AIMS) shown in Table 8.3 was administered and revealed a score of 1

Receptor	Acute ≤1 wk	Consequence	Early <3 mo	Consequence	Late: ≥3 mo	Consequence
α1	Hypotension*	Falls non-adherence	Hypotension*	Falls non-adherence	Hypotension	Falls non-adherence
D 2	Dystonia * Parkinsonism*	Pain non-adherence	Parkinsonism* Akathisia *	↓ Cognition non-adherence	Tardive dyskinesia	Stigma ↓ Socialization ↓ Quality of life
	↑ Prolactin (*)	Sexual dysfunction non-adherence	↑ Prolactin (*)	Sexual dysfunction Hypogonadism non-adherence	↑ Prolactin	Osteoporosis ? CHD ? Breast cancer
H 1	Sedation *	↓ Cognition ↓ Functioning non-adherence	Sedation *	↓ Cognition ↓ Functioning non-adherence	Sedation	↓ Cognition ↓ Functioning non-adherence
	↑ Weight	↑ Lipids/ glucose	↑ Weight	↑ Lipids/glucose non-adherence	Diabetes Dyslipidemia CHD	↓ Functioning ↓ Quality of life Early death
M 1–4	Blurry vision* Dry mouth *	Discomfort non-adherence	↓ Cognition Blurry vision * Dry mouth * Constipation *	↓ Functioning discomfort non-adherence	↓ Cognition Blurry vision * Dry mouth * Constipation *	↓ Functioning Discomfort non-adherence

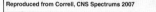

Acute (<1 week)   Early (<3 months)   Late

*= Tolerance may develop; CHD = Coronary heart disease
Reproduced from Correll, CNS Spectrums 2007

Attending physician mental notes (week 1)

- The attending physician selected paliperidone given its efficacy and tolerability in adolescents with schizophrenia (Singh et al. 2011) and is encouraged by the early response. The attending physician is also aware that hallucinations may improve prior to delusions
- Regarding other interventions for early-onset schizophrenia, he considered the evidence base for several interventions – including omega-3 fatty acids – in adolescents at high risk for developing psychosis and noted that there is some evidence for decreasing conversion to psychosis (Bosnjak Kuharic et al. 2019). However, this patient is already expressing significant psychotic symptoms, and therefore a mixed dopamine–serotonin receptor antagonist is indicated
- He is encouraged by the excellent adherence and the absence of extrapyramidal symptoms
- He is reassured by the relative absence of extrapyramidal symptoms (EPS). However, he recognizes that adolescents are at higher risk of developing EPS compared to adults and is aware that, for this patient, who is treated with paliperidone, the risk of EPS and hyperprolactinemia

may be higher than for adolescents treated with other mixed dopamine–serotonin receptor antagonists, despite similar efficacy

- Additionally, as the attending physician considers side effects and monitoring, he will follow the recommended screening shown in Table 8.4

Table 8.4

Assessments	Frequency
Personal and family history	Baseline and annually
Lifestyle monitoring	Every visit
Height, weight, BMI percentile/z-score	Every visit
Somnolence/sedation	Every visit
Sexual symptoms/signs	Baseline, during titration, and every 3 months
Blood pressure, pulse	Baseline, at 3 months, and 6-monthly
HbA1 C and lipids	Baseline, at 3 months, and (6-)12-monthly
Hepatic profile	Baseline, at 3 months, and (6-)12-monthly
Extrapyramidal symptoms, akathisia	Baseline, during titration, at 3 months, and annually
Dyskinesia/TD	Baseline, at 3 months, and annually
Electrolytes, blood count, renal function	On a per case basis (except if on clozapine)
Prolactin	Only when symptomatic
EKG	If on ziprasidone during titration, at max. dose

Question

Given his current symptoms, what would be your next step?

- Titrate paliperidone to 6 mg every night at bedtime
- Begin a long-acting injectable formulation of paliperidone
- Begin adjunctive aripiprazole 5 mg every night at bedtime
- Begin benztropine 1 mg every night at bedtime

Case outcome: third interim follow-up (week 4)

- Since paliperidone was titrated to 6 mg every night at bedtime, he feels that he is thinking more clearly and has not heard the previously described voice in week 1. He denies his prior concerns related to the school staff and continues to deny depressive and manic symptoms. His anxiety is minimal and he is able to concentrate more easily at school
- The family has engaged with a family support group
- He notes occasional restlessness but reports that "I've felt this way before. I don't think it's the medicine." His arm swing is mildly diminished as he walks. His Abnormal Involuntary Movement Scale (AIMS) is shown in Table 8.5

- His weight has increased from 70 to 72 kg over the past week, and his Body Mass Index (BMI) percentile has also increased to the 88th percentile. He shares that he's hungrier than in the past and has been craving more carbohydrates

Rating Scale

Table 8.5

			CODE		
			Pre-Tx	Week 1	Week 4
INSTRUCTIONS:					
MOVEMENT RATINGS: Rate highest severity observed. Rate movements that occur upon activation one less than those observed spontaneously. Circle movement as well as code number that applies.					
Facial and Oral Movements	1.	**Muscles of Facial Expression** e.g. movements of forehead, eyebrows, periorbital area, cheeks, including frowning, blinking, smiling, grimacing	⓪1 2 3 4	⓪1 2 3 4	⓪1 2 3 4
	2.	**Lips and Perioral Area** e.g. puckering, pouting, smacking	⓪1 2 3 4	⓪1 2 3 4	⓪1 2 3 4
	3.	**Jaw** e.g. biting, clenching, chewing, mouth opening, lateral movement	⓪1 2 3 4	⓪1 2 3 4	⓪1 2 3 4
	4.	**Tongue** Rate only increases in movement both in and out of mouth, NOT inability to sustain movement. Darting in and out of mouth.	⓪1 2 3 4	⓪1 2 3 4	⓪1 2 3 4
Extremity Movements	5.	**Upper (arms, wrists, hands, fingers)** Include choreic movements (i.e. rapid, objectively purposeless, irregular, spontaneous), athetoid movements (i.e. slow, irregular, complex, serpentine). DO NOT INCLUDE TREMOR (i.e. repetitive, regular, rhythmic)	⓪1 2 3 4	0①2 3 4	0①2 3 4
	6.	**Lower (legs, knees, ankles, toes)** e.g. lateral knee movement, foot tapping, heel dropping, foot squirming, inversion, and eversion of foot.	⓪1 2 3 4	⓪1 2 3 4	⓪1 2 3 4
Trunk Movements	7.	**Neck, shoulders, hips** e.g. rocking, twisting, squirming, pelvic gyrations	⓪	0	0
Global Judgments	8.	**Severity of abnormal movements overall**	⓪	1	1
	9.	**Incapacitation due to abnormal movements**	⓪	1	1
	10.	**Patient's awareness of abnormal movements** Rate only patient's report No awareness 0 Aware, no distress 1 Aware, mild distress 2 Aware, moderate distress 3 Aware, severe distress 4	⓪	1	1
Dental Status	11.	**Current problems with teeth and/or dentures?**	No	No	No
	12.	**Are dentures usually worn?**	No	No	No
	13.	**Edentia?**	No	No	No
	14.	**Do movements disappear in sleep?**	Yes	Yes	Yes

Question

Given his current symptoms and presentation, what would be your next step?

- Begin metformin 500 mg twice daily
- Recheck weight in 2–4 weeks
- Recheck hemoglobin A1C
- Begin topiramate 25 mg twice daily

Attending physician's mental notes: third interim follow-up (week 4)

- His clinician is pleased with the patient's response, and the family has also engaged with a National Alliance on Mental Health (NAMI) family support group that involves peer-to-peer mentoring
- Also, the clinician has, with permission, spoken with the school staff to evaluate the patient for an IEP. As part of this evaluation, psychoeducational testing has been requested. This will provide a better sense of his current functioning with regard to processing speed, perceptual reasoning, working memory, etc. (see Case 7 for additional descriptions)
- The physician is concerned about the patient's increased risk for EPS, given his age (Pagsberg et al. 2017), although symptoms are very mild currently. At this time, the clinician has chosen not to begin an anticholinergic medication
- The patient's weight has significantly increased over the past several weeks, which is very concerning. There is strong evidence for early intervention in adolescents with mixed dopamine–serotonin receptor antagonist weight gain with metformin
- In the pediatric setting, metformin should be considered particularly in patients who are >85th percentile for BMI and have experienced early mixed dopamine–serotonin receptor agonist-related weight gain. When initiated, metformin is begun at 500 mg twice daily and can be titrated to 1000 mg twice daily over several weeks (DelBello et al. 2017; Strawn and DelBello 2018)
- The attending physician is also aware that topiramate may also attenuate mixed dopamine–serotonin receptor agonist (SGA)-related weight gain in adolescents (Arman and Haghshenas 2022) and that should these interventions be ineffective, trials in adults now suggest the efficacy of glucagon-like peptide-1 (GLP-1) agonists in ameliorating SGA-related weight gain (Siskind et al. 2018, 2019)

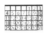

Case outcome: fourth interim follow-up (week 12)

- The patient notes that his appetite is "normal," and his BMI percentile is now 82nd percentile
- His last fasting lipids revealed mild hypertriglyceridemia and the attending physician confirmed that these were fasting. His HbA1C is stable at 4.9 ng/dL
- He denies all psychotic symptoms and has joined the school bowling team. Academically, he is earning Bs and is receiving some nonspecific accommodations at school
- At home, he is doing well, per his parents
- However, his restlessness "has gotten a lot worse," and he sometimes feels stiff. On examination, there is an increased tone in his wrists bilaterally and in his biceps bilaterally. His arm swing is diminished
- He describes excellent adherence with his medication regimen

Attending physician's mental notes: fourth interim follow-up (week 12)

- The patient has developed EPS on his current dose of paliperidone; however, at the lower dose – at which he did not have EPS – his psychotic symptoms were not well controlled
- The clinician has considered standard dosing for paliperidone, which is approved for adolescents with schizophrenia:
  - Adolescents <51 kg: initial 3 mg daily; recommended 3–6 mg daily; maximum 6 mg daily
  - Adolescents >51 kg: initial 3 mg daily; recommended 3–12 mg daily; maximum 12 mg daily
- The clinician is considering switching to another mixed dopamine–serotonin receptor antagonist. However, he recognizes that cross-titration to another agent will need to be done carefully and slowly, and the titration strategy should be informed both by the paliperidone and by the new medication selected
- Regarding the patient's hypertriglyceridemia, which may be related to longer-term use of mixed dopamine–serotonin receptor antagonists, including paliperidone (Pagsberg et al. 2017; Savitz et al. 2015), he is considering adding omega-3 fatty acids, which can reduce hypertriglyceridemia and, in some studies of patients treated with mixed dopamine–serotonin receptor antagonists, have salutary effects (Freeman et al. 2015)

Take-home points

- Prodromal symptoms are nonspecific and vary considerably among adolescents. In general, schizophrenia is characterized by four phases: prodromal, acute, recovery, and residual (McClellan et al. 2013). Prior to the emergence of positive symptoms, patients frequently experience a decline in function, as was the case for this patient. During this prodromal period, social isolation, academic difficulties, odd or idiosyncratic preoccupations, as well as depression and anxiety may be present. This phase may be very short (days to weeks) or chronic (years). In general, adolescent-onset psychotic disorders tend to have a more chronic onset (McClellan et al. 2013)
- For the first episode of psychosis, a comprehensive work-up should include physical and neurologic examination, neuroimaging, and evaluation for autoimmune, metabolic, endocrine, infectious, or other potentially reversible causes of the psychotic symptoms (Sunshine et al. 2023)
- The risk of EPS in children and adolescents is significantly higher than in adults, and these symptoms should be tracked more frequently than in adults. Additionally, when EPS is present, it may be more helpful to consider a switch in medication rather than the addition of an anticholinergic, which may significantly affect learning and produce additional symptoms
- Metformin should be considered early in the course of treatment and should, in adolescents, be titrated up to 2000 mg daily. Extended-release formulations may decrease treatment-related gastrointestinal symptoms

Mechanism of action moment

- Paliperidone, the active metabolite of risperidone, is also known as 9-hydroxy-risperidone and, like risperidone has 5-HT$_{2A}$ and D$_2$ receptor antagonism (Figure 8.2)
- One pharmacokinetic difference, however, between risperidone and paliperidone is that paliperidone, unlike risperidone, is not hepatically metabolized. Still, its elimination is based upon urinary excretion, and thus it has few pharmacokinetic drug interactions
- Another pharmacokinetic difference is that the oral form of paliperidone is provided in a sustained-release oral formulation, which risperidone is not. This actually changes some of the clinical characteristics of paliperidone compared to risperidone, a fact that is not always well recognized and can lead to underdosing of oral paliperidone
- Oral sustained-release means that paliperidone only needs to be administered once a day. In contrast, risperidone, especially when

treatment is initiated and perhaps in younger patients, may need to be given twice daily or three times daily

- Side effects of risperidone may be related in part to the rapid rate of absorption and higher peak doses with greater drug-level fluctuation leading to shorter duration of action, properties that are eliminated by the controlled-release formulation of paliperidone
- Despite the similar receptor binding characteristics of paliperidone and risperidone, paliperidone tends to be more tolerable, with less sedation and less orthostasis
- Paliperidone has a moderate risk for weight gain and metabolic problems. Paliperidone is approved for schizophrenia/maintenance (ages 12 and older)
- Another advantage of paliperidone over risperidone – which may be relevant to this patient as he becomes older, is that the long-acting injectable for paliperidone is easier to load, easier to dose, and has 1-month, 3-month, and 6-month formulations

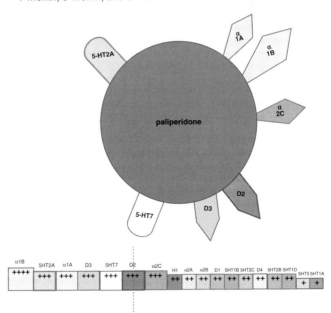

Figure 8.2 Paliperidone's pharmacological and binding profile. This figure portrays a qualitative consensus of current thinking about the binding properties of paliperidone, the active metabolite of risperidone. Paliperidone shares many pharmacological properties with risperidone. As with all agents discussed in this case, binding properties vary greatly with technique and from one laboratory to another; they are constantly being revised and updated. Adapted from *Stahl's Essential Psychopharmacology*, 2021.

Post test question

Which of the following is FDA-approved for the treatment of schizophrenia in adolescents?

A. Haloperidol (Haldol)
B. Molindone (Moban)
C. Paliperidone (Invega)
D. Clozapine (Clozaril)
E. All of the above

Answer: C (Paliperidone, Invega)

Paliperidone (correct answer) has been studied in multiple double-blind, placebo-controlled trials of children and adolescents with schizophrenia and is approved by the FDA for this indication. Molindone was studied in the treatment of early onset schizophrenia study; however, patients were not randomized to this agent if they had a prior history of EPS and there is concern that the risk of EPS is higher, in adolescents, compared to mixed dopamine–serotonin receptor antagonists. Finally, clozapine should not be used as a first-line treatment for mania in adolescents.

References

1. Arman, S., Haghshenas, M. Metabolic effects of adding topiramate on aripiprazole in bipolar patients aged between 6–18 years: a randomized, double-blind, placebo-controlled trial. *J Res Med Sci* 2022; 27(1): 23. https://doi.org/10.4103/jrms.jrms_672_21
2. Bosnjak Kuharic, D., Kekin, I., Hew, J., Rojnic Kuzman, M., Puljak, L. Interventions for prodromal stage of psychosis. *Cochrane Database Syst Rev* 2019; 2019(11): CD012236. https://doi.org/10.1002/14651858.CD012236.pub2
3. DelBello, M. P., Strawn, J. R., Duran, L. P. 1.6 Recognition and management of second-generation antipsychotic-associated adverse effects. *J Am Acad Child Adolesc Psychiatry* 2017; 56(10): S135. https://doi.org/10.1016/j.jaac.2017.07.509
4. Freeman, M. P., McInerney, K., Sosinsky, A. Z., Kwiatkowski, M. A., Cohen, L. S. Omega-3 fatty acids for atypical antipsychotic-associated hypertriglyceridemia. *Ann Clin Psychiatry* 2015; 27(3): 197–202. https://doi.org/10.1016/j.jaac.2016.12.013
5. McClellan, J., Stock, S.; American Academy of Child and Adolescent Psychiatry (AACAP) Committee on Quality Issues (CQI). Practice parameter for the assessment and treatment of children and adolescents with schizophrenia. *J Am Acad Child*

Adolesc Psychiatry 2013; 52(9): 976–90. https://doi.org/10.1016/j.jaac.2013.02.008

6. Pagsberg, A. K., Tarp, S., Glintborg, D., et al. Acute antipsychotic treatment of children and adolescents with schizophrenia-spectrum disorders: a systematic review and network meta-analysis. *J Am Acad Child Adolesc Psychiatry* 2017; 56(3): 191–202. https://doi.org/10.1016/j.jaac.2016.12.013

7. Savitz, A., Lane, R., Nuamah, I., et al. Long-term safety of paliperidone extended release in adolescents with schizophrenia: an open-label, flexible dose study. *J Child Adolesc Psychopharmacol* 2015; 25(7): 548–57. https://doi.org/10.1089/cap.2014.0130

8. Singh, J., Robb, A., Vijapurkar, U., Nuamah, I., Hough, D. A randomized, double-blind study of paliperidone extended-release in treatment of acute schizophrenia in adolescents. *Biological Psychiatry* 2011; 70(12): 1179–87. https://doi.org/10.1016/j.biopsych.2011.06.021

9. Siskind, D., Hahn, M., Correll, C. U., et al. Glucagon-like peptide-1 receptor agonists for antipsychotic-associated cardio-metabolic risk factors: a systematic review and individual participant data meta-analysis. *Diabetes Obes Metab* 2019; 21(2): 293–302. https://doi.org/10.1111/dom.13522

10. Siskind, D. J., Russell, A. W., Gamble, C., et al. Treatment of clozapine-associated obesity and diabetes with exenatide in adults with schizophrenia: a randomized controlled trial (CODEX). *Diabetes Obes Metab* 2018; 20(4): 1050–55. https://doi.org/10.1111/dom.13167

11. Strawn, J. R., DelBello, M. P. 59.4 Recognizing and managing side effects of second-generation antipsychotics. *J Am Acad Child Adolesc Psychiatry* 2018; 57(10): S85. https://doi.org/10.1016/j.jaac.2018.07.358

12. Sunshine, A., McClellan, J. Practitioner Review: psychosis in children and adolescents. *J Child Psychol Psychiatry*. 2023. doi: 10.1111/jcpp.13777. Epub ahead of print. PMID: 36878476.

13. Xu, X., Shao, G., Zhang, X., et al. The efficacy of nutritional supplements for the adjunctive treatment of schizophrenia in adults: a systematic review and network meta-analysis. *Psychiatry Res* 2022; 311: 114500. https://doi.org/10.1016/j.psychres.2022.114500

Case 9: Too much, too little, or just right? Lithium dosing in an adolescent

The Question: How is lithium dosed differently in adolescents compared with adults?

The Psychopharmacological Dilemma: Approaches to monitoring and dosing lithium in pediatric patients differ substantially from the strategies used in adults. This confusion often complicates lithium use and monitoring in adolescents, and represents a significant barrier to using lithium

Pretest self-assessment question

Compared to adults, young adolescents treated with lithium may require higher mg/kg doses because of:

A. Greater renal clearance
B. Increased CYP2D6 activity
C. Faster and more efficient intestinal absorption
D. Enhanced Central Nervous System (CNS) penetration

Answer: A (greater renal clearance)

Patient evaluation on intake

- A 13-year-old adolescent with a history (remote) of antidepressant treatment for a major depressive episode
- She was hospitalized for her first manic episode, and over the past 6 months, she has been treated with aripiprazole 15 mg every night at bedtime
- While treated with aripiprazole, she has experienced significant weight gain but still continues to experience hypomanic symptoms, particularly over the past 8 weeks
- She sleeps 6 hours per night, is struggling at school, and her grades, over the past trimester, have decreased from As to Bs and occasionally a C
- She is irritable in her interactions with peers and with her family members. In addition, she has mildly tangential thought processes and is distractable
- She relates intermittent episodes of tearfulness and guilt but denies suicidal ideation, intent, or plan
- She has no psychotic symptoms and denies anxiety

Psychiatric history

- The onset of depressive symptoms was at age 11, and she was treated with escitalopram 10 mg daily

- She has a history of one prior psychiatric hospitalization for 8 days for her first manic episode. At that time, she had an unsuccessful trial of divalproex extended-release formulation (see below), and aripiprazole was initiated at 5 mg and titrated to 15 mg over the first month of treatment
- During her psychiatric hospitalization, she also had pharmacogenetic testing, which revealed that she was a poor metabolizer for CYP2D6 (*4/*41) and a rapid metabolizer for CYP2C19 (*1/*17)
- She has had Columbia-Suicide Severity Rating Scale (C-SSRS) 1 suicidal ideation in the past but has not experienced this for more than a year. There is no prior history of self-injurious behavior

Social and personal history

- She earns As and Bs in middle school and has "many friends"
- She is active in musical theater and in a school orchestra where she plays the violin
- She denies alcohol and marijuana use, as well as other illicit substances
- She does not vape or use other tobacco-containing products

Medical history

- She was delivered at 40 weeks and had an unremarkable pre- and postnatal course
- Her mother had prenatal care throughout the pregnancy and took a multivitamin
- Developmental milestones were within normal limits
- Menarche was 6 months ago, and periods are irregular. She recently began an oral contraceptive (2 months ago) for acne and worsening mood before her period. Her gynecologist diagnosed her with premenstrual dysphoric disorder (PMDD)
- She has a history of migraine headaches and takes acetaminophen 10 mg/kg approximately twice weekly

Family history

- Maternal aunt with bipolar disorder, type I, and "anxiety"
- There is no family history of suicide
- There is no family history of substance-use disorders or endocrinopathy

Medication history

- Escitalopram was discontinued secondary to her first manic episode
- During her inpatient hospitalization, she had a brief trial of divalproex extended-release formulation, which was titrated to 1 g every night at bedtime (approximately 18 mg/kg). However, she experienced significant sedation, nausea, and several episodes of vomiting with this
- She has been treated with aripiprazole 15 mg every night at bedtime, but experiences akathisia, sedation, stiffness, dry mouth, and orthostatic symptoms

Current medications

- Aripiprazole 15 mg every night at bedtime
- Acetaminophen 10 mg/kg
- Drospirenone/ethinyl estradiol daily

Psychotherapy history

- She is currently working weekly in Mindfulness-Based Therapy for Adolescents (MBT-A). She works with her therapist weekly; sessions are approximately 45 minutes long. The sessions are conducted using a telehealth platform

Attending physician's mental notes: initial psychiatric evaluation

- This patient has persistent manic and depressive symptoms, despite treatment with aripiprazole. However, likely because she is a poor metabolizer for CYP2D6, she would be expected to have significantly elevated aripiprazole serum concentrations. This is likely what is contributing to her current side effects
- In considering alternative agents, the attending clinician is concerned that other CYP2D6 medications will be poorly tolerated (e.g. risperidone). The clinician is concerned about the metabolic profiles of other agents. The family is extremely hesitant to pursue a trial of lurasidone or ziprasidone, given that the patient's aunt experienced "heart problems on that medicine"
- Her attending physician is also aware that she is in a critical developmental period that coincides with the onset of bipolar disorder (Figure 9.1) (Solmi et al. 2022)

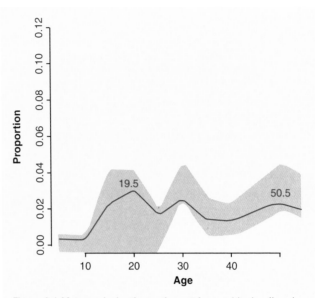

Figure 9.1 Meta-analysis of age of onset for any bipolar disorder diagnosis. Adapted from Solmi, M., Radua, J., Olivola, M., et al. Age at onset of mental disorders worldwide: large-scale meta-analysis of 192 epidemiological studies. *Mol Psychiatry* 2022; 27: 281–95.

Question

What is the next best intervention at this point?

- A trial of low-dose amitryptiline to address both her depressive symptoms and migraine prophylaxis
- A trial of topiramate to address both her manic symptoms and migraine prophylaxis
- A trial of lithium
- Laboratory screening for hypogonadism

Case outcome: first interim follow-up (week 1)

- At her last visit, the patient had a normal thyroid-stimulating hormone (TSH) and free thyroxine (T_4), and a blood urea nitrogen (BUN) and creatinine of 8 ng/dL and 0.4 ng/dL, respectively, and other electrolytes were within normal limits, as was her complete blood count
- Lithium was initiated at 300 mg twice daily, and other medications are unchanged
- With a brief cross-titration from aripiprazole to lithium, the latter has been titrated to 600 mg twice daily after tolerating 300 mg twice daily well for 3 days

- Manic symptoms are improved. However, she continues to endorse racing thoughts, decreased need for sleep, ongoing concentration-related difficulties, and irritability, albeit her irritability has improved
- She denies headaches, nausea, increased thirst, polyuria, and polydipsia and there is no tremor on exam
- Her attending psychiatrist has ordered a trough lithium in 3 days, at which time she will have been treated with lithium 600 mg twice daily for 7 days
- The 12-hour trough lithium concentration is 0.5 mEq/L, and her sodium is 142, potassium is 4.1, BUN is 7, creatinine is 0.6, glucose is 80, calcium is 10.1, and phosphorus is 3.6 (Table 9.1). Her creatinine clearance is (Updated Schwartz formula) 125.8 mL/min/1.73 m^2, and she weighs 56.5 kg

Testing: laboratory results, imaging, EKGs
Table 9.1

Lithium		
	Value	Ref Range
Lithium	0.5 mEq/L	0.6 - 1.1 mEq/L
CBC with Differential		
	Value	Ref Range
WBC	7.8	4.5 - 13.0 K/mcL
RBC	5.1	4.50 - 5.30 M/mcL
HGB	14.6	13.0 - 16.0 gm/dL
HCT	42.7	37.0 - 49.0 %
MCV	87.8	78.0 - 94.0 fL
MCH	30.9	25.0 - 35.0 pg
MCHC	35.2	31.0 - 37.0 gm/dL
RDW	11.5	<14.6 %
PLATELET	224	135 - 466 K/mcL
Comp Metabolic Panel		
	Value	Ref Range
SODIUM	142	136 - 145 mmol/L
POTASSIUM	4.1	3.3 - 4.7 mmol/L
CHLORIDE	111	100 - 112 mmol/L
CO2	22	17 - 31 mmol/L
ANION GAP	9	4 - 15 mmol/L
BUN	7	6 - 21 mg/dL
CREATININE	0.6	0.46 - 1.00 mg/dL
GLUCOSE	80	65 - 106 mg/dL
CALCIUM	10.1	8.3 - 10.6 mg/dL

Attending physician mental notes (week 1)

The attending physician is concerned about persistent hypomanic symptoms with partial response to lithium and a 12-hour lithium level (C_0) of 0.5, no signs of symptoms of lithium toxicity and confirmed adherence from the parent and patient

PATIENT FILE

Question

What's the most appropriate intervention at this time?

- Increase lithium to 600 mg three times daily (31.9 mg/kg) over 2 weeks (increasing by 300 mg/week)
- Discontinue lithium and reattempt treatment with a mixed dopamine–serotonin receptor antagonist
- Convert lithium to a long-acting/extended-release formulation and change dose to 900 mg every night at bedtime (15.9 mg/kg)
- Reintroduce a selective serotonin reuptake inhibitor (SSRI) (e.g. escitalopram 10 mg every morning) to target persistent irritability, dyssomnia and difficulty concentrating

Case outcome second interim follow-up (week 4)

- Lithium was titrated to 600 mg three times daily, and there was a significant reduction in manic symptoms and resolution of functional impairment
- She now sleeps 8.5 hours per night, reports a sleep latency of 20–25 minutes on most nights, is again earning As and Bs at school, and denies depressive symptoms
- She reports no tolerability concerns, does not take any nonsteroidal anti-inflammatories (NSAIDs), and has no tremor, headaches, nausea, or hypothyroid symptoms

Attending physician mental notes (week 4)

- Regarding the prior treatment options, her attending psychiatrist wished to optimize her lithium dose (and exposure) before adding another agent. In general, monotherapy is preferable
- Her clinician chose not to titrate to 900 mg every night at bedtime (15.9 mg/kg) with an extended-release preparation as this would ultimately decrease her lithium dose from approximately 22 mg/kg daily to 15.9 mg/kg daily. Her clinician also targeted the goal lithium dose from many pediatric studies, which has generally been 25–30 mg/kg daily with maximum doses of 40 mg/kg daily
- Finally, her clinician did not consider reintroducing an SSRI, particularly given the persistence of manic symptoms and concerns that the SSRI could destabilize her mood (DelBello et al. 2007)
- Her attending physician rechecked laboratory studies (Table 9.2)
- Her attending physician also continues to consider routine monitoring strategies for lithium-treated patients (Meyer and Stahl 2023) (Box 9.1)

Testing: laboratory results, imaging, EKGs
Table 9.2

Lithium		
	Value	Ref Range
Lithium	0.9 mEq/L	0.6 - 1.1 mEq/L
CBC with Differential		
	Value	Ref Range
WBC	7.8	4.5 - 13.0 K/mcL
RBC	5.1	4.50 - 5.30 M/mcL
HGB	14.6	13.0 - 16.0 gm/dL
HCT	42.7	37.0 - 49.0 %
MCV	87.8	78.0 - 94.0 fL
MCH	30.9	25.0 - 35.0 pg
MCHC	35.2	31.0 - 37.0 gm/dL
RDW	11.5	<14.6 %
PLATELET	224	135 - 466 K/mcL
Comp Metabolic Panel		
	Value	Ref Range
SODIUM	141	136 - 145 mmol/L
POTASSIUM	4.1	3.3 - 4.7 mmol/L
CHLORIDE	111	100 - 112 mmol/L
CO2	22	17 - 31 mmol/L
ANION GAP	10	4 - 15 mmol/L
BUN	12	6 - 21 mg/dL
CREATININE	0.7	0.46 - 1.00 mg/dL
GLUCOSE	93	65 - 106 mg/dL
CALCIUM	9.4	8.3 - 10.6 mg/dL
TSH		
	Value	Ref Range
Thyroid Stimulating Hormone	2.9	0.43 - 4.0 mcIU/mL

Box 9.1 Routine lithium monitoring

1. **Vital signs:** weight at every visit with body mass index (BMI) calculated, and obtain a blood pressure every 6 months
2. **Electrocardiogram (EKG):** a follow-up should be obtained once lithium is at a steady state after initial titration (e.g. week 12), only in those who required an EKG upon lithium initiation (certain patients >40 years old, younger patients with cardiac risk factors, or if required by institutional protocol). In those patients, an annual EKG may be required by local protocol or the presence of pre-existing abnormalities. An annual EKG is not recommended by most treatment guidelines for other patients
3. **Serum calcium and TSH:** every 6 months. An increase in the frequency or the need to add additional laboratory measures (e.g. ionized calcium, parathyroid hormone, T4,

triiodothyronine (T3), free T4 index) will be dictated by the presence of abnormalities

4. **Lithium level:**
   a. **New lithium starts:** a 12 h trough should be obtained approximately 1 week after any dosage change or the introduction or removal of a medication having kinetic interactions with lithium. Through week 24 (6 months) the level should be obtained with the estimated glomerular filtration rate (eGFR)
   b. **Established therapy:** the 12 h trough level should be obtained with the eGFR, and the frequency dictated by the eGFR. For patients with low eGFR values, this may necessitate levels every 6 weeks. For those whose maintenance levels are in the range 0.80–1.00 mEq/L consider increasing the frequency of levels to every 3 months to minimize the occurrence of supratherapeutic levels that might incur risk for renal toxicity (Kirkham et al. 2014; Castro et al. 2016; Heald et al. 2021)

5. **Renal:**
   a. Monitoring for the first 6 months of lithium treatment is shown in Table 9.3
   b. Routine 6-month monitoring during established lithium therapy:
      i. Review medical history for renal dysfunction risk factors and use of nephrotoxic medications
      ii. eGFR

Table 9.3

	6 weeks	12 weeks	18 weeks	6 months
eGFR[a] (baseline eGFR > 60 mL/min)	X	X		X
eGFR[a] (baseline eGFR 45–59 mL/min)	X	X	X	X
24 h fluid intake record[b]	X	X		X
Early morning urine osmolality (EMUO)[c]	X	X		X
Albumin to creatinine ratio (ACR)[d]		X		X

[a] After 6 months the monitoring frequency depends on chronic kidney disease (CKD) stage
[b] Ask the patient to record fluid intake for 2 days (48 hours) and average the result
[c] Should also be added following a new complaint of polyuria/polydipsia
[d] At 3 months and 6 months for those with baseline eGFR < 90 mL/min or risk factors for renal dysfunction. After 6 months the monitoring frequency depends on the ACR stage

iii 24 h fluid intake record (FIR): ask the patient to record fluid intake for 2 days (48 hours) and average the result

iv. EMUO: for those with polyuria complaints, on stable amiloride treatment, or for patients whose most recent EMUO value is 850 mOsm/kg as verified by a repeat specimen

v. ACR: for those with eGFR < 90 mL/min or risk factors for renal dysfunction

c. *Increase frequency of labs to every 3 months during established lithium therapy when one of the following are present (higher risk patients):*

   i. eGFR value: when values are <60 mL/min

   ii. eGFR trends: initial evidence of a decline in eGFR > 2 mL/min over 6 months or > 4 mL/min over 12 months as verified by a repeat specimen

   iii. EMUO: for increased or new complaints of polyuria, when titrating amiloride to manage polyuria, or for urine osmolality values < 300 mOsm/kg

   iv. ACR: if ACR has progressed from stage A1 to A2 as verified by a repeat specimen

d. When to consult a pediatric nephrologist:

   i. eGFR: second decline in eGFR > 2 mL/min over 6 months or > 4 mL/min over 12 months as verified by a repeat specimen

   ii. eGFR < 45 mL/min as verified by a repeat specimen

   iii. ACR: stage A3

   iv. Nephrogenic diabetes insipidus (EMUO values < 300 mOsm/kg) unresponsive to maximal doses of amiloride (10 mg twice daily) for 6 weeks

   v. Hematuria

Take-home points

- Lithium is currently a U.S. Food and Drug Administration (FDA)-approved treatment for bipolar disorder in children and adolescents. However, its use in pediatric patients may be more challenging than in adults because of differences in clearance (Findling et al. 2010, 2011; Landersdorfer et al. 2017)
- Several studies support its efficacy in youth (Findling et al. 2008, 2015) including a double-blind discontinuation study (Findling et al. 2019) (Figure 9.2)
- As noted for this 56.5 kg young adolescent, her calculated creatinine clearance was 125.8 mL/min/1.73 m^2, which makes twice daily lithium dosing challenging in terms of our ability to achieve a lithium level similar to those achieved in the prospective randomized trials of lithium. As such, lithium required three times daily dosing.
- In clinical trials of children and adolescents with bipolar disorder, average lithium levels were near 1.0 mEq/L and were relatively well tolerated (Findling et al. 2015, 2019)
- Data from Collaborative Lithium Trial 1 (CoLT 1) provide weight-based dosing recommendations. As shown in Figure 9.3, kinetic modeling simulation using the dosing recommendation of 25 mg/kg (that best fit all of the parameters) optimizes the balance between efficacy and tolerability. From this dosing strategy of 25 mg/kg (administered as divided twice daily or three times daily doses) and

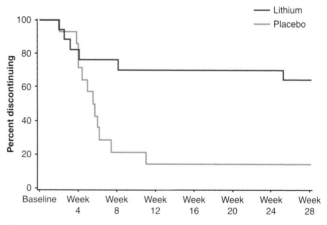

Figure 9.2 Lithium vs. placebo in the maintenance treatment of child/adolescent bipolar 1 disorder (mean age 12.0 years). Adapted from Findling, R. L., McNamara, N. K., Pavuluri, M., et al. Lithium for the maintenance treatment of bipolar I disorder: a double-blind, placebo-controlled discontinuation study. *J Am Acad Child Adolesc Psychiatry* 2019; 58: 287–96.

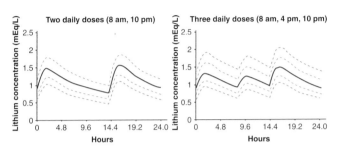

Figure 9.3 Monte Carlo simulations of lithium concentrations for a daily dosage of 25 mg/kg given in two or three divided doses. [NB: The doses administered were rounded to the nearest 300 mg lithium carbonate increment. Where applicable, the higher dose was given in the evening.] Adapted from Landersdorfer, C. B., Findling, R. L., Frazier, J. A., Kafantaris, V., Kirkpatrick, C. M. Lithium in paediatric patients with bipolar disorder: implications for selection of dosage regimens via population pharmacokinetics/ pharmacodynamics. *Clin Pharmacokinet* 2017; 56(1): 77–90.

the response of these manic patients to treatment, two important conclusions were reached:

- ○ The average lithium level required for a 50% reduction in Young Mania Rating Scale (YMRS) was 0.71 mEq/L, but with the caveat that the interindividual variance was 59%
- ○ A daily maintenance lithium carbonate dose of 25 mg/kg divided twice daily may achieve a ≥ 50% reduction in YMRS in 74% of patients, with only 8% of patients expected to have supratherapeutic trough levels > 1.40 mEq/L

- While clinicians must acknowledge that significant interindividual variations in lithium clearance demand close level monitoring when starting treatment, the 25 mg/kg dosing recommendation is more evidence-based than recommendations in lithium carbonate product labeling, when such recommendations exist at all
- When ordering therapeutic drug monitoring in lithium-treated children and adolescents, clinicians should keep several points in mind:
  - ○ Assess concomitant medications and adherence before obtaining lithium concentrations
  - ○ Obtain trough concentrations
  - ○ Random levels are generally unhelpful in terms of therapeutic drug monitoring
  - ○ As shown in Figure 9.4, the average lithium concentration following a single 900 mg dose in pediatric patients varies considerably (Findling et al. 2010). This underscores the importance of obtaining true trough concentrations

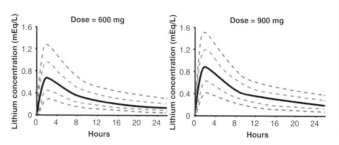

Figure 9.4 Pharmacokinetic single-dose modeling of pediatric lithium clearance from a sample of 39 children and adolescents with mean age 11.9 years. Adapted from Findling, R. L., Landersdorfer, C. B., Kafantaris, V., Pavuluri, M., McNamara, N. K., McClellan, J., Frazier, J. A., Sikich, L., Kowatch, R., Lingler, J., Faber, J., Taylor-Zapata, P., Jusko, W. J. First-dose pharmacokinetics of lithium carbonate in children and adolescents. *J Clin Psychopharmacol* 2010; 30(4): 404–10.

Mechanism of action moment

- Candidates for lithium's mechanism of action include multiple signal transduction sites beyond neurotransmitter receptors (Figure 9.5). This includes second messengers such as the phosphatidyl inositol system, where lithium inhibits the enzyme inositol

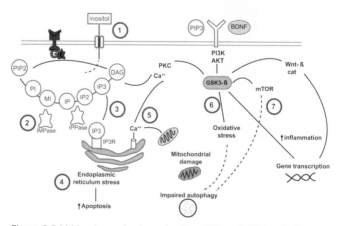

Figure 9.5 Lithium's mechanism of action. Although lithium is the oldest treatment for bipolar disorder, its mechanism of action is still not well understood. Several possible mechanisms exist and are shown here. Lithium may work by affecting signal transduction, perhaps through its inhibition of second-messenger enzymes such as inositol monophosphatase, by modulation of G proteins (left), or by interaction at various sites within downstream signal transduction cascades, including glycogen synthase kinase 3 (GSK-3) (green). Adapted from Meyer and Stahl, *The Lithium Handbook,* 2023.

monophosphatase, modulation of G-proteins, and, most recently, regulation of gene expression for growth factors and neuronal plasticity by interaction with downstream signal transduction cascades, including inhibition of GSK-3 (glycogen synthase kinase 3) and protein kinase C (Figure 9.5)

- Like in adults, the use of lithium has decreased in recent years and the reasons probably include the side effects of lithium, and the monitoring burden, which may be particularly an issue in pediatric patients. Additionally, in pediatric patients, given the clearance-related issues, lithium may need to be dosed three times daily

- Well-known side effects of lithium include gastrointestinal symptoms such as dyspepsia, nausea, vomiting, and diarrhea, as well as weight gain, hair loss, acne, tremor, sedation, decreased cognition, and incoordination

- There are also potential long-term adverse effects on the thyroid and kidney. In pediatric clinical trials, a large proportion of patients experienced increases in TSH over the course of the trial, although weight gain appeared to be less than in adult trials

Two-minute tutorial

- Bipolar disorder frequently emerges in adolescence or young adulthood (Solmi et al. 2022), and the constellation of symptoms is generally similar during manic episodes (e.g. euphoria, pressured speech, grandiose ideation, inappropriate laughter, and occasionally hypersexuality or psychosis, which clearly distinguish this as a mood episode) (Figure 9.6) (van Meter et al. 2016). However, irritability may be more common, and the presence of mixed features is more common in adolescents compared to adults (Birmaher et al. 2009; Hunt et al. 2013)

- Children and adolescents with bipolar disorder often have at least one other lifetime disorder diagnosis (Yen et al. 2016). Anxiety disorders and attention-deficit hyperactivity disorder (ADHD) are common comorbidities, and substance abuse is both a complication and comorbidity in many adolescents with bipolar disorder

- In the *Diagnostic and Statistical Manual of Mental Disorders 5* (*DSM-5*), comorbid conditions in mania must be exacerbated during the manic episode. This represents an attempt to separate "overlap" comorbidity produced by double-counting overlapping symptoms toward the diagnosis of each disorder

- In younger patients, ADHD with comorbid oppositional defiant disorder (ODD) may be confused with bipolar disorder. Some youth with ADHD as well as ODD/conduct disorder, obsessive compulsive disorder (OCD), anxiety disorders, and autism spectrum disorder

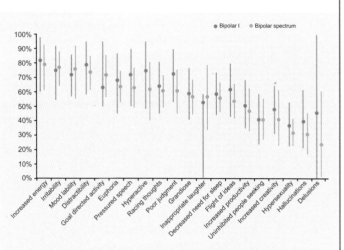

Figure 9.6 Mood symptom prevalence in child-/adolescent-onset mania. Adapted from Van Meter, A. R., Burke, C., Kowatch, R. A., et al. Ten-year updated meta-analysis of the clinical characteristics of pediatric mania and hypomania. *Bipolar Disord* 2016; 18: 19–32.

as well as posttraumatic stress disorder (PTSD) may also have emotional dysregulation and outbursts. Further, disruptive mood dysregulation disorder (DMDD) is characterized by such outbursts, although this is in the context of chronic irritability

- Evaluating pediatric patients with bipolar disorder should involve multiple informants, including a parent. Clinical course, developmental history, and context also need to be considered, and comorbidities should be systematically evaluated

- Treatment response differs in pediatric patients and adults with bipolar disorder. Many traditional mood stabilizers (e.g. divalproex, carbamazepine, oxcarbazepine, lamotrigine) have failed to demonstrate efficacy in pediatric patients with bipolar disorder, whereas most studies of mixed dopamine–serotonin receptor antagonists have demonstrated superiority to placebo (Correll et al. 2010)

- Currently approved mixed dopamine–serotonin receptor antagonists with FDA indications in children and adolescents ages 10–17 with mixed/manic episodes are aripiprazole, asenapine, olanzapine, quetiapine, and risperidone. Additionally, lurasidone and olanzapine/fluoxetine combination have been approved for children and adolescents with bipolar depression

- Most bipolar adolescents experience syndromic recovery after their first episode; however, symptomatic and functional recoveries are lower and just over one-third of children and adolescents with bipolar disorder have full medication adherence (DelBello et al. 2007)

- Predictors of poor syndromic recovery in adolescents with bipolar disorder include comorbid ADHD, anxiety disorders, and disruptive behavior disorders as well as nonadherence to psychotropic medication and lower socioeconomic status (DelBello et al. 2007)
- Adolescents with bipolar disorder who have alcohol-use disorders, are treated with antidepressants, and do not receive psychotherapy are more likely to have a relapse (DelBello et al. 2007)

Another 2-minute tutorial

- Twice daily or three times daily lithium regimens are more common in pediatric populations compared to adults, as discussed earlier. However, as patients approach adulthood, the lithium dose could be consolidated to every night at bedtime, starting initially by converting three times daily to twice daily dosing, and then slowly transitioning to every night at bedtime. The eventual goal by late adolescence is every night at bedtime dosing, with a 12 h trough of 0.6–0.8 ideally, but up to 1.0 as needed. The rationale for this approach, as described in detail in Meyer and Stahl's *Lithium Handbook*, is that high lithium concentrations over time are nephrotoxic and that it may be advantageous to avoid excursions above 1.0 mEq/L
- In adults, despite the modest duration of lithium exposure in the final sample, after adjustment for all patient, demographic, and other treatment-related risk factors, there were two patterns of lithium treatment associated with significantly increased renal disease risk: use of lithium more than once daily and having even one lithium level >1.20 mEq/L (Meyer and Stahl 2023)
- In adults, the debate over the renoprotective effect of once-daily lithium dosing originated in the early 1980s, with papers noting a greater degree of polyuria in patients receiving twice daily dosing compared to those on every night at bedtime dosing. It later became clear that polyuria is the earliest clinical manifestation of intracellular lithium accumulation in collecting duct principal cells and of the ensuing processes that combine with chronic kidney disease risks to accelerate age-related glomerular filtration rate (GFR) declines (Meyer and Stahl 2023)
- While not directly addressing the question of polyuria, the 2016 Massachusetts General Hospital (MGH) case-control analysis provided the best evidence from a large methodologically sound study that once-daily dosing reduces renal insufficiency risk by

20%, even with modest lithium exposure duration (Castro et al. 2016). In adults, there was also no difference in renal insufficiency risk between standard or extended-released lithium preparations. Still, periods of lithium toxicity are a clear risk factor for lithium-related nephropathy (Clos et al. 2015)

- The underlying reason for the association between once-daily dosing in adults and decreased renal dysfunction risk is unknown, but two plausible hypotheses are advanced (Meyer and Stahl 2023):
  - The first rests on the concept that many clinicians may unwittingly expose patients to more lithium when it is prescribed twice daily due to the distorting effect on morning trough values from divided dosages
  - The second hypothesis is that prolonged higher trough lithium levels from divided daily dosing may lead to a sufficiently high lithium concentration in tubular fluid

Post test question

Compared to adults, young adolescents treated with lithium may require higher mg/kg doses because of:

A. Greater renal clearance
B. Increased cytochrome CYP2D6 activity
C. Faster and more efficient intestinal absorption
D. Enhanced CNS penetration

Answer: A (Greater renal clearance)

Greater renal clearance (correct answer) accounts for greater clearance of lithium in pediatric patients compared to adults. In general, CYP2D6 activity reaches adult levels early in life and intestinal absorption in pediatric patients – for lithium – is similar to adults. However, of relevance to other medications, intestinal transit time will be increased in younger patients which for some delayed-release preparations may result in incomplete absorption. Finally, after the neonatal period, central nervous system (CNS) penetration is relatively constant over the lifespan.

References

1. Birmaher, B., Axelson, D., Goldstein, B., et al. Four-year longitudinal course of children and adolescents with bipolar spectrum disorders: the course and outcome of bipolar youth (COBY) study. *Am J Psychiatry* 2009; 166(7): 795–804. https://doi.org/10.1176/appi.ajp.2009.08101569

2. Castro, V. M., Roberson, A. M., McCoy, T. H., et al. Stratifying risk for renal insufficiency among lithium-treated patients: an electronic health record study. *Neuropsychopharmacology* 2016; 41(4): 1138–43. https://doi.org/10.1038/npp.2015.254

3. Clos, S., Rauchhaus, P., Severn, A., Cochrane, L., Donnan, P. T. Long-term effect of lithium maintenance therapy on estimated glomerular filtration rate in patients with affective disorders: a population-based cohort study. *Lancet Psychiatry* 2015; 2(12): 1075–83. https://doi.org/10.1016/S2215-0366(15)00316-8

4. Correll, C. U., Sheridan, E. M., DelBello, M. P. Antipsychotic and mood stabilizer efficacy and tolerability in pediatric and adult patients with bipolar I mania: a comparative analysis of acute, randomized, placebo-controlled trials. *Bipolar Disord* 2010; 12(2): 166–41. https://doi.org/10.1111/j.1399-5618.2010.00798.x

5. DelBello, M. P., Hanseman, D., Adler, C. M., Fleck, D. E., Strakowski, S. M. Twelve-month outcome of adolescents with bipolar disorder following first hospitalization for a manic or mixed episode. *Am J Psychiatry* 2007; 164(4): 582–90. https://doi.org/10.1176/ajp.2007.164.4.582

6. Findling, R. L., Frazier, J. A., Kafantaris, V., et al. The Collaborative Lithium Trials (CoLT): specific aims, methods, and implementation. *Child Adolesc Psychiatry Mental Health* 2008; 2: 21. https://doi.org/10.1186/1753-2000-2-21

7. Findling, R. L., Kafantaris, V., Pavuluri, M., et al. Dosing strategies for lithium monotherapy in children and adolescents with bipolar I disorder. *J Child Adolesc Psychopharmacol* 2011; 21(3): 195–205. https://doi.org/10.1089/cap.2010.0084

8. Findling, R. L., Landersdorfer, C. B., Kafantaris, V., et al. First-dose pharmacokinetics of lithium carbonate in children and adolescents. *J Clin Psychopharmacol* 2010; 30(4): 404–10. https://doi.org/10.1097/JCP.0b013e3181e66a62

9. Findling, R. L., McNamara, N. K., Pavuluri, M., et al. Lithium for the maintenance treatment of bipolar I disorder: a double-blind, placebo-controlled discontinuation study. *J Am Acad Child Adolesc Psychiatry* 2019; 58(2): 287–96. https://doi.org/10.1016/j.jaac.2018.07.901

10. Findling, R. L., Robb, A., McNamara, N. K. Lithium in the acute treatment of bipolar I disorder: a double-blind, placebo-controlled study. *Pediatrics* 2015; 136(5): 885–94. https://doi.org/10.1542/peds.2015-0743

11. Heald, A. H., Holland, D., Stedman, M., et al. Can we check serum lithium levels less often without compromising patient safety? *BJPsych Open* 2021; 8: e18. https://doi.org10.1192/bjo.2021.1027

12. Hunt, J. I., Case, B. G., Birmaher, B., et al. Irritability and elation in a large bipolar youth sample: relative symptom severity and clinical outcomes over 4 years. *J Clin Psychiatry* 2013; 74(1): e110–17. https://doi.org/10.4088/JCP.12m07874

13. Kirkham, E., Skinner, J., Anderson, T., et al. One lithium level >1.0 mmol/L causes an acute decline in eGFR: findings from a retrospective analysis of a monitoring database. *BMJ Open* 2014; 4: e006020. https://doi.org/10.1136/bmjopen-2014-006020

14. Landersdorfer, C. B., Findling, R. L., Frazier, J. A., Kafantaris, V., Kirkpatrick, C. M. J. Lithium in paediatric patients with bipolar disorder: implications for selection of dosage regimens via population pharmacokinetics/pharmacodynamics. *Clinical Pharmacokinetics* 2017; 56(1): 77–90. https://doi.org/10.1007/s40262-016-0430-3

15. Meyer, J. M., Stahl, S. M. *The Lithium Handbook.* Cambridge, UK: Cambridge University Press, 2023.

16. Solmi, M., Radua, J., Olivola, M., et al. Age at onset of mental disorders worldwide: large-scale meta-analysis of 192 epidemiological studies. *Mol Psychiatry* 2022; 27(1): 281–95. https://doi.org/10.1038/s41380-021-01161-7

17. van Meter, A. R., Burke, C., Kowatch, R. A., Findling, R. L., Youngstrom, E. A. Ten-year updated meta-analysis of the clinical characteristics of pediatric mania and hypomania. *Bipolar Disord* 2016; 18(1): 19–32. https://doi.org/10.1111/bdi.12358

18. Yen, S., Stout, R., Hower, H., et al. The influence of comorbid disorders on the episodicity of bipolar disorder in youth. *Acta Psychiatr Scand* 2016; 133(4): 324–34. https://doi.org/10.1111/acps.12514

Case 10: Tic, tic, tic: motor and vocal tics in a boy

The Question: What is the role of pharmacotherapy in Tourette syndrome?

The Psychopharmacological Dilemma: Although tics can be common in children and adolescents, choosing among pharmacological approaches to management of Tourette syndrome is complex

Pretest self-assessment question

Which of the following represents an evidence-based intervention for a child with Tourette syndrome?

A. Aripiprazole (Abilify)
B. Methylphenidate osmotic controlled-release oral delivery system (OROS) (Concerta)
C. Mixed amphetamine salt (Adderall)
D. Diazepam (Valium)
E. All of the above

Answer: A (Aripiprazole, Abilify)

Patient evaluation on intake

- 10-year-old boy with attention-deficit hyperactivity disorder (ADHD), combined presentation, and motor and vocal tics
- The patient's tics consist of eye blinking and shoulder shrugging, and he has repetitive vocalizations, including short, high-pitched barking noises, as well as sniffing
- He is able to suppress these tics in some situations, but it becomes increasingly difficult to resist the urge as time progresses
- His parents first noted the tics at the age of 8 and they seem to have progressed in frequency and severity
- His tics occur multiple times per day and the longest period during which he has not had tics on a typical day is 40–60 minutes
- Parents, teachers, and peers have noticed the tics and his mother believes that the patient's tics are worse when he is excited and when he is under stress or feeling anxious, particularly around strangers

Psychiatric history

- History of ADHD, combined presentation since age 4
- In addition to atomoxetine (Strattera) 60 mg each morning for ADHD, his parents have given low-dose melatonin every night at bedtime (1.5 mg) on an as-needed basis to help with insomnia

Social and personal history

- Lives with both parents in a suburban community and is active with his family in their local non-denominational church
- Attends the third grade at a public elementary school and does not have an Individualized Education Plan (IEP) or 504 Plan. His grades are mostly As and occasional Bs and he enjoys art and recess
- Has a small group of friends and enjoys playing video games and baseball as well as soccer
- There is no history of physical or sexual abuse

Medical history

- His mother smoked throughout the first and second trimesters of pregnancy, although she attempted to decrease her smoking, with intermittent success
- He was delivered at 40 weeks to a 30-year-old mother and 30-year-old father. There were concerns related to low birth weight and intrauterine growth restriction. He was observed for 2 days in the "special care nursery," but the parents do not recall any specific interactions
- Developmental milestones are as shown in Table 10.1

Table 10.1

Gross Motor – Patient	Average typical milestone
Roll over, 5 months	Roll over, 5–6 months
Sitting, 8 months	Sitting, 7 months
Walking, 14 months	Walking, 15 months
Runs, "about 2," parents unsure	Runs, 20 months
Jump, 3 years of age	Jump, 2 ½ years
Fine motor/adaptive	
Reaches, 6 months	Reaches, 6 months
Scribbles, 16 months	Scribbles,16–17 months
Two cube towers, unable to recall	Two cube towers, 12 months
Language	
Making sounds, 1 month	Make sounds, 1 month
Laughing, 3 months	Laughing, 3 months
Mama/dada specific, 14–15 months	Mama/dada specific, 13–14 months
Personal/social	
Smile, 2–3 months	Smile, 2 months
Feeding self, 6 months	Feeding self, 6 months
Indicate wants, 1 year, perhaps earlier, parents unsure	Indicate wants, 13 months
Remove garment, 2 years, approximate	Remove garment, 2 years
Dress independently, 5 years, approximate	Dress independently, 4 years, 9 months

Family history

- Father with obsessive compulsive disorder (OCD)
- Mother with a history of multiple sclerosis and ADHD as well as chronic fatigue syndrome

- Sister, age 22, has a history of ADHD and developed severe cognitive symptoms after her second course of COVID-19 and had to drop out of college during her junior year

Medication history

- Atomoxetine (Strattera) 60 mg daily
- History of methylphenidate OROS (Concerta), titrated to 36 mg daily (approximately 1 mg/kg and at the time of treatment), which was associated with worsening of both motor and vocal tics
- Melatonin 1.5 mg every evening at bedtime as needed – insomnia

Current medications

- Atomoxetine 40 mg daily
- Melatonin 1.5 mg every night at bedtime as needed – insomnia

Psychotherapy history

- The family worked with an online psychoeducational program that his parents located through a family friend who has worked with the Tourette Association of America
- He also tried psychotherapy using Habit Reversal Therapy for 12 sessions. This was conducted in person, and he reports excellent compliance with homework

Further investigation

Is there anything else that you would like to know about the patient? What about details related to obsessive compulsive disorder symptoms?

- He has some mild obsessions per his father. However, the patient denies hearing songs or sentences in his head over and over, having thoughts of hurting himself or hurting someone else
- He occasionally worries that bad things might happen to someone or that he might get contaminated by germs or dirt
- With regard to compulsions, he and his parents do not report repeated washing or cleaning, checking, counting, hoarding, or collecting, repeating, or ordering/arranging
- Additionally, regarding ritualistic behavior, he denies touching, tapping, or rubbing things in a certain way, repeatedly asking about the correctness of behavior, feeling that he has to tell on himself, trichotillomania, repeatedly having to say the same words, prayers, or sentences over and over, or eating and drinking in a special order

What about additional physical symptoms and vital signs?

- No reports of depressed mood, guilt, anhedonia, or suicidal ideation
- Vital signs are within normal limits; his BMI is in the 50th percentile for age and sex
- He denies cardiac symptoms, including palpitations
- Physical examination is unremarkable and his neurologic examination is summarized as:
  - On mental status exam, he is alert, and his speech is clear and fluent
  - On cranial nerve exam, pupils are equal, round, and reactive to light bilaterally. He has no afferent pupillary defect. Extraocular movements are intact. There is no nystagmus. Smile, eye closure, and palatal elevation are symmetric. Facial sensation and hearing are intact. Shoulder shrug is normal bilaterally. Tongue protrusion is in the midline
  - On motor exam, he has normal muscle bulk and tone. Motor strength is 5/5 bilaterally. Deep tendon reflexes are 2/4 throughout. No Babinski sign
  - Sensation is intact to light touch, vibration, and temperature
  - There is no tremor, dysdiadochokinesia, dysmetria, chorea, dystonia, or myoclonus
  - Gait is narrow-based. He is able to toe-walk, heel-walk, and tandem walk. No Romberg sign

What about recent infections?

- The family reports no history of recent infections, including streptococcal infections. His mother and sister have had SARS-CoV-2 infections, but neither required immunotherapy, steroids, or antiviral therapy

What about rating scales?

- The Tourette Impairment – Child self-report results are shown in Table 10.2

Rating scales

Table 10.2

In the past month, how much trouble have YOU had doing the following … :	Problems due to tics				Problems due to ADHD, OCD, Anxiety, Rages, Other			
	Not at all	Just a little	Pretty much	Very much	Not at all	Just a little	Pretty much	Very much
Being prepared for class (having books, homework)			✓		✓			

Writing in class		✓	✓
Taking tests or exams		✓	✓
Doing homework		✓		✓
Concentrating on work		✓		✓
Doing household chores	✓			✓
Getting ready for bed	✓		✓
Getting along with parents	✓		✓
Visiting relatives	✓		✓
Being teased by other kids		✓	✓
Going to a friend's house			✓	✓
Having a friend over		✓		✓
Being with friends on phone/social media	✓			✓
Doing sports/music/ extra-curriculars	✓			✓

Attending physician's mental notes: initial psychiatric evaluation

- This patient has significant symptoms of Tourette syndrome and there is a history of worsening with stimulant treatment. He has not had improvement with Habit Reversal Therapy (HRT) and has not tried Comprehensive Behavioral Intervention for Tics (CBIT)
- The child and adolescent psychiatrist is particularly interested in the past medical history and family history, given that a family history of tic disorders is common. Additional risk factors for this boy include being low birth weight (Brander et al. 2018) and having a history of maternal autoimmune disease (Dalsgaard et al. 2015)
- The clinician has also enquired about recent streptococcal infections, which might be associated with pediatric autoimmune neuropsychiatric disorders associated with streptococcal infections, and other infectious or noninfectious conditions in pediatric acute-onset neuropsychiatric syndrome (Swedo et al. 2015). Tics have increasingly been observed following streptococcal infections (Swedo et al. 2015). The clinician also noted nicotine exposure during pregnancy, and the absence of cannabis exposure. This is important, given that dose-dependent gestational exposure risks to tobacco (Browne et al. 2016) and cannabis (Mathews et al. 2014) have been described
- Regarding sleep, the child and adolescent psychiatrist notes that this patient has initial and middle insomnia. This is not surprising

clinically, given that sleep disorders frequently occur in patients with Tourette syndrome. In fact, in one study of patients with Tourette syndrome, two-thirds met *Diagnostic and Statistical Manual of Mental Disorders* (*DSM-5*) criteria for a sleep disorder (Ghosh et al. 2014)

- Given the presence of tics and ADHD, the child and adolescent psychiatrist has enquired carefully about OCD symptoms, given that OCD-ADHD-tic disorders commonly co-occur
- Regarding his current medication treatment, the treating clinician will need to explore ADHD symptoms and potentially consider a therapy that targets both his ADHD and tics
- Regarding psychotherapy, it is noteworthy that the psychotherapy does not appear to have had a significant impact on his symptoms. However, the child and adolescent psychiatrist notes that is an evidence-based psychotherapy for tic disorders
- The child and adolescent psychiatrist is aware that some patients suppress tics during an evaluation, and others have increased tics due to the anxiety. Sometimes having the patient focus on reading or another cognitively engaging activity will reduce tics. Ultimately, the diagnosis of a tic disorder is based on very typical history and observations, and an extensive work-up is unnecessary. However, concerning features on examination include unilateral tics or clinical suggestions of seizures

Question

Given his prior psychotherapy and current pharmacologic treatment, which of the following would be your next step?

- Discontinue atomoxetine
- Begin clonidine
- Begin haloperidol
- Begin aripiprazole
- Refer to CBIT

Case outcome: first interim follow-up (week 14)

- At his last visit, he was referred to CBIT and has completed 10 sessions. The child and adolescent psychiatrist has had several discussions with the therapist who reports that there have been some improvements in terms of tics and in terms of identification of stressors. However, his tics remain in the moderate range and cause embarrassment at school and continue to affect interactions with peers

- He continues to deny depressive symptoms and there are no new OCD symptoms
- His ADHD symptoms are mild and primarily consist of hyperactivity and occasional impulsivity. However, his teacher is generally working with him to address this in a way that does not disrupt the classroom

Given his prior psychotherapy and current pharmacologic treatment, which of the following would be your next step?

- Discontinue atomoxetine (Straterra)
- Begin clonidine (Catapres)
- Begin haloperidol (Haldol)
- Begin aripiprazole (Abilify)
- Refer to Cognitive Processing Therapy (CPT)

Case outcome: second interim follow-up (week 16)

- The family began clonidine (immediate release, 0.1 mg tablets), using the titration shown in Table 10.3. However, he is aware that clonidine is also available as a transdermal formulation and can be compounded by many pharmacies as a suspension
- Since beginning clonidine and titration to 0.1 mg twice daily, both his motor and vocal tics have improved. His parents have observed similar improvements. At school, his teachers note that he has been less "fidgety" and has had fewer tics as well. However, he occasionally feels tired and notes that he does not have as much energy when he is playing soccer
- His blood pressure and heart rate are decreased compared to baseline; both are 35th percentile for age, sex, and height

Table 10.3

Week	Morning	Evening
1	0 tablets	½ tablet (0.05 mg)
2	0 tablets	1 tablet (0.1 mg)
3	½ tablet (0.05 mg)	1 tablet (0.1 mg)
4	1 tablet (0.1 mg)	1 tablet (0.1 mg)

Attending physician's mental notes: second interim follow-up (week 16)

- Several studies have demonstrated the efficacy of clonidine in pediatric patients with tic disorders, including Tourette syndrome, and include studies of both oral and transdermal formulations (Shapiro et al. 1983; Gancher et al. 1990; Leckman et al. 1991). By contrast, the α_{2A}-selective agonist guanfacine has positive (Scahill et al. 2001) and negative (Murphy et al. 2017) trials

- The attending physician is concerned by the decrease in heart rate and by the patient's decreased exercise tolerance
- The patient's blood pressure is still within the normal range, however, the attending physician knows that orthostatic intolerance or orthostatic symptoms are less common in pediatric patients treated with α_2 agonists compared to adults, given how blood pressure is differentially regulated in pediatric vs. adult patients
- The physician is concerned about the possibility of α_2 agonist-related bradycardia which is a side effect of α_2 agonists in some pediatric patients and orders an electrocardiogram (EKG)

Testing: laboratory results, imaging, EKGs

The EKG shown in Figure 10.1 reveals a second-degree atrioventricular (AV) block and bradycardia with a heartrate of 47 beats per minute

Figure 10.1

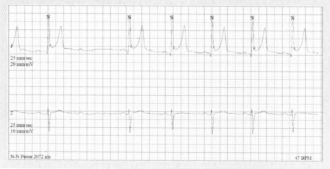

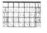

Case outcome: third interim follow-up (week 18)

- After consultation with a pediatric cardiologist, clonidine is discontinued and the patient's tiredness improves; however, there is relatively rapid recrudescence of both his motor and vocal tics
- Alternative medications are discussed with the family and the patient, including aripiprazole
- Aripiprazole is initiated at 2 mg every night at bedtime

Attending physician's mental notes: third interim follow-up

- The attending physician agrees with the pediatric cardiologist and is aware of the U.S. Food and Drug Administration (FDA) approval for aripiprazole for Tourette syndrome in pediatric patients
- However, the physician also considers the patient's atomoxetine and considers potential CYP2D6-related interactions

- However, based on the current dose and the low dose of aripiprazole that he has chosen, he elects not to obtain pharmacogenetic testing

Case outcome: fourth interim follow-up (week 20)

- Two weeks after beginning aripiprazole, the patient's motor and vocal tics improve significantly and the clinician obtains another Tourette Impairment – Child self-report measure (Table 10.4)

Table 10.4

In the past month, how much trouble have YOU had doing the following … :	Problems due to tics				Problems due to ADHD, OCD, Anxiety, Rages, Other			
	Not at all	Just a little	Pretty much	Very much	Not at all	Just a little	Pretty much	Very much
Being prepared for class (having books, homework)	✓				✓			
Writing in class		✓			✓			
Taking tests or exams		✓			✓			
Doing homework	✓				✓			
Concentrating on work	✓				✓			
Doing household chores	✓				✓			
Getting ready for bed	✓				✓			
Getting along with parents	✓				✓			
Visiting relatives	✓				✓			
Being teased by other kids					✓			
Going to a friend's house	✓				✓			
Having a friend over	✓				✓			
Being with friends on phone/social media		✓			✓			
Doing sports/music/extra-curriculars	✓				✓			

Take-home points

- Whether transient or persistent, tics are common, particularly in young children. When tics include both movements and vocalizations and have been present for at least 1 year, *DSM-5* criteria for Tourette syndrome have been met
- Tourette syndrome is often comorbid with OCD and ADHD. When a patient presents with two of these syndromes, he or

she should carefully explore symptoms associated with the third

- Tic disorders can be highly disabling
- The first-line psychotherapeutic treatment for tics and Tourette syndrome is CBIT; however, HRT can also be helpful
- Pharmacotherapy is generally reserved for patients with tic disorders or Tourette syndrome who experience moderate to severe symptoms
- First-line pharmacotherapy includes α_2 agonists, although there is evidence for mixed dopamine–serotonin recent antagonists. Among the mixed dopamine–serotonin receptor antagonists, aripiprazole (5–20 mg daily) is approved by the FDA for the treatment of Tourette syndrome. In general, for pediatric patients with Tourette syndrome weighing <50 kg, dosing should be initiated at 2 mg daily with a target dose of 5 mg daily after 2 days. The dose can be increased to 10 mg daily in patients who do not achieve optimal control of tics. Dosage adjustments should occur gradually at intervals of no less than 1 week. For children or adolescents weighing 50 kg or more, dosing should be initiated at 2 mg daily for 2 days, and then increased to 5 mg daily for 5 days, with a target dose of 10 mg daily on day 8. The dose can be increased up to 20 mg daily for patients who do not achieve optimal control of tics. Dosage adjustments should occur gradually in increments of 5 mg daily at intervals of no less than 1 week
- While not first- or second-line agents for the treatment of Tourette syndrome, haloperidol is FDA-approved for treating "tics and vocal utterances of Tourette Disorder," and pimozide is FDA-approved for "suppression of motor and phonic tics in patients with Tourette Disorder who have failed to respond satisfactorily to standard treatment."
- In terms of outcome and course, tics begin in childhood, on average between ages 4 and 6 years, and typically follow a rostral–caudal progression
- Motor tics generally precede vocal tics, and wax and wane
- Tics generally peak between 8 and 12 years of age and tend to decrease in late adolescence (Leckman et al. 1998). When tics persist into adulthood, they are generally mild (Bloch and Leckman 2009)
- Predictors of worse outcome in adulthood include severe tics, having been teased in childhood, having a family history of tics, and having co-occurring ADHD and OCD (Groth et al. 2019)
- Presence of premonitory urges during childhood may predict worse cognition and psychiatric outcomes as the patient ages (Cavanna et al. 2012)
- Comorbid ADHD (Groth 2018), OCD (Leckman et al. 2014), and depressive symptoms (Goto et al. 2019), as well as anxiety (Nissen et al. 2019; Rizzo et al. 2017), are associated with worse outcomes

Tips and pearls

- Tourette syndrome is a highly heritable condition. A population cohort multigenerational study calculated a heritability of 0.77 (Mataix-Cols et al. 2015), with offspring of a parent with Tourette syndrome or chronic tics having a nearly 20% chance of developing either condition. The sibling recurrence rate is 10% (Browne et al. 2015). Earlier genetic models proposed autosomal dominant inheritance, more recent studies support a highly complicated polygenetic architecture
- In assessing tics, parents are the best source of history for younger children, whereas older children can provide more information themselves (Frankel et al. 2012). Important questions include:
  - Does the child make repetitive movements such as eye blinking or shoulder shrugging?
  - What about repetitive sounds such as coughing or sniffing?
  - Are these tics difficult to control or suppress?
  - When did the tics start?
  - How often do the tics occur?
  - How intense or noticeable are the tics?
  - Are there any urges, sensations, or thoughts that precede the movements or sounds?
  - What increases or decreases the frequency of the tics?
  - What is the timing? Are the tics constant? Waxing and waning?
  - Have you tried any intervention to address the tics?
  - Is there a family history of tics?

Mechanism of action moment

- Aripiprazole is a D_2/5-HT_{1A} partial agonist and has only moderate affinity for 5-HT_{2A} receptors (Figure 10.2) but higher affinity for 5-HT_{1A} receptors
- Aripiprazole lacks the pharmacological properties normally associated with sedation, namely, muscarinic cholinergic and H_1 histamine antagonist properties (Figure 10.2), and thus is not generally sedating
- A major differentiating feature of aripiprazole is that it has, like ziprasidone and lurasidone, less of a risk of weight gain, although weight gain can be a problem for some, including children and adolescents. Additionally, there is some concern that weight gain may be related to dose and may be increased in patients who are slower CYP2D6 metabolizers

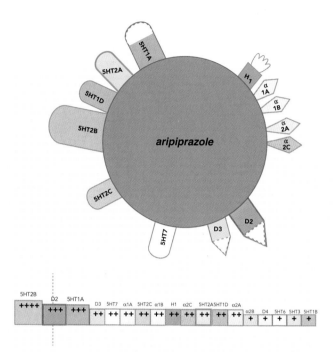

Figure 10.2 Aripiprazole's pharmacological and binding profile. This figure portrays a qualitative consensus of current thinking about the binding properties of aripiprazole. Aripiprazole is a partial agonist at D_2 receptors rather than an antagonist. Additional important pharmacological properties that may contribute to its clinical profile include 5-HT$_{2A}$ antagonist actions, 5-HT$_{1A}$ partial agonist actions, 5-HT$_7$ antagonist actions, and 5-HT$_{2C}$ antagonist actions. Aripiprazole lacks or has weak binding potency at receptors usually associated with significant sedation.

Another mechanism of action moment

- Atomoxetine increases both norepinephrine (NE) and dopamine (DA) in the prefrontal cortex. Importantly, in the prefrontal cortex, clearance of both NE and DA is largely due to the norepinephrine transporter (NET). However, agents such as norepinephrine do not increase NE or DA in the nucleus accumbens because there are few NETs present there (Figure 10.3)
- Atomoxetine's effects are very specific for the norepinephrine transporter and it does not appear to be pharmacologically active at dopaminergic receptors
- It is well absorbed, no interindividual differences in absorption

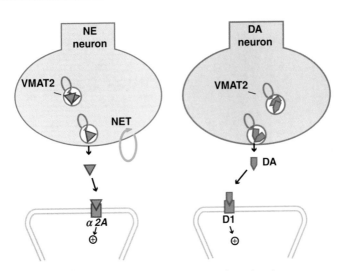

Figure 10.3 Atomoxetine effects within the prefrontal cortex.
Inhibitors of the NET, such as atomoxetine, can have therapeutic
effects in ADHD without abuse liability. This is because they can
increase both NE and dopamine DA in the prefrontal cortex, where
clearance of both is largely due to NET, yet do not increase NE or DA
in the nucleus accumbens because there are few NETs present there.

- Atomoxetine's penetration of the CNS is passive
- Atomoxetine is highly metabolized by CYP2D6. In normal CYP2D6
  metabolizers, atomoxetine is excreted within 24 h ($t_{1/2}$ = 5 h);
  however, in poor metabolizers, excretion time is 72 h ($t_{1/2}$ = 20 h).
  Additionally, medication exposure (area under the curve [AUC]) is
  significantly higher in patients who are poor CYP2D6 metabolizers
  and requires dose adjustment (Figure 10.4)

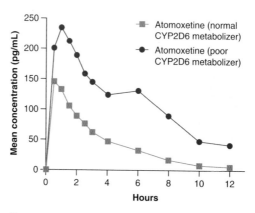

Figure 10.4 Atomoxetine concentrations in normal and poor CYP2D6 metabolizers. Peak concentrations of atomoxetine and total exposure to the medication are significantly higher in CYP2D6 poor metabolizers. Adapted from Trzepacz, P. T., Williams, D. W., Feldman, P. D., et al. CYP2D6 metabolizer status and atomoxetine dosing in children and adolescents with ADHD. *European Neuropsychopharmacology* 2008; 18(2): 79–86.

Post test question

Which of the following represents an evidence-based intervention for a child with Tourette syndrome?

A. Aripiprazole (Abilify)
B. Methylphenidate OROS (Concerta)
C. Mixed amphetamine salt (Adderall)
D. Diazepam (Valium)
E. All of the above

Answer: A (Aripiprazole, Abilify)

Aripiprazole (A) has multiple pediatric indications: schizophrenia/ maintenance (age 13 and older), bipolar mania/maintenance (ages 10 and older), autism-related irritability (ages 5 to 17), and Tourette syndrome (ages 6 to 18). Methylphenidate OROS (B) is approved for the treatment of ADHD in pediatric patients. Also, relevant to this case, methylphenidate medications may be better tolerated relative to mixed amphetamine salts (C) in terms of their likelihood of worsening tics. Diazepam has been used to treat spasticity and other neuromotor symptoms in pediatric patients, but has not been systematically evaluated in pediatric patients with Tourette syndrome.

Resources for parents

- The Tourette Association of America, www.tourette.org
- *Managing Tourette Syndrome: A Behavioral Intervention Workbook, Parent Workbook*, Douglas W. Woods, John Piacentini, Susanna Chang, Thilo Deckersbach, Golda Ginsburg, Alan Peterson, Lawrence D. Scahill, John T. Walkup and Sabine Wilhelm, Oxford University Press.
- *Nix Your Tics! Eliminate Unwanted Tic Symptoms: A How-To Guide for Young People*, B. Duncan McKinley PhD

References

1. Bloch, M. H., Leckman, J. F. Clinical course of Tourette syndrome. *J Psychosom Res* 2009; 67(6): 497–501. https://doi.org/10.1016/j.jpsychores.2009.09.002
2. Brander, G., Rydell, M., Kuja-Halkola, R., et al. Perinatal risk factors in Tourette's and chronic tic disorders: a total population sibling comparison study. *Mol Psychiatry* 2018; 23(5): 1189–97. https://doi.org/10.1038/mp.2017.31
3. Browne, H. A., Hansen, S. N., Buxbaum, J. D., et al. Familial clustering of tic disorders and obsessive-compulsive disorder. *JAMA Psychiatry* 2015; 72(4): 359–66. https://doi.org/10.1001/jamapsychiatry.2014.2656
4. Browne, H. A., Modabbernia, A., Buxbaum, J. D., et al. Prenatal maternal smoking and increased risk for Tourette syndrome and chronic tic disorders. *J Am Acad Child Adolesc Psychiatry* 2016; 55(9): 784–91. https://doi.org/10.1016/j.jaac.2016.06.010
5. Cavanna, A. E., David, K., Orth, M., Robertson, M. M. Predictors during childhood of future health-related quality of life in adults with Gilles de la Tourette syndrome. *Eur J Paediatr Neurol* 2012; 16(6): 605–12. https://doi.org/10.1016/j.ejpn.2012.02.004
6. Dalsgaard, S., Waltoft, B. L., Leckman, J. F., Mortensen, P. B. Maternal history of autoimmune disease and later development of Tourette syndrome in offspring. *J Am Acad Child Adolesc Psychiatry* 2015; 54(6): 495–501.e1. https://doi.org/10.1016/j.jaac.2015.03.008
7. Frankel, J., Abdullayeva, N., Mavrides, N., Coffey, B. Tic disorders. In Dulcan, M. (ed.), *Dulcan's Textbook of Child and Adolescent Psychiatry*, 3rd edn. Washington DC: American Psychiatric Publishing, 2021.
8. Gancher, S., Conant-Norville, D., Angell, R. Treatment of Tourette syndrome with transdermal clonidine: a pilot study.

J Neuropsychiatry Clin Neurosci 1990; 2(1): 66–69. https://doi
.org/10.1176/jnp.2.1.66

9. Ghosh, D., Rajan, P. V., Das, D., et al. Sleep disorders in children
with Tourette syndrome. *Pediatr Neurol* 2014; 51(1): 31–35.
https://doi.org/10.1016/j.pediatrneurol.2014.03.017

10. Goto, R., Fujio, M., Matsuda, N., et al. The effects of comorbid
Tourette symptoms on distress caused by compulsive-like
behavior in very young children: a cross-sectional study. *Child
Adolesc Psychiatry Ment Health* 2019; 13: 28. https://doi
.org/10.1186/s13034-019-0290-3

11. Groth, C., Skov, L., Lange, T., Debes, N. M. Predictors of the
clinical course of Tourette syndrome: a longitudinal study.
J Child Neurol 2019; 34(14): 913–21. https://doi
.org/10.1177/0883073819867245

12. Leckman, J. F., Hardin, M. T., Riddle, M. A., et al. Clonidine
treatment of Gilles de la Tourette syndrome. *Arch
GenPsychiatry* 1991; 48(4): 324–28. https://doi.org/10.1001/
archpsyc.1991.01810280040006

13. Leckman, J. F., King, R. A., Bloch, M. H. Clinical features of
Tourette syndrome and tic disorders. *J Obsessive Compuls
Relat Disord* 2014; 3(4): 372–79. https://doi.org/10.1016/
j.jocrd.2014.03.004

14. Leckman, J. F., Zhang, H., Vitale, A., et al. Course of tic severity in
Tourette syndrome: the first two decades. *Pediatrics* 1998; 102(1
Pt 1): 14–19. https://doi.org/10.1542/peds.102.1.14

15. Mataix-Cols, D., Isomura, K., Pérez-Vigil, A., et al. Familial risks of
Tourette syndrome and chronic tic disorders: a population-based
cohort study. *JAMA Psychiatry* 2015; 72(8): 787–93. https://doi
.org/10.1001/jamapsychiatry.2015.0627

16. Mathews, C. A., Scharf, J. M., Miller, L. L., et al. Association
between pre- and perinatal exposures and Tourette syndrome or
chronic tic disorder in the ALSPAC cohort. *Br J Psychiatry* 2014;
204(1): 40–45. https://doi.org/10.1192/bjp.bp.112.125468

17. Murphy, T. K., Fernandez, T. V., Coffey, B. J. Extended-release
guanfacine does not show a large effect on tic severity in children
with chronic tic disorders. *J Child Adolesc Psychopharmacol* 2017;
27(9): 762–70. https://doi.org/10.1089/cap.2017.0024

18. Nissen, J. B., Partner, E. T., Thomsen, P. H. Predictors of
therapeutic treatment outcome in adolescent chronic tic disorders.
BJPsych Open 2019; 5(5): e74. https://doi.org/10.1192/
bjo.2019.56

19. Rizzo, R., Gulisano, M., Martino, D., Robertson, M. M. Gilles
de la Tourette syndrome, depression, depressive illness, and

correlates in a child and adolescent population. *J Child Adolesc Psychopharmacol* 2017; 27(3): 243–49. https://doi.org/10.1089/cap.2016.0120

20. Scahill, L., Chappell, P. B., Kim, Y. S., et al. A placebo-controlled study of guanfacine in the treatment of children with tic disorders and attention deficit hyperactivity disorder. *Am J Psychiatry* 2001; 158(7): 1067–74. https://doi.org/10.1176/appi.ajp.158.7.1067

21. Shapiro, A. K., Shapiro, E., Eisenkraft, G. J. Treatment of Gilles de la Tourette syndrome with clonidine and neuroleptics. *Arch Gen Psychiatry* 1983; 40(11): 1235–40. https://doi.org/10.1001/archpsyc.1983.01790100081011

22. Swedo, S. E., Seidlitz, J., Kovacevic, M., et al. Clinical presentation of pediatric autoimmune neuropsychiatric disorders associated with streptococcal infections in research and community settings. *J Child Adolesc Psychopharmacol* 2015; 25(1): 26–30. https://doi.org/10.1089/cap.2014.0073

Case 11: How slow can you go? Selective serotonin reuptake inhibitor (SSRI) withdrawal and discontinuation in an adolescent

The Questions: When should SSRIs be discontinued in adolescents? How should SSRIs be discontinued in adolescents? What are the strategies for managing SSRI-related discontinuation symptoms?

The Psychopharmacological Dilemma: Stopping SSRIs after remission is certainly a goal of treating adolescents with depressive and anxiety disorders, although clinicians vary in their thresholds for discontinuing these medications, and disagree about approaches to discontinuation of SSRIs

Pretest self-assessment question

When discontinuing an SSRI in an adolescent with major depressive disorder following 12 months of treatment, the highest risk of relapse occurs:

A. In the first month after discontinuation
B. In the first 3 months after discontinuation
C. In the first 6 months after discontinuation
D. In the first 12 months after discontinuation

Answer: B (In the first 3 months after discontinuation)

Patient evaluation on intake

- 15-year-old adolescent with a history of major depressive disorder (MDD) who has been in remission for 15 months presents with his parents
- The patient and his parents are interested in a consultation regarding the discontinuation of his antidepressant medication
- The patient denies current depressive symptoms. He enjoys spending time with friends, plays lacrosse, and enjoys spending time with his girlfriend and her friends
- He denies anxiety and denies psychotic symptoms as well as substance use
- He denies any side effects associated with his sertraline, although he notes that he has had nausea, headaches, and mild increases in anxiety symptoms when he misses his medication

Psychiatric history

- His mother recalls that from an early age, the patient was preoccupied with anxiety around separation, especially from his mother and grandmother. Often the patient protested his mother's full-time work

- Major depressive episode with anxious distress with onset at age 13
- No psychotic symptoms have been present, and there is no history of suicide attempts or self-injurious behavior

Social and personal history

- The patient is the middle of three children who live with their biological parents
- His mother is an infectious disease physician, and his father is an engineer
- He is a sophomore and takes two advanced placement (AP) courses. There is no Individualized Education Plan (IEP) or 504 Plan
- He is in a relationship and has not been sexually active
- There is no history of trauma

Medical history

- He was delivered at 39 weeks to a 35-year-old mother and 41-year-old father
- Normal developmental milestones

Family history

- Father with generalized anxiety disorder (GAD) and MDD
- There is no family history of completed suicide

Medication history

- Sertraline (Zoloft) 150 mg daily
- Multivitamin daily

Current medications

- Sertraline (Zoloft) 150 mg daily
- Multivitamin daily

Psychotherapy history

- The patient was seen in cognitive behavior therapy (CBT) for 16 weeks early in the course of his depressive episode and began medication and psychotherapy concurrently

Further investigation

Is there anything else that you would like to know about the patient? What about details related to his symptoms that emerge when he misses a dose or how often he misses doses?

- He misses doses approximately once per week but will only miss two consecutive doses once per month

Testing: laboratory results, imaging, EKGs

- CYP2D6 genotype: *4/*4 | CYP2D6 phenotype: poor metabolizer
- CYP2C19 genotype: *17/*17 | CYP2C19 phenotype: ultrarapid metabolizer
- CYP2C9 genotype: *1/*1 | CYP2C9 phenotype: normal metabolizer
- CYP3A4 genotype: *3/*3 | CYP3A4 phenotype: normal
- SLC6A4 genotype: long/long
- MTHFR (C677T) genotype: C/C | MTHFR (C677T) phenotype: normal
- COMT: Homozygous for the Met allele of the Val158Met polymorphism in the catechol-o-methyltransferase gene

Attending physician's mental notes: initial psychiatric evaluation

- This patient has significant withdrawal symptoms following several missed doses of his medication and records from his pediatrician reveal that he is a poor CYP2D6 metabolizer and an ultrarapid metabolizer for CYP2C19
- Given his CYP2C19 phenotype, the child and adolescent psychiatrist is concerned that his withdrawal symptoms – even after just two missed doses – may have related to his significantly increased metabolism (Figure 11.1)
- Additionally, the patient's clinician is aware that CYP2C19 genotype significantly affects sertraline concentrations in pediatric patients (Figure 11.2)

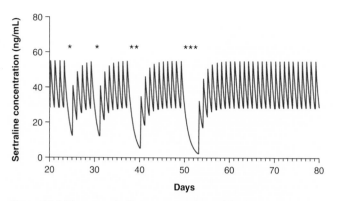

Figure 11.1 Plasma sertraline concentrations with missed doses. The effect of missed doses (*) can be seen in an adolescent treated with 150 mg daily of sertraline who is an ultrarapid CYP2C19 metabolizer. Reproduced from Strawn et al. Adverse effects of antidepressant medications and their management in children and adolescents. *Pharmacotherapy* 2023;43(7):675–690.

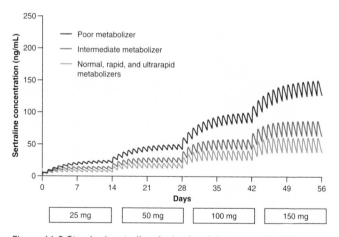

Figure 11.2 Standard sertraline dosing in adolescents with differing CYP2C19 activities. For sertraline-treated adolescents, the C_{max} is higher in poor metabolizers and intermediate metabolizers compared to normal, rapid and ultra-rapid metabolizers. Reproduced from Strawn et al. CYP2C19-guided escitalopram and sertraline dosing in pediatric patients: a pharmacokinetic modeling study. *Journal of Child and Adolescent Psychopharmacology* 2019.

Question

Which of the following would be most appropriate regarding the decision to discontinue the patient's sertraline?

- No attempts should be made to discontinue sertraline
- Sertraline should be cross-titrated to fluoxetine and then fluoxetine should be discontinued once he is on a stable dose of 20 mg daily
- Sertraline should be decreased to 75 mg for 3 days and then discontinued
- Sertraline should be decreased to 75 mg daily and then decreased to 50 mg daily and then decreased to 25 mg daily and then discontinued with approximately 1 month at each dose

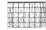

Case outcome: follow-up visits

- Sertraline was decreased to 75 mg daily and then decreased to 50 mg daily and then decreased to 25 mg daily and then discontinued with approximately 1 month at each dose. This produced plasma sertraline concentrations shown in Figure 11.3
- The patient maintained excellent adherence during this period and used an app to track adherence. Additionally, he did not experience significant withdrawal symptoms

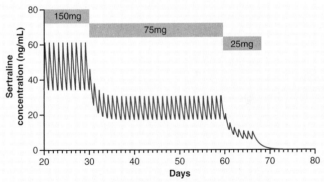

Figure 11.3 Sertraline concentrations in an adolescent during discontinuation. Reproduced from Strawn et al. Adverse effects of antidepressant medications and their management in children and adolescents. *Pharmacotherapy* 2023.

- After sertraline was discontinued, he checked in with his clinician monthly for 3 months and during this time, his Quick Inventory of Depressive Symptomatology (QIDS) scores (see Case 4) remained at 2, 1, and 2, respectively, and he denied any recrudescence of depressive or anxiety symptoms

PATIENT FILE

Attending physician's mental notes: follow-up visits

- The timing of antidepressant discontinuation in children and adolescents has received much attention in the literature, although these discussions are largely based on studies in adults and expert opinion
- The decision to discontinue an antidepressant should consider the adolescent's current environment and stressors (Hathaway et al. 2017)
- Antidepressants may be discontinued during lower-stress periods, recognizing the importance of incorporating factors such as school or separation-related events (e.g. leaving for summer camp) into the decision to stop an antidepressant
- Additionally, clinicians should consider the type, frequency, and duration of psychotherapy. Long-term data in children and adolescents with MDD and anxiety disorders suggest more rapid improvement associated with combined therapy (i.e. SSRI + psychotherapy) relative to antidepressant treatment or psychotherapy alone (Strawn et al. 2022). A patient who has successfully engaged in psychotherapy during the course of pharmacologic treatment or a patient with a more rapid response to acute treatment (more likely with combined treatment) might require a briefer psychopharmacologic intervention. However, no prospective, randomized controlled trials have evaluated this possibility

Take-home points

- Withdrawal symptoms have been described with SSRIs and serotonin–norepinephrine reuptake inhibitors (SNRIs) in children, adolescents, and adults over the past several decades and generally emerge when antidepressants are discontinued abruptly, although they can occur with missed doses and, in some patients, following significant dose reductions
- SSRI-related withdrawal symptoms generally include gastrointestinal and flu-like symptoms, dysesthesias, dyssomnia, increasing anxiety, agitation, or irritability and must be distinguished from recrudescence of symptoms associated with the disorder being treated
- The general approach to managing antidepressant withdrawal is ensuring: (1) adherence and (2) slow discontinuation when stopping an antidepressant is necessary (Fava et al. 2015; Harvey et al. 2003)
- Regarding adherence, pharmacokinetic modeling studies suggest significant decreases in serum concentrations of several

antidepressants used in children and adolescents (e.g. sertraline and escitalopram), even following one or two missed doses (Strawn et al. 2021). These effects may be accentuated in children and adolescents with increased CYP2C19 metabolism (Figure 11.1)

- Slow discontinuation has been consistently recommended; however, few studies have evaluated slow vs. rapid discontinuation of antidepressants although some studies suggest that titration to lower doses may mitigate withdrawal symptoms in adults (Shapiro 2018)
- Several studies have examined the risk of relapse in children and adolescents with depressive disorders (Emslie et al. 2008; Kennard et al. 2014). In the first, fluoxetine-treated children and adolescents were randomized to either continue fluoxetine (n = 20) or switched to placebo (n = 20) (Emslie et al. 2004). In a follow-up study of children and adolescents 7–18 years of age with major depressive disorder, adolescents who responded to acute fluoxetine treatment were randomized to continue fluoxetine or placebo for an additional 6 months (Emslie et al. 2008). In a separate study, children and adolescents aged 8–17 years who acutely responded to fluoxetine were randomized to continued fluoxetine or fluoxetine + CBT for 6 months (Kennard et al. 2014) with long-term follow-up assessments at weeks 52 and 78. These trials provide a glimpse into predictors of relapse and reveal that the risk of relapse is highest in the first 3 months after discontinuing treatment and that children and adolescents at highest risk for relapse are those with comorbid dysthymia, those with more depressive symptoms, and those who continue to experience ongoing insomnia. Additionally, those who had the greatest response to acute treatment were less likely to relapse. Finally, having received CBT decreased the likelihood of relapse

Two-minute tutorial

- Antidepressant withdrawal has been evaluated from both pharmacokinetic and pharmacodynamic perspectives. In general, pharmacodynamic aspects of antidepressant withdrawal have focused on the 5-HT transporter (Horowitz and Taylor, 2019)
- Regarding pharmacokinetics, withdrawal symptoms are more common with antidepressants with shorter half-lives (e.g. paroxetine) than antidepressants with longer half-lives (e.g. fluoxetine) (Rosenbaum et al. 1998)

Tips and pearls

- Recently, hyperbolic discontinuation has been proposed as an alternative to more rapid discontinuations in adults (Horowitz and Taylor 2019) and in pediatric patients (Strawn et al. 2023). This approach leverages the hyperbolic relationship between SSRI concentration and receptor occupancy
- Hyperbolic dose reductions, which occur as a fixed percentage, produce exponential decreases in total dose, as opposed to a linear reduction
- Hyperbolic discontinuation is based mainly on positron emission tomography (PET) imaging data of serotonin transporter occupancy by SSRIs in adults and supports the notion that hyperbolically reducing SSRI doses decreases serotonin transporter inhibition linearly. This approach also recommends tapering more slowly, which is frequently done in the discontinuation components of most clinical trials and drops to doses lower than typical "therapeutic minimums" (Horowitz and Taylor 2019)
- While debate remains regarding the optimal duration of antidepressant treatment for children and adolescents with MDD or anxiety disorders, the overarching goal of treatment is obvious: remission. Any discussion regarding treatment discontinuation is predicated on the patient having achieved remission of depressive or anxiety symptoms; remission status indicates clinical relief is linked to functional recovery (Hathaway et al. 2017)
- Current data suggest that 9–12 months of SSRI treatment is recommended for pediatric patients with MDD (Hathaway et al. 2017). For children and adolescents with generalized separation and social anxiety disorders, 6–9 months of SSRI treatment may be sufficient (Ginsburg et al. 2018; Hathaway et al. 2017)
- Many clinicians extend treatment to 12 months, based on extrapolation of data from adults with anxiety disorders (Rickels et al. 2010). Such extended treatment periods may decrease the risk of long-term morbidity and recurrence; however, the goal of treatment is ultimately remission (Strawn et al. 2020) rather than the duration of antidepressant pharmacotherapy
- A prospective trial of fluoxetine-treated adolescents examined double-blind discontinuation of medication and found that fluoxetine prevented relapse. However, when fluoxetine was discontinued, the highest risk of relapse was in the first 3 months after discontinuation. Additionally, in a study comparing relapse in pediatric patients with MDD who were receiving standard medication management or medication management + CBT, those who received combination treatment had a lower likelihood of relapsing (Figure 11.4)

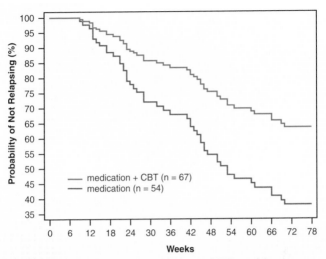

Figure 11.4 Relapse in pediatric patients with MDD receiving either medication management or medication management + CBT. Reproduced from Emslie et al. Continued effectiveness of relapse prevention cognitive-behavioral therapy following fluoxetine treatment in youth with major depressive disorder. *Journal of the American Academy of Child & Adolescent Psychiatry* 2015.

Mechanism of action moment

- Sertraline has two candidate mechanisms that distinguish it from other SSRIs: dopamine transporter (DAT) inhibition and σ_1 receptor binding (Figure 11.5)
- The DAT inhibitory actions are controversial since they are weaker than the serotonin transporter (SERT) inhibitory actions, thus leading some experts to suggest that there is not sufficient DAT occupancy by sertraline to be clinically relevant
- As described above, sertraline concentrations in pediatric patients are related to CYP2C19 variation. However, overall, in pediatric populations, there is a direct relationship between sertraline concentrations and dose (Figure 11.6)

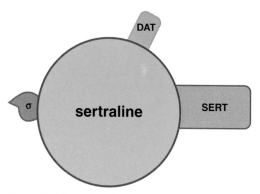

Figure 11.5 Sertraline. Sertraline has dopamine transporter (DAT) inhibition and σ_1 receptor binding, in addition to serotonin reuptake inhibition (SRI). The clinical relevance of sertraline's dopamine transporter inhibition is unknown, although it may improve anergia, amotivation, and concentration. Its sigma properties may contribute to anxiolytic actions, and it has been studied extensively in pediatric anxiety disorders and obsessive compulsive disorder (OCD).

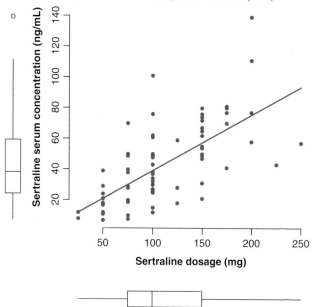

Figure 11.6 Sertraline concentrations in children and adolescents. Sertraline concentrations are generally related to dose, although some variation is related to CYP2C19 variation. Reproduced from Tini et al. Therapeutic drug monitoring of sertraline in children and adolescents: a naturalistic study with insights into the clinical response and treatment of obsessive-compulsive disorder. *Comprehensive Psychiatry* 2022.

Post test question

When discontinuing an SSRI in an adolescent with major depressive disorder following 12 months of treatment, the highest risk of relapse occurs:

A. In the first month after discontinuation
B. In the first 3 months after discontinuation
C. In the first 6 months after discontinuation
D. In the first 12 months after discontinuation

Answer: B (In the first 3 months after discontinuation)

Several studies have examined the risk of relapse in children and adolescents with depressive disorders (Emslie et al. 2008; Kennard et al. 2014) and revealed that the highest likelihood of relapse occurs during the first 3 months (B) following discontinuation. It is of interest that in this study, children and adolescents were treated with fluoxetine, which has the longest half-life of SSRIs currently used in adolescents, yet many patients relapsed within the first 2–4 weeks following discontinuation of fluoxetine.

References

1. Emslie, G. J., Heiligenstein, J. H., Hoog, S. L., et al. Fluoxetine treatment for prevention of relapse of depression in children and adolescents: a double-blind, placebo-controlled study. *J Am Acad Child Adolesc Psychiatry* 2004; 43(11): 1397–405. https://doi.org/10.1097/01.chi.0000140453.89323.57

2. Emslie, G. J., Kennard, B. D., Mayes, T. L., et al. Fluoxetine versus placebo in preventing relapse of major depression in children and adolescents. *Am J Psychiatry* 2008; 165(4): 459–67. https://doi.org/10.1176/appi.ajp.2007.07091453

3. Fava, G. A., Gatti, A., Belaise, C., Guidi, J., Offidani, E. Withdrawal symptoms after selective serotonin reuptake inhibitor discontinuation: a systematic review. *Psychother Psychosom* 2015; 84(2): 72–81. https://doi.org/10.1159/000370338

4. Ginsburg, G. S., Becker-Haimes, E. M., Keeton, C., et al. Results from the Child/Adolescent Anxiety Multimodal Extended Long-Term Study (CAMELS): primary anxiety outcomes. *J Am Acad Child Adolesc Psychiatry* 2018; 57(7): 471–80. https://doi.org/10.1016/j.jaac.2018.03.017

5. Harvey, B. H., McEwen, B. S., Stein, D. J. Neurobiology of antidepressant withdrawal: implications for the longitudinal outcome of depression. *Biol Psychiatry* 2003; 54(10): 1105–17. https://doi.org/10.1016/s0006-3223(03)00528-6

6. Hathaway, E. E., Walkup, J. T., Strawn, J. R. Antidepressant treatment duration in pediatric depressive and anxiety disorders: how long is long enough? *Curr Probl Pediatr Adolesc Health Care* 2017; 48(2): 31–39. https://doi.org/10.1016/j.cppeds.2017.12.002

7. Horowitz, M. A., Taylor, D. Tapering of SSRI treatment to mitigate withdrawal symptoms. *Lancet Psychiatry* 2019; 6(6): 538–46. https://doi.org/10.1016/S2215-0366(19)30032-X

8. Kennard, B. D., Emslie, G. J., Mayes, T. L., et al. Sequential treatment with fluoxetine and relapse-prevention CBT to improve outcomes in pediatric depression. *Am J Psychiatry* 2014; 171(10): 1083–90. https://doi.org/10.1176/appi.ajp.2014.13111460

9. Rickels, K., Etemad, B., Khalid-Khan, S., et al. Time to relapse after 6 and 12 months' treatment of generalized anxiety disorder with venlafaxine extended release. *Arch Gen Psychiatry* 2010; 67(12): 1274–81. https://doi.org/10.1001/archgenpsychiatry.2010.170

10. Rosenbaum, J. F., Fava, M., Hoog, S. L., Ascroft, R. C., Krebs, W. B. Selective serotonin reuptake inhibitor discontinuation syndrome: a randomized clinical trial. *Biol Psychiatry* 1998; 44(2): 77–87. https://doi.org/10.1016/s0006-3223(98)00126-7

11. Shapiro, B. B. Subtherapeutic doses of SSRI antidepressants demonstrate considerable serotonin transporter occupancy: implications for tapering SSRIs. *Psychopharmacology (Berl)* 2018; 235(9): 2779–81. https://doi.org/10.1007/s00213-018-4995-4

12. Strawn, J. R., Lu, L., Peris, T. S., Levine, A., Walkup, J. T. Research review: pediatric anxiety disorders – what have we learnt in the last 10 years? *J Child Psychol Psychiatry Allied Discipl* 2021; 62(2): 114–39. https://doi.org/10.1111/jcpp.13262

13. Strawn, J. R., Mills, J. A., Poweleit, E. A., Ramsey, L. B., Croarkin, P. E. Adverse effects of antidepressant medications and their management in children and adolescents. *Pharmacotherapy* 2023. https://doi.org/10.1002/phar.2767. Epub ahead of print. PMID: 36651686.

14. Strawn, J. R., Mills, J. A., Suresh, V., et al. Combining selective serotonin reuptake inhibitors and cognitive behavioral therapy in youth with depression and anxiety. *J Affect Dis* 2022; 298(Pt A): 292–300. https://doi.org/10.1016/j.jad.2021.10.047

15. Strawn, J. R., Poweleit, E. A., Uppugunduri, C. R. S., Ramsey, L. B. Pediatric therapeutic drug monitoring for selective serotonin reuptake inhibitors. *Front Pharmacol* 2021; 12: 749692. https://doi.org/10.3389/fphar.2021.749692

Case 12: The adolescent who doesn't eat: anorexia nervosa in an adolescent

The Questions: What is the "medical" workup in a child or adolescent with an eating disorder? When should a child or adolescent with anorexia nervosa be hospitalized? What is the psychopharmacological approach to treating eating disorders and related behaviors in children and adolescents?

The Psychopharmacological Dilemma: Eating disorders can create anxiety for many clinicians as a result of confusion related to the medical workup for these patients, treatment decisions, and special considerations related to using pharmacotherapy in this population

Pretest self-assessment question

Which of the following may reduce binging and purging in adolescents with eating disorders, including anorexia nervosa?

A. Paroxetine (Paxil)

B. Selegeline (Emsam)

C. Olanzapine (Zyprexa)

D. Naltrexone (Revia)

Answer: D (Naltrexone, Revia)

Patient evaluation on intake

- A 15-year-old adolescent with a history of separation and social anxiety disorders and major depressive disorder, and recent weight loss
- The patient endorses numbness and disinterest in soccer as well as significant fatigue
- She had been having worsening depressive symptoms and dyssomnia, including initial and middle insomnia
- Over the past month, she has had more restrictive eating behavior and has been restricting to 500–700 kcal/day
- She reports fatigue, more difficulty with concentration, less endurance, and, over the past week, had to stop multiple activities secondary to her fatigue and orthostatic symptoms and also canceled her volunteer activities
- She feels tired, has dry skin, and has dizziness but denies significant hair loss. She reports three syncopal episodes over the past 2 weeks
- Denies chest pain or palpitations but notes gastroesophageal reflux symptoms as well as nausea and constipation
- Her last bowel movement was 9 days ago, and her last menstrual period was 12 weeks prior

- She has lost weight primarily by restriction, counts calories, and shared that there has been a steeper decline in intake over the last week after having eaten half of a doughnut 1 week prior while at a market with her family
- She also reports self-induced vomiting with a maximum frequency of twice daily. Her vomit appears as partially digested food
- She has lost 13 lb (5.9 kg) over the last month
- Her exercise regimen includes running for 1 hour daily, approximately 4 miles per day, but she hasn't been able to run for the last 2 weeks

Psychiatric history

- Previously diagnosed with anorexia nervosa binge purge type (AN-P)
- One prior psychiatric admission (7 days) for suicidal ideation 2 years ago. During this admission, her eating disorder symptoms which had previously been overshadowed by her depressive and anxiety disorders, were identified
- She completed an intensive outpatient program focused on anorexia nervosa with family-based treatment 18 months ago
- Major depressive disorder (two episodes) with onset at age 13
- No psychotic symptoms have been present and there is a remote history of superficial cutting

Social and personal history

- She lives with her parents and her brother who is taking a semester off from college
- Her mother is an executive and works 70–80 hours weekly and her father is an attorney. She describes a limited relationship with both parents, although had a closer relationship with her maternal grandmother until the family moved to her current city 4 years ago
- She is not in a relationship and is not interested in relationships, commenting, "that would just be too much work"
- She is not currently involved in extracurricular activities
- Academically, she is in the ninth grade and does well academically and shares that she has a weighted grade point average (GPA) of 4.25. She does not have an Individualized Education Plan (IEP) or 504 Plan

Medical history

- She was delivered at 39 weeks to a 30-year-old mother and 32-year-old father
- Normal developmental milestones

PATIENT FILE

Family History
- Father with "depression"
- Brother with alcohol-use disorder
- There is no family history of completed suicide

Medication history
- Fluoxetine (Prozac) 40 mg daily
- Multivitamin daily
- Norgestimate-ethinyl estradiol triphasic 0.18/0.215/0.25/0.35 mg daily

Current medications
- Fluoxetine (Prozac) 40 mg daily
- Multivitamin daily

Psychotherapy history
- The patient was seen in cognitive behavior therapy (CBT) for 12 months and completed family-based therapy for eating disorders previously

Further investigation

Is there anything else that you would like to know about the patient? What about vital signs and laboratory studies?

- Vital signs were repeated, including orthostatic vital signs. She is bradycardic at 45 bpm and hypotensive with a blood pressure of 84/50 mmHg. Her blood pressure percentiles are 1st percentile for systolic and 8th percentile diastolic
- Orthostatic vital signs reveal a blood pressure 85/50 mmHg and heart rate of 44 bpm while seated and 80/45 mmHg and 58 bpm while standing
- Her body mass index (BMI) is 16.2 kg/m^2
- An electrocardiogram (EKG) was obtained and reveals sinus bradycardia and a corrected QT interval (QTc) of 445 ms
- Routine laboratory studies that are recommended in the acute work-up were obtained (Table 12.1):
  - Complete blood count (CBC)
  - Comprehensive metabolic panel, including magnesium and phosphorus
  - Pre-albumin
  - Urinalysis

What about a physical examination?

- General: Tired appearing but alert, cooperative
- Skin: warm and dry
- Head, eye, ears, nose, and throat: normocephalic and atraumatic, extraocular movements intact, eyes sunken. Mucous membranes appear dry, and her lips are dry and cracked
- Neck: neck is supple, and there is full active range of motion
- Lungs: respiratory effort normal, clear to auscultation, normal breath sounds bilaterally
- Cardiac: regular rate and rhythm, normal S1 and S2, II/VI flow murmur
- Abdomen: Soft but with tenderness in lower quadrants with palpable stool present
- Back: inspection of the back is normal
- Lymphadenopathy: normal, and no adenopathy noted
- Musculoskeletal/Ext: reduced muscle mass, no contractures, or deformities
- Neurologic: cranial nerves II–XII grossly intact, gross motor exam normal by observation, strength normal and symmetric

Testing: laboratory results, imaging, EKGs
Table 12.1

CBC with Differential		
	Value	Ref Range
WBC	4.0	4.5–13.0 K/mcL
RBC	4.67	4.50–5.30 M/mcL
HGB	12.9	13.0–16.0 gm/dL
HCT	37.0	37.0–49.0 %
MCV	82.8	78.0–94.0 fL
MCH	28.1	25.0–35.0 pg
MCHC	33.9	31.0–37.0 gm/dL
RDW	14.5	<14.6 %
PLATELET	105	135–466 K/mcL
Comp Metabolic Panel		
	Value	Ref Range
SODIUM	136	136–145 mmol/L
POTASSIUM	2.8	3.3–4.7 mmol/L
CHLORIDE	90	100–112 mmol/L
CO2	39	17–31 mmol/L
ANION GAP	11	4–15 mmol/L
BUN	13	6–21 mg/dL
CREATININE	1.45	0.5–1.0 mg/dL
GLUCOSE	76	65–106 mg/dL
CALCIUM	8.9	8.3–10.6 mg/dL
PHOSPHORUS	1.6	2.8–5.1 mg/dL
ALBUMIN	3	3.3–4.8 gm/dL

	TSH	
	Value	Ref Range
Thyroid Stimulating Hormone	4.3	0.43-4.0 mcIU/mL
	Magnesium	
	Value	Ref Range
Magnesium	1.0 mg/dL	1.7-2.4 mg/dL
	Vitamin D	
	Value	Ref Range
25-OH-Vit-D	19 mg/dL	30-60 mg/dL
	Pre-Albumin	
	Value	Ref Range
Pre-albumin	19 mg/dL	30-60 mg/dL

Attending physician's mental notes: initial psychiatric evaluation

- This adolescent meets criteria for anorexia nervosa, binge-purge subtype, and presents with medical complications, including acute kidney injury with elevated creatinine, bradycardia, significant electrolyte disturbances, and an inability to maintain minimum caloric intake
- Her metabolic profile reveals mild acute kidney injury with a creatinine of 1.45 (baseline 0.84). Her metabolic panel reveals a hypokalemic, hypochloremic metabolic alkalosis consistent with her purging, and she has hypophosphatemia and hypomagnesemia
- Her CBC shows trilinear hypoplasia (leukopenia, anemia, and thrombocytopenia), which is common in anorexia nervosa (Sabel et al. 2013)
- She has a low vitamin D which is consistent with decreased intake of calorically dense dairy-based foods
- She will require admission for a refeeding protocol, and her electrolytes will need to be monitored as she is at risk for developing refeeding syndrome. Specifically, her severe electrolyte disturbances, including hypophosphatemia, increase her risk of refeeding syndrome. Her electrolyte imbalances are likely related to excessive purging and increase her risk of cardiac arrhythmias and seizures
- Regarding refeeding, there is an acute shift from catabolic to anabolic metabolism. The associated hyperparathyroidism potentially contributes to hypophosphatemia (Ornstein et al. 2003). Phosphate and thiamine supplementation during refeeding of severely malnourished patients with anorexia nervosa can be lifesaving

- Monitoring and managing electrolyte disturbances is one of the most important aspects of the initial diagnosis and management of eating disorders (Mehler et al. 2018)
- Bradycardia is common in patients with anorexia nervosa and tends to normalize with weight restoration (Cotter et al. 2019; Sachs et al. 2016). Additionally, QTc-interval prolongation may be observed in addition to nonspecific T-wave (Frederiksen et al. 2018) abnormalities related to electrolyte disturbances and has implications for the coadministration of psychotropic medications
- Gastrointestinal symptoms are prevalent in eating disorders, and the constipation reported in this patient is consistent. However, even after refeeding, gastrointestinal symptoms, including functional gastrointestinal disorders, are more common in patients with anorexia (Mehler et al. 2018) compared to the general population (Kessler et al. 2020; Schalla and Stengel 2019)
- She will require medical hospitalization for ongoing monitoring for complications of her anorexia nervosa. In general, the National Institute for Health and Clinical Excellence guidelines can be used to identify patients at high risk of refeeding problems (Table 12.2)

Table 12.2 National Institute for Health and Clinical Excellence recommendations for identifying patients at high risk of developing refeeding syndrome and medical findings in eating disorders

Hospitalization is recommended if the patient has:

One or more of the following:	Or two or more of the following:
• Body mass index (kg/m^2) <16	• Body mass index <18.5
• Little or no nutritional intake for >10 days	• Little or no nutritional intake for >5 days
• Unintentional weight loss >15% in the past 3–6 months	• Unintentional weight loss >10% in the past 3–6 months
• Low potassium, phosphate, or magnesium before feeding	• History of alcohol misuse or drugs, including insulin, chemotherapy, antacids, or diuretics

Medical findings Laboratory abnormalities	Eating disorder	Management	Severe physical complications
Hyponatremia	Anorexia nervosa (AN), bulimia nervosa (BN)	Periodic monitoring; careful sodium supplementation	Pontine myelinolysis in case of rapid normalization
Hypokalemia	BN, AN-P	Periodic monitoring; cessation of purging behaviors; potassium supplementation	Seizures, cardiac arrhythmias; nephropathy, Pseudo-Bartter syndrome after cessation of purging
Hypophosphatemia	AN	Periodic monitoring; phosphate supplementation	Refeeding syndrome
Hypoglycemia	AN	Rapid refeeding; glucose	Seizures, coma
Leucopenia (neutropenia)	AN	Weight restoration	Infections comparatively rare

Anemia (typically macrocytic)	AN	Weight restoration	Rare
Thrombocytopenia purpura	AN	Weight restoration	Bleeding risk
Low	AN	Weight restoration	Contributes to edemas
Elevated liver enzymes	AN	Periodic monitoring; weight restoration	Starvation hepatitis, liver necrosis
Elevated creatinine kinase	AN	Periodic monitoring; weight restoration	Rhabdomyolysis
Vitamin D deficiency	AN, BN	Vitamin D supplementation	Contributes to reduction of bone mineral density
Thiamine deficiency	AN	Supplementation of vitamin B1, weight restoration	Wernicke's encephalopathy
Inflammation, oxidative stress	AN	Weight restoration	Contributes to overall physical morbidity
Renal functioning (see also lab abnormalities)			
Renal failure	AN	Cessation of purging; normalization of drinking behavior	Hypokalemic nephropathy
Peripheral edema	AN	Weight restoration; for excessive edemas: diuretics if necessary	–
Cardiac functioning			
Sinus bradycardia	AN	Telemetry when <35 bpm	Severe complications rare
QT-prolongation	AN, BN	Check electrolytes, cessation of medications prolonging QTc (e.g. amisulpride, ziprasidone, citalopram)	Arrhythmias
Pericardial effusion	AN	Diuretics for severe effusion; weight restoration	Severe complications rare
Mitral and iricuspidal valve prolapse	AN	Weight restoration	Severe complications rare
GI functioning			
Slowed GI motility, prolonged gastric emptying, abdominal complaints	AN, BN, binge eating disorder (BED)	Prokinetic and motility agents, unavoidable	Gastric dilatation, gastric necrosis, gastric perforation
Constipation	AN	Weight restoration; laxatives, if necessary; dose reduction or cessation of medications with anticholinergic potential (e.g. olanzapine, quetiapine]	(Toxic) Ileus in rare cases, rectal prolapse
Cathartic colon, melanosis coli	AN, BN with laxative abuse	Cessation of laxative abuse	–
Esophageal: esophaghitis, Mallory–Weiss syndrome	BN, AN-P	Cessation of purging; proton pump inhibitors	Esophageal rupture, bleeding; adenocarcinoma
Endocrine functioning			

Multiple endocrine dysregulation, i.e. low estrogen, low testosterone, elevated cortisol, low leptin, low T3, low T4	AN, (BN), (BED)	Weight restoration, cessation of purging; estrogen supplementation	Amenorrhea, delayed puberty, growth deceleration, reduction of bone mineral density
Osteopenia, osteoporosis	AN	Weight restoration and light physical activity, moderate evidence for transdermal estrogen, calcium, vitamin D	Pathological fractures

Other

Hair loss	AN	Weight restoration	–
Skin: dry skin, acrocyanosis, nail fragility, lanugo hair	AN	Weight restoration	Cold injuries
Russel sign	BN, AN-P	Cessation of vomiting	–
Dental erosion, caries	BN, AN-P	Cessation of vomiting	–
Subconjunctival hemorrhage, epistaxis	BN, AN-P	Cessation of vomiting	–
Sialadenosis (swelling of parotid)	BN, AN-P	Cessation of vomiting	–
Neuromusculoskeletal: weakness of muscles diffuse gray and white matter atrophy	AN	Weight restoration	Extreme muscle weakness, cognitive deficits
Hypothermia	AN	Weight restoration; warming	–
Multiple micronutrient deficiencies		Micronutrient supplementation	–

Reproduced from Voderholzer, Haas, Correll, Körner. Medical management of eating disorders: an update. *Curr Opin in Psychiatry* 2020; 33(6): 542–53. In considering the medical examination of patients with eating disorders.

Inpatient hospitalization

- The patient was admitted to a pediatric hospital for malnutrition, and she began a meal plan with calorie counts and a 1500 kcal goal
- She received intravenous (IV) fluids, given her acute kidney injury
- Daily weights were obtained, and her metabolic panel and magnesium were monitored daily. Additionally, she was kept on telemetry
- At discharge, she was tolerating a goal of a 1750 kcal nasogastric diet with additional oral (PO) feeds that remained variable and at least 2000 mL of fluids, although she would drink PO fluid on top of that without limitations
- Her vitals stabilized, and her lowest heart rate and blood pressure over the 24 hours before discharge were 62 bpm and 94/77 mmHg. Her orthostatic vitals were stabilized at a 35-bpm increase in heart rate from sitting to standing without symptoms

- She was also referred to a dietician with whom she would meet weekly after discharge, and she and her family were referred for family-based therapy. She was also asked to follow up with an adolescent medicine clinic

Testing: laboratory results, imaging, EKGs (discharge)

CBC with Differential

	Value	Ref Range
WBC	4.5	4.5-13.0 K/mcL
RBC	4.67	4.50-5.30 M/mcL
HGB	**12.9**	**13.0-16.0 gm/dL**
HCT	37.0	37.0-49.0 %
MCV	82.8	78.0-94.0 fL
MCH	28.1	25.0-35.0 pg
MCHC	33.9	31.0-37.0 gm/dL
RDW	14.5	<14.6 %
PLATELET	**129**	**135-466 K/mcL**

Comp Metabolic Panel

	Value	Ref Range
SODIUM	140	136-145 mmol/L
POTASSIUM	4.4	3.3-4.7 mmol/L
CHLORIDE	107	100-112 mmol/L
CO2	28	17-31 mmol/L
ANION GAP	5	4-15 mmol/L
BUN	11	6-21 mg/dL
CREATININE	0.69	0.5-1.0 mg/dL
GLUCOSE	76	65-106 mg/dL
CALCIUM	8.9	8.3-10.6 mg/dL
PHOSPHORUS	4.6	2.8-5.1 mg/dL

Magnesium

	Value	Ref Range
Magnesium	2.1 mg/dL	1.7-2.4 mg/dL

Vitamin D

	Value	Ref Range
25-OH-Vit-D	**28 mg/dL**	**30-60 mg/dL**

Albumin

	Value	Ref Range
Albumin	3.4 mg/dL	3.4-5.0 mg/dL

Interim visit: post-discharge week 4

- The patient has been discharged from a partial hospitalization program and "weight restored"
- Her depressive symptoms have improved. However – now 4 weeks after discharge – she is struggling with more distorted thoughts related to her body image and feeling more intense thoughts

related to her eating and is very fixated on an unrealistic ideal body weight
- Additionally, she has continued to binge and purge and has struggled with caloric restriction
- Over the 4 weeks since discharge, her weight has decreased by 1.5 kg. However, her other vital signs are stable
- She meets with her dietician and her family-based eating disorder therapist weekly, and there is a close collaboration relationship within her treatment team

Question

Which of the following would be the most appropriate intervention at this point?

- Continue to monitor her symptoms
- Add cyproheptadine to assist with appetite stimulation
- Discontinue fluoxetine (Prozac) and begin paroxetine (Paxil)
- Add low-dose olanzapine (Zyprexa)

Attending physician's mental notes: interim visit post-discharge week 4

- Her attending physician is concerned by her weight loss, despite an intensive outpatient program, and by the degree of fixation on her body image
- Several studies of olanzapine have produced conflicting reports in patients with anorexia nervosa (Han et al. 2022; Spettigue et al. 2018). However, one placebo-controlled trial in adults with anorexia nervosa (N = 152) with a mean BMI of 16.7 kg/m^2 revealed that 5–10 mg of olanzapine was superior to placebo in improving BMI
- Interestingly, in several studies of patients with anorexia nervosa, olanzapine was not associated with dyslipidemia or altered glucose metabolism

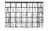

Case outcome: interim visit post-discharge week 5

- Since olanzapine 2.5 mg twice daily was begun 1 week ago, the patient's mood has improved. Specifically, her depressive and anxiety symptoms are contemporaneously improved, and she has been spending more time with friends
- Her parents, therapist, and dietician note that she has been more engaged in treatment
- She has gained 0.5 kg over the past week and reports being more flexible in her thinking

- She continues to meet with her dietician and with her family-based eating disorder therapist weekly, and there is a close collaboration relationship within her treatment team
- However, she has continued to binge and purge several times per week and based on this, her physician has obtained laboratory studies (Table 12.3)
- She denies any orthostatic symptoms

Testing: laboratory results, imaging, EKGs (post-discharge week 5)

Table 12.3

Comp Metabolic Panel		
	Value	Ref Range
SODIUM	140	136–145 mmol/L
POTASSIUM	3.9	3.3–4.7 mmol/L
CHLORIDE	99	100–112 mmol/L
CO2	27	17–31 mmol/L
ANION GAP	5	4–15 mmol/L
BUN	11	6–21 mg/dL
CREATININE	0.69	0.5–1.0 mg/dL
GLUCOSE	80	65–106 mg/dL
CALCIUM	8.9	8.3–10.6 mg/dL
PHOSPHORUS	4.5	2.8–5.1 mg/dL
ALBUMIN	**3.2**	**3.3–4.8 gm/dL**
Magnesium		
	Value	Ref Range
Magnesium	2.0 mg/dL	1.7–2.4 mg/dL

Attending physician's mental notes: post-discharge week 5

- Her attending physician is encouraged by her improved mood and appropriate weight gain over this short period and consults with her dietician and therapist in addition to speaking with the patient's parents. This approach is essential in avoiding splitting amongst treatment team members and ensuring that the treatment team remains cohesive
- Her physician is reassured by her laboratory studies and will observe the patient with the treatment team over the next 2 weeks
- Finally, her tolerability with regard to olanzapine is encouraging

Interim visit: post-discharge week 7

- She has been treated with olanzapine 2.5 mg twice daily for 3 weeks in addition to her fluoxetine, and her mood and depressive symptoms remain stable. Additionally, there is less rumination

- Her parents, therapist, and dietician continue to report that she is engaged in treatment and speaks openly about her urges and difficulty resisting the urge to binge and purge. She has continued to binge and purge approximately three times per week
- She has gained an additional 0.5 kg over the past 2 weeks
- She continues meeting with her dietician and her family-based eating disorder therapist

Question

Which of the following would be the most appropriate intervention at this point?

- Continue to monitor her symptoms
- Discontinue low-dose olanzapine (Zyprexa)
- Add adjunctive naltrexone (Revia)
- Add interpersonal psychotherapy for adolescents (IPT-A)

Interim visit: post-discharge week 9

- At her last visit, secondary to concerns about the persistent frequency of her binging and purging, naltrexone was added
- There has been a significant reduction in her binging and purging; she reports that she has neither binged nor purged over the past week
- Her weight has returned to her discharge weight
- She has no tolerability concerns, and her vital signs have remained within normal limits
- She continues to meet with her dietician and her family-based eating disorder therapist, and her treatment team has relaxed some exercise restrictions

Take-home points

- The history of a patient with an eating disorder should also consider the following:
  ° Weight history: including the highest, lowest, and when, preferred weight, weighing patterns, fear of gaining weight
  ° Eating behavior: it is helpful to include a 24-hour recall, where the patient eats and with whom, binges, compulsive or emotional eating, night eating, nocturnal eating, grazing, and orthorexia drives
  ° Purging behavior modes: inquire regarding self-induced vomiting, laxatives, diuretics, diet pills, fat absorbers, enemas, ipecac, etc., frequency, effects
  ° Body image: helpful questions can include "What percentage of your day do you think about weight, shape, size, and food?"

Also, enquire as to body image distress, relationship with the body, body checking, and comparison
- ○ Preoccupations and rituals: include questions related to table behaviors, calorie counting, frequency, and patterns of weighing
- ○ Activity: obtain a history of exercise, including frequency, presence of compulsive properties, pacing, or standing
- Consider and actively screen for psychiatric and medical comorbidity
- Consider the risk of the refeeding syndrome and laboratory studies as appropriate (Table 12.4)
- In considering psychotropic medication use, particularly selective serotonin-reuptake inhibitors (SSRIs), remember that SSRIs will not be effective until the patient is 80–85% of ideal body weight

Table 12.4

Medical examinations in eating disorders

- Height and body weight (BMI for adults or percentiles for children and adolescents)
- Blood pressure and pulse, body temperature
- Inspection of peripheral body areas (blood circulation, edema, acrocyanosis, lanugo hair)
- Auscultation of the heart, orthostasis test
- EKG (in case of abnormalities in the long-term EKG), possibly echocardiography to exclude pericardial effusion.
- For enduring eating disorders: bone density measurement
- Abdominal palpation and auscultation
- Dual-energy radiograph absorptiometry of bone, for patients who have been underweight for longer than 6 months. MRI or computed tomography of the brain and neuropsychological assessment for patients with atypical features, such as hallucinations, delusions, delirium, and persistent cognitive impairment, despite weight restoration.
- Before and during refeeding of extremely underweight patients: abdominal sonography and echocardiography assessing dehydration, edema, and effusion as well as organ changes related to AN (e.g. renal, hepatic, pancreatic)
- Laboratory parameters: complete blood count, C-reactive protein; fasting glucose values; serum electrolytes (sodium, potassium, calcium, magnesium, phosphate); renal status: creatinine; liver status: ALT, AST, AP, CK, GGT, total and direct bilirubin, PTT; amylase, lipase; urine status; TSH. In selected patients also iron, ferritin, vitamin A, vitamin E, vitamin B12, vitamin D, folic acid, β-carotene, zinc, copper, selenium as well as drug screening, EKG (before initiation of atypical antipsychotic medications) in case of elevated creatinine: creatinine clearance recommended
- In case of low BMI (BMI less than 12 kg/m^2) and at the beginning of renutrition: control of sodium, potassium, and phosphate (at least weekly) recommended

ALT, alanine transaminase; AN, anorexia nervosa; AP, alkaline phosphatase; AST, aspartate transferase; CK, creatine kinase; GGT, gamma-glutamyl transferase; MRI, magnetic resonance imaging; PTT, partial thromboplastin time; TSH, thyroid stimulating hormone. Reproduced from Voderholzer, Haas, Correll, Körner. Medical management of eating disorders: an update. *Curr Opin Psychiatry* 2020; 33(6): 542–53.

Two-minute tutorial

- Refeeding syndrome is a potentially fatal condition that may be precipitated by rapid refeeding after undernutrition (Birmingham 2006; Mehanna et al. 2008)

- ◦ Refeeding syndrome is characterized by hypophosphatemia, fluid and electrolyte shifts, and metabolic and clinical complications
- ◦ Patients at high risk for refeeding syndrome include chronically undernourished patients and patients with little or no caloric intake for >5 days (Mehanna et al. 2008)
- ◦ Vitamin supplementation should also be started with refeeding and continued for at least 10 days (Mehanna et al. 2008)

Tips and pearls

- Management of co-occurring psychiatric disorders is critical in eating disorders. However, the underlying eating disorder may interfere with the efficacy and tolerability of psychotropic medications. For example, antidepressant medications may be relatively ineffective until weight is restored, secondary to overall monoamine depletion due to total protein malnutrition
- In patients with severe electrolyte disturbances, the effects of some medications on QTc-interval may be accentuated, while in patients with hypovolemia, bradycardia, or orthostatic symptoms, the adverse hemodynamic effects of some medications may be more likely
- Finally, while screening for suicidality is critical in all psychiatric disorders, it is especially so in patients with eating disorders, and suicide represents a leading cause of death in this population (Kask et al. 2016)
- The medical evaluation of the patient with anorexia is essential (Table 12.2)

Mechanism of action moment

- Naltrexone, an opioid antagonist, initially developed in the 1960s, was approved by the U.S. Food and Drug Administration (FDA) for treating adults with opioid addiction in 1984 and later alcohol-use disorder
- In children and adolescents, naltrexone is used off-label for compulsive and impulsive behavior disorders driven by the opioid reward circuit, such as binge eating, impulsiveness, and nonsuicidal self-injury. In some open-label studies, it reduces binging and purging in adolescents with eating disorders (Stancil et al. 2019)
- Oral naltrexone is rapidly and nearly completely absorbed after oral administration, suggesting translocation from the gut to the portal venous circulation. However, despite its nearly complete absorption, its absolute bioavailability is low (~5–40%) because of extensive first-pass metabolism. Developmental and genetic factors contribute to variability in bioavailability. In a prospective pharmacokinetic study of 21 adolescents with eating disorders the increase in exposure associated with food for $AUC_{0-\infty}$ was large (Cohen's d = 2.6) (Stancil et al. 2021)

- Exposure to naltrexone in adolescents with eating disorders varies significantly, and food slows its absorption considerably (Figure 12.1) (Stancil et al. 2021)
- While the exact mechanism of naltrexone in reducing binging and purging behaviors is unclear, it is hypothesized that the reinforcing effects of binging and purging may be mediated – through the release of endogenous opioids – by action at µ receptors and increases in dopamine release to the nucleus accumbens. Naltrexone is a µ-opioid receptor antagonist; thus, it blocks the pleasurable effects of these behaviors and the subsequent dopamine release and reinforcement (Figure 12.2)

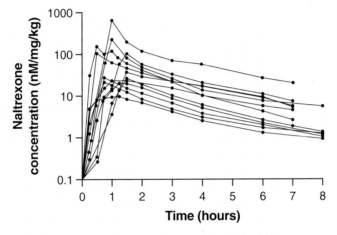

Figure 12.1 Concentration–time curves in adolescents with eating disorders following single-dose naltrexone. Reproduced from Stancil et al. Developmental considerations for the use of naltrexone in children and adolescents. *Journal of Pediatric Pharmacology and Therapeutics* 2021.

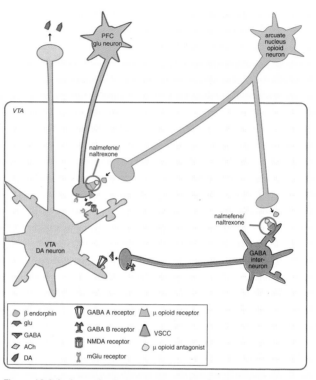

Figure 12.2 Actions of naltrexone in the ventral tegmental area (VTA). Opioid neurons form synapses in the VTA with GABAergic interneurons and with presynaptic nerve terminals of glutamate neurons. Potentially the reinforcing effects of binging and purging are mediated – through the release of endogenous opioids – by action at μ receptors and increases dopamine release to the nucleus accumbens. Naltrexone is a μ-opioid receptor antagonist; thus, it blocks the pleasurable effects of these behaviors. ACh, acetylcholine; DA, dopamine; GABA, γ-aminobutyric acid; glu, glutamine; mGluR, metabotropic glutamate receptor; NMDA, N-methyl-D-aspartate; PFC, prefrontal cortex; VSCC, voltage-sensitive calcium channel.

Post test question

Which of the following may reduce binging and purging in adolescents with eating disorders, including anorexia nervosa?

A. Paroxetine (Paxil)

B. Selegeline (Emsam)

C. Olanzapine (Zyprexa)

D. Naltrexone (Revia)

Answer: D (Naltrexone, Revia)

There are no studies of the efficacy of paroxetine (A) in adolescents with eating disorders, and SSRIs –and potentially monoamine oxidase inhibitors (MAOIs) (B) – are generally less effective when the patient is less than 80–85% of their ideal body weight and acutely malnourished. Olanzapine (C) has demonstrated efficacy in improving weight, and some open-label studies and clinical experiences suggest that it may help address meal-related anxiety and obsessional thinking related to disordered eating. Naltrexone (D, correct answer) is hypothesized to block the reinforcing effects of binging and purging that are putatively mediated – through the release of endogenous opioids – by action at μ receptors (Figure 12.2). Several studies suggest that naltrexone may reduce binging and purging behavior in adolescents with eating disorders, although its absorption is variable (Figure 12.1).

References

1. Birmingham, C. L. Assessment and treatment of acute medical complications during the refeeding process. In Jaffa, T. (ed.), *Eating Disorders in Children and Adolescents*. Cambridge, UK: Cambridge University Press, 2006. https://doi.org/10.1017/CBO9780511543890.016
2. Frederiksen, T. C., Christiansen, M. K., Østergaard, P. C., et al. QTc interval and risk of cardiac events in adults with anorexia nervosa. A long-term follow-up study. *Circ Arrhyth Electrophysiol* 2018; 11(8): e005995. https://doi.org/10.1161/CIRCEP.117.005995
3. Cotter, R., Lyden, J., Mehler, P. S., et al. A case series of profound bradycardia in patients with severe anorexia nervosa: thou shall not pace? *HeartRhythm Case Rep* 2019; 5(10): 511–15. https://doi.org/10.1016/j.hrcr.2019.07.011
4. Han, R., Bian, Q., Chen, H, Effectiveness of olanzapine in the treatment of anorexia nervosa: a systematic review and meta-analysis. *Brain Behav* 2022; 12(2): e2498. https://doi.org/10.1002/brb3.2498
5. Kask, J., Ekselius, L., Brandt, L., et al. Mortality in women with anorexia nervosa: the role of comorbid psychiatric disorders. *Psychosom Med* 2016; 78(8): 910–19. https://doi.org/10.1097/PSY.0000000000000342
6. Kessler, U., Rekkedal, G., Rø, Ø., et al. Association between gastrointestinal complaints and psychopathology in patients with anorexia nervosa. *Int J Eating Disord* 2020; 53(5): 802–06. https://doi.org/10.1002/eat.23243

7. Mehanna, H. M., Moledina, J., Travis, J. Refeeding syndrome: what it is, and how to prevent and treat it. *BMJ* 2008; 336(7659): 1495. https://doi.org/10.1136/bmj.a301

8. Mehler, P. S., Blalock, D. V., Walden, K., et al. Medical findings in 1,026 consecutive adult inpatient–residential eating disordered patients. *Int J Eating Disord* 2018; 51(4): 305–13. https://doi.org/10.1002/eat.22830

9. Ornstein, R. M., Golden, N. H., Jacobson, M. S., Shenker, I. R. Hypophosphatemia during nutritional rehabilitation in anorexia nervosa: implications for refeeding and monitoring. *J Adolesc Health* 2003; 32(1): 83–88. https://doi.org/10.1016/S1054-139X(02)00456-1

10. Sabel, A. L., Gaudiani, J. L., Statland, B., Mehler, P. S. Hematological abnormalities in severe anorexia nervosa. *Ann Hematol* 2013; 92(5): 605–13. https://doi.org/10.1007/s00277-013-1672-x

11. Sachs, K. V., Harnke, B., Mehler, P. S., Krantz, M. J. Cardiovascular complications of anorexia nervosa: a systematic review. *Int J Eating Disord* 2016; 49(3): 238–48. https://doi.org/10.1002/eat.22481

12. Schalla, M. A., Stengel, A. Gastrointestinal alterations in anorexia nervosa: a systematic review. *Eur Eating Disord Rev* 2019; 27(5): 447–61. https://doi.org/10.1002/erv.2679

13. Spettigue, W., Norris, M. L., Maras, D., et al. Evaluation of the effectiveness and safety of olanzapine as an adjunctive treatment for anorexia nervosa in adolescents: an open-label trial. *J Can Acad Child Adolesc Psychiatry* 2018; 27(3): 197–208. PMID: 30038658

14. Stancil, S. L., Abdel-Rahman, S., Wagner, J. Developmental considerations for the use of naltrexone in children and adolescents. *J Pediatr Pharmacol Ther* 2021; 26(7): 675–95. https://doi.org/10.5863/1551-6776-26.7.675

15. Stancil, S. L., Adelman, W., Dietz, A., Abdel-Rahman, S. Naltrexone reduces binge eating and purging in adolescents in an eating disorder program. *J Child Adolesc Psychopharmacol* 2019; 29(9): 721–24. https://doi.org/10.1089/cap.2019.0056

16. Strawn J. R., Mills J. A., Poweleit E. A., Ramsey L. B., Croarkin P. E. Adverse effects of antidepressant medications and their management in children and adolescents. *Pharmacotherapy* 2023; 43(7): 675–690.

Case 13: High or higher antidepressant concentrations? Cannabis-related drug interactions in an adolescent

The Questions: How does cannabis affect outcomes in adolescents with depressive disorders? What is the impact of cannabis on selective serotonin reuptake inhibitor (SSRI) pharmacokinetics in adolescents?

The Psychopharmacological Dilemma: Cannabis use is increasingly common in adolescents, yet the pharmacological implications are unclear for many clinicians

Pretest self-assessment question

Cannabis increases the concentrations of which medication in adolescents?

A. Vilazodone (Viibryd)
B. Aripiprazole (Abilify)
C. Fluoxetine (Prozac)
D. Sertraline (Zoloft)
E. All of the above

Answer: D (Sertraline, Zoloft)

Patient evaluation on intake

- 16-year-old adolescent with major depressive disorder (*Diagnostic and Statistical Manual of Mental Disorders, DSM-5* criteria) who has been treated with sertraline for 6 months and complains of increased sedation, nausea, and severe amotivation
- Moderate to severe depressive symptoms, which are accompanied by significant anxiety symptoms, and there is no suicidal ideation, intent, or plan currently
- He denies any recent stressors, although he is concerned about his academic performance, and his parents share this concern
- However, over the past 8 months, he has smoked cannabis. Initially, he smoked once or twice per week. However, this increased and he now smokes twice daily most days
- During this time when he has been smoking, he notes that his motivation has significantly worsened but does not think that this is related to his cannabis. Additionally, he does not see his cannabis use as problematic and shares that several friends smoke cannabis regularly
- He denies nicotine or alcohol use

Psychiatric history

- History of depressive symptoms beginning at age 13
- Over the past 12 months, he developed increasing withdrawal and irritability and worsening academic performance, which has resulted in significant conflict with his parents
- He experiences significant irritability, initial insomnia, and daytime tiredness
- He now naps daily, generally for 1–2 hours after school
- As mentioned above, he has increasingly experienced sedation, nausea, severe amotivation, some "spinning feelings," and frequent xerostomia

Social and personal history

- He lives with his mother, father, and adopted younger brother, age 12
- His academic performance has deteriorated, and he has had more struggles with motivation which has also affected friendships
- He is not in a relationship and is not sexually active
- There is no history of abuse or trauma

Medical history

- Delivered at 40 weeks to a 25-year-old mother and 25-year-old father
- Prenatal exposure to nicotine, but no cannabis was used during his mother's pregnancy
- Normal developmental milestones
- Seasonal allergies
- Obesity

Family History

- Father with no psychiatric history
- Mother with a history of major depressive disorder (MDD), and she has done well with sertraline 100 mg daily
- His mother used cannabis "for a few years during college" and notes that she stopped this prior to graduation from college and has smoked cannabis several times per year for the last decade

Medication history

- Sertraline (Zoloft) 150 mg daily

Current medications (and substances)

- Sertraline (Zoloft) 150 mg daily
- Cannabis – two joints twice daily on most days

Psychotherapy history

- He was treated with cognitive behavioral therapy (CBT) weekly for 6 months and now sees his therapist every 4–6 weeks
- Psychotherapy sessions generally involve a brief check-in with his parents at the beginning and end of every other session, and most of the appointment is spent alone with his therapist

Further investigation

Is there anything else that you would like to know about the patient? What about accompanying symptoms?

- He notes increased anxiety over the past 4 months and has felt sluggish, and has been having panic attacks approximately once weekly, but he denies agoraphobia, social anxiety, or separation anxiety
- He denies any psychotic symptoms, including perceptual disturbances (e.g. illusions)

What about additional physical symptoms and vital signs?

- Vital signs are within normal limits; his BMI is in the ninety-fifth percentile for age and sex
- He denies cardiac symptoms, including palpitations, although he has felt lightheaded at times and describes orthostatic symptoms and several episodes of presyncopal symptoms

What about tolerance?

- He notes that when he first began smoking cannabis with his friends, he would feel a euphoric "high" with some degree of dissociation. However, he notes that, even when smoking for longer periods now, he does not feel "the same way as when I first did"

Attending physician's mental notes: initial psychiatric evaluation

- Provisionally, this patient has MDD, moderate to severe with anxious distress, and a cannabis use disorder, severe. However, his anxiety symptoms – which emerged as his cannabis use increased – may be related to a cannabis-induced anxiety disorder
- Regarding the side effects he experiences (e.g. sedation/tiredness, dry mouth, insomnia, intermittent orthostatic symptoms), the attending physician is concerned that these have intensified since he began smoking cannabis more regularly. These "side effects" may relate to both cannabis use (Zuurman et al. 2009), worsening of his underlying depressive disorder, or even a pharmacodynamic interaction between $\Delta 9$-tetrahydrocannabinol (THC) and sertraline

(Vaughn et al. 2021). Additionally, cannabis (specifically THC) increases sertraline exposure (e.g. blood concentrations) in patients, including adolescents (Vaughn et al. 2021) (Figure 13.1)

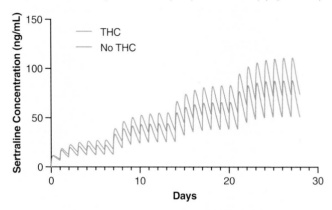

Figure 13.1 Simulated time course of sertraline plasma concentrations in adolescent CYP2C19 normal metabolizers consuming THC or low-dose cannabidiol (CBD) versus not consuming. In this model, sertraline was initiated at 50 mg daily and increased by 50 mg each subsequent week until reaching 200 mg daily. Concurrent THC or low-dose CBD (5–15 mg daily) use with sertraline was simulated, with the total body clearance reduced by 25%. Adapted from Vaughn, S. E., Strawn, J. R., Poweleit, E. A., Sarangdhar, M., Ramsey, L. B. The impact of marijuana on antidepressant treatment in adolescents: clinical and pharmacologic considerations. *J Pers Med* 2021;11(7): 615.

- The attending physician attempts to quantify how much cannabis he is smoking and knows that THC content varies considerably from one strain of cannabis to another. Additionally, the physician is aware that THC content has, in general, increased significantly over time (Cascini et al. 2012). Additionally, he is aware that patients frequently are unaware of how much THC they ingest and that the way in which the cannabis is consumed, the type of product, route of administration, the patient's body composition, and tolerance all affect exposure (Grotenhermen 2003)
- In considering the patient's cannabis use, his attending physician is aware that when the patient smokes, approximately ~50% of the THC content is converted to smoke and up to 50% of inhaled smoke is exhaled again. Further, some inhaled cannabis undergoes localized metabolism in the lung. Thus, the bioavailability of an inhaled dose of THC is between 10–25% of the content in the cannabis. The clinician is also aware that the patient likely perceives

effects within seconds and that the duration of effect is probably about 3 hours (Strougo et al. 2008)

- Based on the patient's reported use (two joints [0.4 g] per episode of smoking), his attending physician has calculated the following using an online calculator (www.latimes.com/projects/la-me-weed-101-thc-calculator) (Figure 13.2):

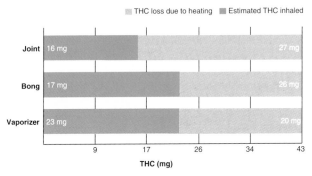

Figure 13.2 Approximate amount of THC to which this patient is exposed based on his reported use. *Data source: LA Times, Accessed December 4, 2022.*

- The attending physician knows that medium doses of THC are associated with the effect shown in Table 13.1 (Zuurman et al. 2009):

Table 13.1

THC	Inconsistent user (studied doses)	Frequent user (extrapolated doses)	Experienced effects
low	<1–5 mg daily	<3–20 mg daily	Consistently experience: • Increased heart rate • Intensified visual and auditory perception • Decreased attention • Impaired cognition on sequential tasks
medium	5–15 mg daily	15–60 mg daily	Reliably experience the effects listed above, and potentially: • Dry mouth • Reduced nausea and vomiting (anti-emetic action) • Impaired decision-making • Decreased blood pressure • Reduced or increased anxiety • Increased α brain wave activity • Reduced rapid eye movement (REM) sleep • Blood glucose drop – "munchies"
high	>15–30 mg daily	>45–120 mg daily	Toxicity or undesirable effects listed above and: • Delusions • Hallucinations • Paranoia • Confused, disorganized thought • Anxiety and panic • Derealization

Adapted from Zuurman, L., et al., *Br J Clinical Pharmacology* 2009.

- Regarding his sleep difficulties, these could – like other symptoms – relate to increased concentrations of sertraline or to the effects of the cannabis. Acutely, THC decreases sleep onset latency and REM sleep; however, chronically, THC produces habituation and daytime sleepiness as well as negative effects on mood and memory (Babson et al. 2017)
- The patient has described tolerance which develops quickly in frequent smokers and results in a significant attenuation of the subjective "high" that patients experience (Desrosiers et al. 2014) (Figure 13.3)

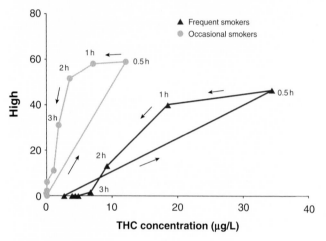

Figure 13.3 Experiences of being high relative to plasma THC concentrations in frequent (blue triangles) and occasional (light blue circles) cannabis smokers. Adapted from Desrosiers et al. Phase I and II cannabinoid disposition in blood and plasma of occasional and frequent smokers following controlled smoked cannabis. *Clin Chem* 2014; 60(4): 631–43.

Question

Which of the following would be your next step in addition to referring to a substance-use treatment program?

- Discontinue sertraline (Zoloft)
- Decrease sertraline (Zoloft) to 100 mg daily
- Begin naltrexone (Revia) 50 mg daily
- Add bupropion XL (Wellbutrin XL) 150 mg every morning

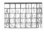

Case outcome: second interim follow-up (week 4)

- Since his initial consultation, he has begun an intensive outpatient program to address his heavy cannabis use. His parents have been engaged in treatment with him and increased the frequency of his psychotherapy
- At his initial visit, sertraline was decreased to 100 mg daily, and he experienced a significant improvement in his tiredness and is no longer napping daily. He has had contemporaneous improvement in his nausea
- He has decreased his cannabis use to two to three times weekly, and the intensive outpatient program therapist is working with his parents, who have seen this frequency of use as "normal"
- He reports fewer depressive symptoms, less insomnia, and resolution of his orthostatic symptoms and xerostomia. However, he continues to struggle in school and with motivation, rarely completes his homework, and wishes to drop out of school. He has only noted a mild improvement in his anxiety symptoms

Attending physician's mental notes: first interim follow-up (week 4)

- His depressive symptoms are partially improving and there have been very mild improvements in anxiety
- Many of the symptoms that either represent cannabis-related increased sertraline exposure or direct effects of cannabis have improved
- However, he continues to experience significant amotivation
- His attending physician is concerned that given his obesity, the effects of months of moderate-to-heavy cannabis use will persist and that the amotivation may represent a lasting effect of this heavy cannabis use
- His attending physician recalls studies of adults in which heavy cannabis users had decreased dopamine synthesis in several brain areas (Figure 13.4), and individuals with greater cannabis use had reduced dopamine synthesis capacity ($r = -0.77$, $p < 0.001$) (Bloomfield et al. 2014). In other studies, dopamine synthesis capacity, based on positron emission tomography (PET) imaging, in cannabis users predicts apathy (Figure 13.4)
- Data from three large, long-running longitudinal studies suggest strong relationships between the maximum frequency of cannabis use before age 17 years (i.e. never, less than monthly, monthly or more, weekly or more, or daily) and high-school completion (Figure 13.5). There is a dose-response relationship between

the frequency of adolescent cannabis use and a lower likelihood of completing high school, graduating from college, and a higher likelihood of developing a cannabis-use disorder or other substance-use disorder (Silins et al. 2014)

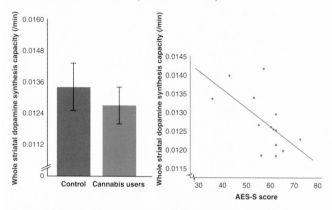

Figure 13.4 Cannabis users have reduced dopamine synthesis capacity in the striatum (effect size = 0.85) (left). Adapted from data presented in Bloomfield et al. Dopaminergic function in cannabis users and its relationship to cannabis-induced psychotic symptoms. *Biol Psychiatry* 2014; 75(6): 470–78. Importantly, cannabis users with decreased dopamine synthesis capacity have less motivation (right) reflected by scores on the Apathy Evaluation Scale (AES-S). Adapted from Bloomfield et al. The link between dopamine function and apathy in cannabis users: an [18 F]-DOPA PET imaging study. *Psychopharmacology (Berl)* 2014; 231(11): 2251–59.

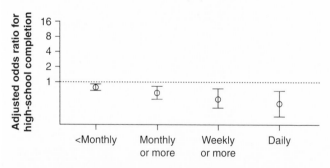

Figure 13.5 Adjusted odds ratios (log scale) between maximum frequency of cannabis use before age 17 years and the likelihood of completing high school, compared with individuals who have never used cannabis. Error bars show 95% CIs. Adapted from Silins, E., et al.; Cannabis Cohorts Research Consortium. Young adult sequelae of adolescent cannabis use: an integrative analysis. *Lancet Psychiatry* 2014; 1(4): 286–93.

Question

Given his current psychotherapy and pharmacologic treatment (sertraline 100 mg daily), which of the following would be your next step?

- Return to sertraline (Zoloft) 150 mg daily
- Add adjunctive bupropion XL (Wellbutrin XL) 150 mg daily
- Cross-titrate sertraline (Zoloft) to paroxetine (Paxil)
- Begin adjunctive atomoxetine (Strattera)

Case outcome: interim follow-up (week 10)

- At his last visit, bupropion XL was added, and he noted improved motivation and less fatigue
- He has had some improvement in terms of his academic performance; however, he still struggles to complete homework and feels unmotivated at school and with friends. That said, he denies most neurovegetative symptoms of depression
- He also notes that he no longer experiences any significant anxiety
- He continues in outpatient psychotherapy and in the intensive outpatient substance-use program, although this has been stepped down to once weekly

Question

Given his current pharmacologic treatment (sertraline 100 mg daily and bupropion XL 150 mg daily), which of the following would be your next step?

- Return to sertraline (Zoloft) 150 mg daily
- Titrate adjunctive bupropion extended-release formulation (Wellbutrin XL) from 150 mg daily to 300 mg daily
- Cross-titrate sertraline (Zoloft) to paroxetine (Paxil)
- Begin adjunctive methylphenidate osmotic controlled-release oral delivery system (OROS) (Concerta) 18 mg daily

Attending physician's mental notes: interim follow-up (week 10)

- The addition of bupropion has been helpful, and the attending physician assumes that this effect is primarily related to the dopaminergic effects of bupropion
- The attending physician believes the persistent amotivation to be a residual effect of his heavy cannabis use rather than to a symptom of depression and he is concerned that the patient's increased adipose tissue may potentiate this effect. The physician selected bupropion not as an "antidepressant" but rather to boost dopaminergic tone and in doing so to increase motivation

Case outcome: interim follow-up (week 12)

- At his last visit, bupropion XL was titrated, and he again notes improved motivation
- He continues to deny any significant anxiety or use of substances other than cannabis. However, his cannabis use has increased from once weekly to three times weekly, and he continues to smoke approximately one joint with each use

Question

Given his current pharmacologic treatment (sertraline 100 mg daily and bupropion XL 300 mg daily), which of the following would be your next step?

- Titrate adjunctive bupropion XL from 300 mg daily to 450 mg daily
- Discontinue sertraline
- Begin adjunctive N-acetylcysteine 600 mg twice daily with a goal dose of 1200 mg twice daily
- Begin adjunctive methylphenidate OROS 18 mg daily

Attending physician's mental notes: interim follow-up (week 12)

- The addition of bupropion has been helpful; however, titration to 450 mg daily may not provide additional benefit for his motivation – which has largely normalized. Similarly, the addition of methylphenidate may have little benefit, particularly given his lack of inattentive symptoms. Discontinuing sertraline would potentially increase his risk of recrudescence of depressive symptoms and increasing anxiety symptoms could further increase his risk of continued or increased cannabis use
- The attending physician is very concerned about the increase in cannabis use and considers specific pharmacotherapy. In a study of adolescents with cannabis-use disorder, administration of *N*-acetylcysteine (NAC) more than doubled the odds, compared to placebo participants, of submitting negative urine cannabinoid tests during treatment (odds ratio = 2.4, p = 0.029) (Gray et al. 2012). In this study, NAC was well tolerated and dosing involved 1200 mg twice daily

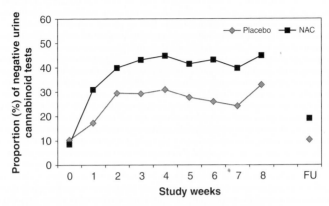

Figure 13.6 Proportion of negative urine cannabinoid tests in patients participating in a double-blind, placebo-controlled trial of N-acetylcysteine (NAC) or placebo. NAC was associated with more than doubling the likelihood of a negative urine drug screen. Reproduced from Gray et al. A double-blind randomized controlled trial of N-acetylcysteine in cannabis-dependent adolescents. *Am J Psychiatry* 2012; 169(8): 805–12.

Performance in practice: confessions of a psychopharmacologist

- In working with this adolescent with significant substance use, the attending physician tried to maintain an alliance with the patient and his parents; however, in doing so he may not have been as direct as needed in helping the parents to understand that their normalization of his cannabis use pharmacokinetically and pharmacodynamically undermined his antidepressant treatment
- An intensive outpatient program, as well as NAC or other substance use-focused pharmacotherapy could have been implemented earlier

Take-home points

- Adolescents with depression are twice as likely to report cannabis use and use amongst depressed teens has increased more rapidly over the past 15 years compared to their peers (Weinberger et al. 2020)
- One in three twelfth graders (17–18 years old) used cannabis in the past year, and 6% of these adolescents used cannabis on a daily basis. Similarly, among eighth and tenth graders, daily use increased since 2018, with 1.3% of eighth graders (an 85.7% increase in 13–14-year-olds) and 4.8% of tenth graders (a 41.2% increase in 15–16-year-olds) reporting daily use

- THC and CBD have clinically significant pharmacokinetic interactions – through CYP2C19 – with es/citalopram and sertraline, and this increases the likelihood of side effects with these medications
- THC and CBD have pharmacodynamic interactions with SSRIs which potentially decrease SSRI efficacy (Figure 13.7) (Vaughn et al. 2021)

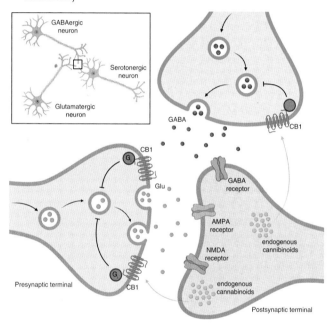

Figure 13.7 Cannabinoid-mediated impact on monoamine, GABAergic, and glutamatergic signaling in the brain. Cannabinoid-mediated stimulation of CB_1 receptors on monoaminergic neurons leads to delayed transport of monoamines to the synapse, decreasing monoamines in the synapse. These effects may be mediated though binding at CB1 which alters excitatory–inhibitory balance. Abbreviations: GABA, gamma aminobutyric acid; Glu, glutamate; AMPA, α-amino-3-hydroxy-5-methyl-4-isoxazolepropionic acid; NMDA, N-methyl-D-aspartate; CB_1, cannabinoid-1 receptor. Reproduced from Vaughn, S. E., et al. The impact of marijuana on antidepressant treatment in adolescents: clinical and pharmacologic considerations. *J Pers Med* 2021; 11(7): 615.

- There is also a direct link between serotonin (5-HT) signaling and the endocannabinoid system. Long-term cannabinoid administration alters the 5-HT receptor signaling, upregulating 5-HT_{2A} activity and down-regulating 5-HT_{1A} activity (Hill et al. 2006)

- THC is an agonist at CB_1 receptors, which may result in increased appetite, decreased working memory, and the euphoria associated with intoxication, whereas THC also agonizes CB_2 and 5-HT_3, potentially conferring antiemetic properties (Pertwee 2008)
- Cannabis use decreases dopamine synthesis, and this effect may persist and manifest clinically as amotivation. Dopaminergic interventions may be helpful in addressing this
- N-acetylcysteine has demonstrated efficacy in adolescents and young adults with cannabis-use disorders and is generally well tolerated
- Concomitant medications can affect CYP2D6 activity, and these include strong inhibitors such as fluoxetine. This is important when considering adjunctive medications such as aripiprazole which is metabolized by CYP2D6

Tips and pearls

- Cannabis use is prevalent in adolescents with depressive disorders and is increasing (Weinberger et al. 2020). Screening for substance use is critical in adolescents presenting with affective, anxiety, and psychotic symptoms
- For patients treated with sertraline and es/citalopram, clinicians should consider the impact of cannabinoids on SSRI exposure, given interactions with CYP2C19
- In patients who are heavily using cannabis, side effects may be confounded by the effects of cannabis use or withdrawal, as well as interactions with SSRI pharmacotherapy
- Amotivation is common in adolescents who are heavily using cannabis. Clinicians should attempt to disentangle how amotivation relates to the side-effect profile of the medication or cannabis use. Motivational enhancement therapy may be helpful here. However, for many adolescents, secondary to delays in prefrontal cortical development, insight into substance-use-related impairment, complications, and effects is often impaired

Mechanism of action moment

- Bupropion has weak blocking properties for the dopamine transporter (DAT) and for the norepinephrine transporter (NET) (Foley et al. 2006). Some of its effects may be explained in part by the more potent inhibitory properties of its metabolites:
  - Bupropion is metabolized to multiple active metabolites, some of which are not only more potent NET inhibitors than

bupropion itself and equally potent DAT inhibitors, but are also concentrated in the brain. The most potent of these is the + enantiomer of the 6-hydroxy metabolite of bupropion, also known as radafaxine

- Norepinephrine–dopamine reuptake inhibitors (NDRIs), like bupropion, block the transporters for both NETs and DATs. However, depending on the site of action, they have differing effects. In the prefrontal cortex, NET blockade increases synaptic norepinephrine. But, because the prefrontal cortex lacks dopamine transporters, norepinephrine transporters transport dopamine. Because of this, NET blockade also increases synaptic dopamine in the prefrontal cortex (Figure 13.8)

NDRI action in prefrontal cortex: NET blockade increases NE and DA

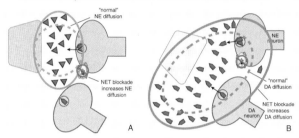

**NDRI action in striatum:
DAT blockade increases DA**

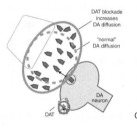

Figure 13.8 Norepinephrine–dopamine reuptake inhibitor actions in prefrontal cortex and striatum. Norepinephrine–dopamine reuptake inhibitors (NDRIs) block the transporters for both norepinephrine (NETs) and dopamine (DATs). (A) NET blockade in the prefrontal cortex leads to an increase in synaptic norepinephrine (NE), thus increasing its diffusion radius. (B) Because the prefrontal cortex lacks DATs, and NETs transport dopamine (DA) as well as NE, NET blockade also leads to an increase in synaptic DA in the prefrontal cortex, further increasing its diffusion radius. Thus, despite the absence of DAT in the prefrontal cortex, NDRIs still increase DA there. (C) DAT is present in the striatum, and thus DAT inhibition increases DA diffusion there. Reproduced from *Stahl's Essential Psychopharmacology*, 2021.

- Bupropion is generally activating and lacks a significant serotonergic component to its mechanism of action
- Given its dopaminergic effects – as were leveraged in this case – bupropion is especially targeted at the symptoms of the "dopamine deficiency syndrome" and "reduced positive affect" (e.g. symptoms of loss of happiness, motivation, joy, interest, pleasure, energy, enthusiasm, and alertness)

Two-minute tutorial

- The brain makes its own cannabis-like neurotransmitters – anandamide and 2-arachidonoylglycerol (2-AG) – which bind to CB_1 and CB_2 and make up the "endocannabinoid" system – the endogenous cannabinoid system (Figure 13.9)

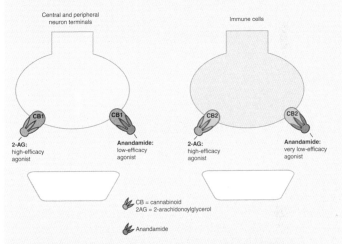

Figure 13.9 The endocannabinoid system: cannabinoid (CB) receptors and ligands. CB_1 receptors are the most abundant and are present at neuron terminals throughout the central and peripheral nervous systems. CB_2 receptors are not expressed as widely in the brain, although they are present in glial cells and in the brainstem. Instead, CB_2 receptors are primarily found in immune cells, where they modulate cell migration and cytokine release. Of the multiple endogenous cannabinoids, the best understood are anandamide and 2-arachidonoylglycerol (2-AG). Anandamide is a low-efficacy agonist at CB_1 receptors and a very low-efficacy agonist at CB_2 receptors. 2-AG is a high-efficacy agonist at both CB_1 and CB_2 receptors. Reproduced from *Stahl's Essential Psychopharmacology*, 2021.

- Both CB_1 receptors and CB_2 receptors are localized in the brain, with CB_1 receptors present in greater density. Both receptors bind both endocannabinoids, 2-AG with high efficacy and anandamide with low efficacy. CB$_2$ receptors are also in the periphery, mostly on immune cells, and bind the same two endocannabinoids

- The endocannabinoid system is tightly linked with neurotransmitter regulation and, in particular, dopaminergic functioning (Bloomfield et al. 2016) (Figure 13.10)

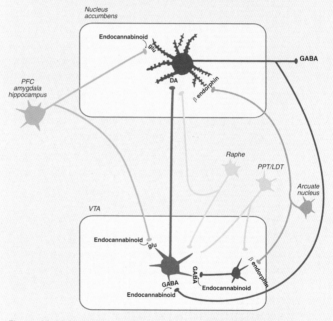

Figure 13.10 Neurotransmitter regulation of mesolimbic reward. The mesolimbic dopamine pathway is modulated by many naturally occurring substances in the brain to deliver normal reinforcement to adaptive behaviors – "natural highs." These neurotransmitter inputs to the reward system include endorphins, endocannabinoids (e.g. anandamide), acetylcholine, and others. Cannabinoids bypass the brain's endocannabinoid system and directly stimulate the brain's receptors in the reward system, causing dopamine release and a consequent "artificial high." Thus, alcohol, opioids, stimulants, cannabis, benzodiazepines, sedative-hypnotics, hallucinogens, and nicotine affect this mesolimbic dopaminergic system. Abbreviations: 5-HT, serotonin; ACh, acetylcholine; DA, dopamine; GABA, gamma-aminobutyric acid; glu, glutamine; mGluR, metabotropic glutamate receptor; NMDA, N-methyl-D-aspartate; PFC, prefrontal cortex; PPT/LDT, pedunculopontine tegmentum/laterodorsal tegmentum; VTA, ventral tegmental area. Reproduced from *Stahl's Essential Psychopharmacology*, 2021.

- ○ The mesolimbic dopamine pathway is modulated by multiple naturally occurring substances in the brain (e.g. endocannabinoids) in order to deliver normal reinforcement to adaptive behaviors – "natural highs"
- ○ In a small PET study, the availability of CB_1 receptors in the prefrontal cortex is a significant determinant of DA release within both the ventral and dorsal reward corticostriatal circuit (Ceccarini et al. 2022)
- Cannabis is a mixture of hundreds of chemicals and over 100 alkaloid cannabinoids
  - ○ The most important of these are THC and CBD
  - ○ THC interacts with CB_1 and CB_2 receptors and has psychoactive properties. CBD is an isomer of THC and relatively inactive at CB_1 and CB_2 receptors
  - ○ CBD does not have psychoactive properties, and its mechanism of action is unknown. Cannabis comes in various mixtures of THC and CBD. Higher CBD content generally has a lower risk of hallucinations, delusions, and memory impairment
- Over time, cannabis has become more potent in terms of more THC and less CBD (Cascini et al. 2012)
- Recent years have led to a search for potential therapeutic uses of cannabis in general and THC and CBD (Incze et al. 2021). However, the problem with "medical marijuana" is that it is not a prescription option that can be developed according to the standards of prescription medication. Those standards require the therapeutic agent's consistent, pure, well-defined chemical formulation, whereas medical marijuana is an unprocessed plant containing 500 chemicals with 100+ cannabinoids. Prescription drugs require a consistent, well-defined pharmacokinetic profile, safety and efficacy data from double-blind, placebo-controlled, randomized clinical trials, and warnings for all potential side effects. However, medical marijuana contains compounds that vary from plant to plant, with residual impurities such as pesticides and fungal contaminants. Further, dosing is not well regulated

Post test question

Cannabis increases the concentrations of which medication in adolescents?

A. Vilazodone (Viibryd)
B. Aripiprazole (Abilify)
C. Fluoxetine (Prozac)

D. Sertraline (Zoloft)

E. All of the above

Answer: D (Sertraline, Zoloft)

CBD and THC increase concentrations of CYP2C19-metabolized SSRIs, including es/citalopram and sertraline (D). Using CBD and/ or THC likely increases sertraline and es/citalopram concentrations in adolescents and may increase the risk of concentration-related SSRI side effects (Vaughn et al. 2021). Paroxetine (A) and fluoxetine (C) are metabolized primarily by CYP2D6 and are less likely to be affected by THC or CBD. Venlafaxine (B) is also primarily metabolized by CYP2D6 and does not appear to be substantially influenced by concomitant THC or CBD.

References

1. Babson, K. A., Sottile, J., Morabito, D. Cannabis, cannabinoids and sleep: a review of the literature. *Curr Psychiatry Rep* 2017; 19(4): 23. https://doi.org/10.1007/s11920-017-0775-9

2. Bloomfield, M. A. P., Ashok, A. H., Volkow, N. D., et al. The effects of δ9-tetrahydrocannabinol on the dopamine system. *Nature* 2016; 539(7629): 369–77. https://doi.org/10.1038/nature20153

3. Bloomfield, M. A. P., Morgan, C. J. A., Kapur, S., et al. The link between dopamine function and apathy in cannabis users: an [18 F]-DOPA PET imaging study. *Psychopharmacology (Berl)* 2014; 231(11): 2251–59. https://doi.org/10.1007/s00213-014-3523-4

4. Cascini, F., Aiello, C., Di Tanna, G. Increasing delta-9-tetrahydrocannabinol (δ -9-THC) content in herbal cannabis over time: systematic review and meta-analysis. *Curr Drug Abuse Rev* 2012; 5(1): 32–40. https://doi.org/10.2174/1874473711205010032

5. Ceccarini, J., Koole, M., Van Laere, K. Cannabinoid receptor availability modulates the magnitude of dopamine release in vivo in the human reward system: a preliminary multitracer positron emission tomography study. *Addict Biol* 2022; 27(3): e13167. https://doi.org/10.1111/adb.13167

6. Desrosiers, N. A., Himes, S. K., Scheidweiler, K. B., et al. Phase I and II cannabinoid disposition in blood and plasma of occasional and frequent smokers following controlled smoked cannabis. *Clin Chem* 2014; 60(4): 631–43. https://doi.org/10.1373/clinchem.2013.216507

7. Foley, K. F., DeSanty, K. P., Kast, R. E. Bupropion: pharmacology and therapeutic applications. *Expert Rev Neurother* 2006; 6(9): 1249–65. https://doi.org/10.1586/14737175.6.9.1249

8. Gray, K. M., Carpenter, M. J., Baker, N. L., et al. A double-blind randomized controlled trial of N-acetylcysteine in cannabis-dependent adolescents. *Am J Psychiatry* 2012; 169(8): 805–12. https://doi.org/10.1176/appi.ajp.2012.12010055

9. Grotenhermen, F. Pharmacokinetics and pharmacodynamics of cannabinoids. *Clin Pharmacokinet* 2003; 42(4): 327–60. https://doi.org/10.2165/00003088-200342040-00003

10. Hill, M. N., Sun, J. C., Tse, M. T. L., et al. Altered responsiveness of serotonin receptor subtypes following long-term cannabinoid treatment. *Int J Neuropsychopharmacol* 2006; 9(3): 277–86. https://doi.org/10.1017/S1461145705005651

11. Incze, M. A., Kelley, A. T., Singer, P. M. Heterogeneous state cannabis policies: potential implications for patients and health care professionals. *JAMA* 2021; 326(23): 2363–64. https://doi.org/10.1001/jama.2021.21182

12. Pertwee, R. G. The diverse CB1 and CB2 receptor pharmacology of three plant cannabinoids: delta9-tetrahydrocannabinol, cannabidiol and delta9-tetrahydrocannabivarin. *Br J Pharmacol* 2008; 153(2): 199–215. https://doi.org/10.1038/sj.bjp.0707442

13. Silins, E., Horwood, L. J., Patton, G. C., et al. Young adult sequelae of adolescent cannabis use: an integrative analysis. *Lancet Psychiatry* 2014; 1(4): 286–93. https://doi.org/10.1016/S2215-0366(14)70307-4

14. Strougo, A., Zuurman, L., Roy, C., et al. Modelling of the concentration-effect relationship of THC on central nervous system parameters and heart rate: insight into its mechanisms of action and a tool for clinical research and development of cannabinoids. *J Psychopharmacol* 2008; 22(7): 717–26. https://doi.org/10.1177/0269881108089870

15. Vaughn, S. E., Strawn, J. R., Poweleit, E. A., et al. The impact of marijuana on antidepressant treatment in adolescents: clinical and pharmacologic considerations. *J Pers Med* 2021a; 11(7): 615. https://doi.org/10.3390/jpm11070615

16. Weinberger, A. H., Zhu, J., Lee, J., et al. Cannabis use among youth in the United States, 2004–2016: faster rate of increase among youth with depression. *Drug Alcohol Depend* 2020; 209: 107894. https://doi.org/10.1016/j.drugalcdep.2020.107894

17. Zuurman, L., Ippel, A. E., Moin, E., et al. Biomarkers for the effects of cannabis and THC in healthy volunteers. *Br J Clin Pharmacol* 2009; 67(1): 5–21. https://doi.org/10.1111/j.1365-2125.2008.03329.x

Case 14: The boy whose bed was always wet: nocturnal enuresis in a child

The Question: What is the role of pharmacotherapy in managing nocturnal enuresis in children?

The Psychopharmacological Dilemma: Views on when and how to use pharmacotherapy in children with nocturnal enuresis vary considerably among clinicians

Pretest self-assessment question

Which of the following represents a first-line evidence-based pharmacologic intervention for a child with nocturnal enuresis?

A. Fluoxetine (Prozac)
B. Desvenlafaxine (Pristiq)
C. Desmopressin (DDAVP)
D. Imipramine (Tofranil)
E. All of the above

Answer: Desmopressin (DDAVP)

Patient evaluation on intake

- 10-year-old boy with attention-deficit hyperactivity disorder (ADHD), combined presentation (*Diagnostic and Statistical Manual of Mental Disorders, DSM-5* criteria), and frequent bedwetting
- He is having difficulty as his friends were able to attend an overnight camp last year and are going again this year, and he continues to be unable to spend the night at friends' houses because of his bedwetting
- He wets the bed approximately five or six nights per week
- There is no daytime enuresis, and he denies irritative voiding symptoms
- ADHD symptoms are well controlled
- He denies depressive and anxiety symptoms
- He denies nightmares

Psychiatric history

- History of attention-deficit hyperactivity disorder (ADHD), combined presentation, has been stably treated for 2 years, and experiences minimal symptoms currently
- He does well at school, although he takes tests in a quiet room with several other individuals because of his ADHD
- He takes viloxazine 200 mg each morning for his ADHD
- His parents have used a "bell and pad" system to address his nocturnal enuresis. However, this has been ineffective

Social and personal history

- He lives with his mother, father, and an older brother, who will be leaving for college later this year. He reports a close relationship with his older brother
- He is in the third grade and earns Bs. He has no Individualized Education Plan (IEP) or 504 Plan
- He plays video games and enjoys watching YouTube videos in his free time. He participates in limited physical activity
- There is no history of abuse or trauma

Medical history

- Delivered at 40 weeks to a 36-year-old mother and 38-year-old father
- Developmental milestones were within normal limits
- He has occasional headaches, but these are not migraines
- There is no history of urinary tract infections, neurogenic bladder, sleep disorder, genitourinary malformation or obstruction

Family history

- Father with no psychiatric history, although he had nocturnal enuresis as a child and was treated with amitriptyline in the 1980s for his enuresis
- Mother with a history of adjustment-related depressive symptoms when in high school
- No family history of diabetes mellitus or insipidus

Medication history

- Extended-release viloxazine (200 mg each morning)

Current medications

- Extended-release viloxazine (200 mg each morning)

Psychotherapy history

- He has never been in psychotherapy

Further investigation

Is there anything else that you would like to know about the patient? What about details related to caffeine intake?

- His parents allow him to have one caffeinated beverage daily, and he generally drinks this in the evening. Each can contains approximately 55 mg of caffeine

What about additional physical symptoms and vital signs?

- Vital signs are within normal limits; his weight is 36 kg; his body mass index (BMI) is in the 75th percentile for age and sex

Attending physician's mental notes: initial psychiatric evaluation

- The patient has nocturnal enuresis (enuresis, nocturnal only [*DSM-5*]) and secondary withdrawal from normal age-related activities, including overnights with friends and summer camp
- The attending physician enquired about anxiety and fear of the dark (specific phobia, environmental type). In some patients, fear of the dark may prevent them from leaving their beds to go to the bathroom
- Caffeine decreases the release of vasopressin (antidiuretic hormone) and viloxazine inhibits CYP1A2, which results in a sixfold increase in caffeine concentrations (Figure 14.1). The physician is concerned that this could potentiate his nocturnal enuresis

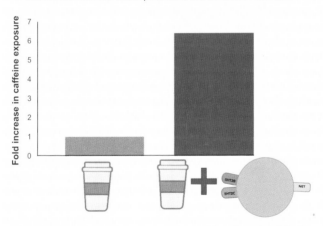

Figure 14.1 Caffeine exposure in patients taking viloxazine (blue) and those not taking viloxazine (green).

Question

Given his prior psychotherapy and current pharmacologic treatment, which of the following would be your next step?

- Discontinue viloxazine
- Begin imipramine 25 mg every night at bedtime
- Begin sublingual desmopressin 0.2 mg for one week, then 0.4 mg every night at bedtime
- Obtain a computed tomography (CT) scan of the abdomen, and pelvis and renal ultrasound

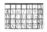

Case outcome: first follow-up (week 4)

- Since beginning desmopressin 0.4 mg every night at bedtime, he has done markedly better
- He has also stopped drinking caffeinated beverages following a discussion about the interaction between viloxazine and caffeine
- He has been adherent in limiting fluid intake to a minimum from 1 hour before administration until the next morning or at least 8 hours after desmopressin administration
- He is excited to spend the night at his cousin's house next week

Attending physician's mental notes: first follow-up (4 weeks)

- The attending physician selected desmopressin based on multiple double-blind, placebo-controlled trials of patients with primary nocturnal enuresis (Glazener and Evans 2002; Keten et al. 2020). In the first of these studies, patients (N = 329) were 5–17 years old and 72% male. Following a 2-week baseline in which the average number of wet nights was 10 (range 4–14), patients were randomized to receive 0.2, 0.4, or 0.6 mg of desmopressin or placebo (Table 14.1). The second study involved intranasal desmopressin and was positive. However, intranasal desmopressin is no longer recommended for pediatric patients secondary to reports of hyponatremic seizures

Table 14.1 Response to desmopressin acetate tablets and placebo at 2 weeks of treatment: mean (SE) number of wet nights/2 weeks

	Placebo (n = 85)	0.2 mg (n = 79)	0.4 mg (n = 82)	0.6 mg (n = 83)
Baseline	10 (0.3)	11 (0.3)	10 (0.3)	10 (0.3)
Reduction from baseline	1 (0.3)	3 (0.4)	3 (0.4)	4 (0.4)
Percentage reduction from baseline	10%	27%	30%	40%
p-Value vs. placebo	–	<0.05	<0.05	<0.05

Patients treated with desmopressin acetate tablets showed a statistically significant reduction in the number of wet nights compared to placebo-treated patients. A greater response was observed with increasing doses up to 0.6 mg.

- The attending physician did not choose to prescribe imipramine or another tricyclic antidepressant (TCA) as these are no longer first-line medication treatments for enuresis, although he is aware that double-blind, placebo controlled trials for imipramine suggest its efficacy in nocturnal enuresis (Caldwell et al. 2016; Shaffer et al. 1968). Additionally, the attending physician is aware of several tragic fatal overdoses in children who took the entire bottle of imipramine, hoping that, unlike several tablets which would work for a night, the whole bottle might cure their nocturnal enuresis (Mikkelsen 2021)

Take-home points

- In most patients, nocturnal enuresis typically has a high rate of spontaneous remission and remits between ages 5 and 7. Most affected children experience spontaneous remission, and cases of nocturnal enuresis persisting into adolescence are generally rare
- When evaluating a child with enuresis, obtain a thorough history paying particular attention to developmental milestones and behavioral interventions. This evaluation should also focus on anxiety. For example, in some children, fear of the dark may produce nocturnal enuresis, given that the child is afraid to get up from bed to go to the bathroom
- In evaluating nocturnal enuresis, many clinicians use a calendar tracking method to record the frequency of these events. This is also helpful in establishing a baseline before beginning treatment
- Behavioral interventions (e.g. bell and pad conditioning) are effective and may have persistent effects after discontinuation, unlike pharmacologic interventions, wherein enuresis will typically reoccur when the medication is stopped
- Pharmacologic treatment for nocturnal enuresis began in the 1960s with imipramine. Typically, this involved 25 mg every night at bedtime and titration in 25 mg increments each week until the patient was no longer experiencing nocturnal enuresis. In general, the maximum dosage was 5 mg/kg daily. However, secondary to safety concerns, TCAs are no longer recommended
- Desmopressin is the first-line pharmacologic intervention for children with nocturnal enuresis; however, the U.S. Food and Drug Administration (FDA) alert has called attention to the potential risk of hyponatremia and seizures as well as some deaths related to intranasal desmopressin. This formulation should no longer be used in pediatric patients. Also, care should be taken not to use desmopressin in patients who are predisposed to electrolyte imbalances, and if a patient is ill with a condition that acutely may cause electrolyte imbalances, desmopressin should be held

Tips and pearls: desmopressin

- Desmopressin is FDA-approved for children and adolescents 6 years and older for primary nocturnal enuresis and is available for subcutaneous, intranasal, or sublingual administration (dissolvable sublingual strip)
- Patients should limit fluid intake to a minimum from 1 hour before administration until the next morning or at least 8 hours after administration

- The recommended starting dose is 0.2 mg orally daily at bedtime and may be titrated up to the maximum dose of 0.6 mg daily at bedtime. The desired response is typically achieved with dosages of 0.2 mg or 0.4 mg daily
- Sublingual desmopressin (Dossche et al. 2021)
  - Generally used in the pediatric population due to the ease of administration and the increased bioavailability over tablets
  - Taking desmopressin sublingually in the fasted state increases concentrations over time by 50% and similarly increases the effect on diuresis by about 50% (Dossche et al. 2021; Michelet et al. 2020)
  - Sublingual desmopressin produces peak concentrations quickly (within 1 hour, Figure 14.2 left), and its effects on diuresis can also be seen quickly. Additionally, the duration of action is approximately 8 hours compared to 6 hours with the tablet formulation (Figure 14.2 right) (Michelet et al. 2020)
- Because desmopressin increases urine concentration, it can produce hyponatremia. This risk appears to be higher with intranasal formulations, and this formulation is no longer recommended for children
- Minor adverse effects of desmopressin include headaches, tachycardia, and facial flushing
- Hyponatremia is an absolute contraindication to desmopressin, and desmopressin is also contraindicated in patients with renal impairment
- DDAVP-related diuresis varies by age (Figure 14.3)
- DDAVP's bioavailability is significantly affected by food

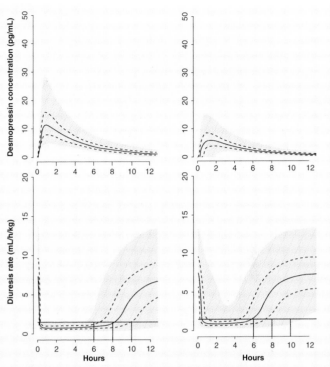

Figure 14.2 Simulation results after desmopressin sublingual formulation (left) or tablet (right). On top, the plasma concentration–time profiles are shown, whereas the pharmacodynamic response, depicted as the diuresis rate per kilogram body weight, is shown below. The horizontal line marks the target of 1.5 mL/h/kg, and the solid line marks the median response, with the shaded area representing the 90% prediction interval and the dashed lines representing the 25th–75th percentiles. Vertical lines mark the targets of 6 h effect, 8 h effect, and no more than 10 h effect. Adapted from Michelet et al. An integrated paediatric population PK/PD analysis of dDAVP: how do PK differences translate to clinical outcomes? *Clin Pharmacokinet* 2020; 59(1): 81–96.

Tips and pearls: viloxazine

- Viloxazine is an effective treatment for children and adolescents with ADHD (Johnson et al. 2020; Nasser et al. 2021)
- Viloxazine dosing varies by age:
  - Ages 6–11: 100–400 mg once daily
- Initial dose 100 mg once daily; can increase by 100 mg each week; maximum recommended dose 400 mg once daily
  - Ages 12–17: 200–400 mg once daily
  - Adults: 200–600 mg once daily

- Viloxazine is metabolized by CYP2D6, UGT1A9, and UGT2B15, has a half-life of 7 hours, and is a potent inhibitor of CYP1A2, which significantly increases caffeine exposure. Additionally, viloxazine is a weak inhibitor of CYP2D6 and CYP3A4 (Findling et al. 2021; Yu et al. 2020)

Mechanism of action moment

- Arginine vasopressin (AVP), which is also known as antidiuretic hormone (ADH), stimulates the kidneys to conserve water, but not sodium. In effect, urine is concentrated, and urine volume is reduced. However, caffeine decreases the release of vasopressin
- Desmopressin acts as an agonist at the renal collecting duct by binding to Vasopressin$_2$ (V$_2$) receptor. These receptors trigger the translocation of aquaporin channels to the apical membrane of the collecting duct and these channels increase water reabsorption from the urine

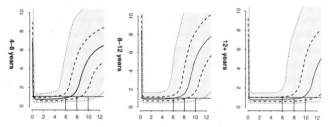

Figure 14.3 Desmopressin-related diuresis by age. Note desmopressin was administered at time '0' and the y-axis is diuresis (mL/kg/h); the horizontal line represents the target urine output (1 mL/h/kg for children older than 2 years of age), and the solid line represents the median response. Shading represents the 90% prediction interval, and the dashed lines are the 25th–75th percentiles. The targets of 6 h effect, 8 h effect, and no more than 10 h effect are shown by vertical lines. Adapted from Michelet et al. An integrated paediatric population PK/PD analysis of dDAVP: how do PK differences translate to clinical outcomes? *Clin Pharmacokinet* 2020; 59(1): 81–96.

Two-minute tutorial

- Nocturnal enuresis is common in children and decreases with increased age
- Children with nocturnal enuresis fail to decrease urine production (Figure 14.4) and fail to concentrate their urine overnight (Figure 14.4) (Rittig et al. 1989), which potentially is the pathophysiologic target of DDAVP, the synthetic analog of vasopressin first developed four decades ago

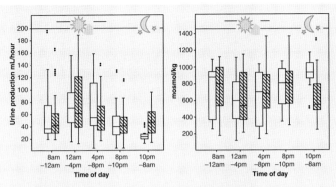

Figure 14.4 Diurnal variation in urine production (left) and urinary osmolality (right) in patients with nocturnal enuresis (shaded) and those without (open bars). Adapted from Rittig, S., et al. Abnormal diurnal rhythm of plasma vasopressin and urinary output in patients with enuresis. *Am J Physiol* 1989; 256(4 Pt 2): F664-71.

Post test question

Which of the following represents a first-line evidence-based pharmacologic intervention for a child with nocturnal enuresis?

A. Fluoxetine (Prozac)

B. Desvenlafaxine (Pristiq)

C. Desmopressin (DDAVP)

D. Imipramine (Tofranil)

E. All of the above

Answer: C (Desmopressin)

Fluoxetine (A) and desvenlafaxine (B) have not been evaluated as treatments for nocturnal enuresis. Desmopressin has demonstrated efficacy in multiple placebo-controlled trials and is approved by the FDA for the treatment of primary nocturnal enuresis in children aged 6 years and older. While imipramine (D) has efficacy for the treatment of enuresis in pediatric patients, its safety profile limits its use. Additionally, fatal imipramine overdoses have been observed in children with enuresis, and TCAs require baseline and follow-up electrocardiogram (EKG) monitoring in children and adolescents.

References

1. Caldwell, P. H. Y., Sureshkumar, P., Wong, W. C. F. Tricyclic and related drugs for nocturnal enuresis in children. *Cochrane Database Syst Rev* 2016; 2016(1): CD002117. https://doi.org/10.1002/14651858.CD002117.pub2

2. Dossche, L., Michelet, R., de Bruyne, P., et al. Desmopressin oral lyophilisate in young children: new insights in pharmacokinetics

and pharmacodynamics. *Arch Dis Childhood* 2021; 106: 597–602. https://doi.org/10.1136/archdischild-2019-318225

3. Findling, R. L., Candler, S. A., Nasser, A. F., et al. Viloxazine in the management of CNS disorders: a historical overview and current status. *CNS Drugs* 2021; 35(6): 643–53. https://doi.org/10.1007/s40263-021-00825-w

4. Glazener, C. M. A., Evans, J. H. C. Desmopressin for nocturnal enuresis in children. *Cochrane Database Syst Rev* 2002; 2010(1): CD002112. https://doi.org/10.1002/14651858.CD002112

5. Johnson, J. K., Liranso, T., Saylor, K., et al. A phase II double-blind, placebo-controlled, efficacy and safety study of SPN-812 (extended-release viloxazine) in children with ADHD. *J Atten Disord* 2020; 24(2): 348–58. https://doi.org/10.1177/1087054719836159

6. Keten, T., Aslan, Y., Balci, M., et al. Comparison of the efficacy of desmopressin fast-melting formulation and enuretic alarm in the treatment of monosymptomatic nocturnal enuresis. *J Pediatr Urol* 2020; 16(5): P645.E1–E7. https://doi.org/10.1016/j.jpurol.2020.07.018

7. Michelet, R., Dossche, L., van Herzeele, C. An integrated paediatric population PK/PD analysis of dDAVP: how do PK differences translate to clinical outcomes? *Clin Pharmacokin* 2020; 59(1): 81–96. https://doi.org/10.1007/s40262-019-00798-6

8. Mikkelsen, E. J. Elimination disorders. In Dulcan, M. (ed.), *Dulcan's Textbook of Child and Adolescent Psychiatry*, 3rd edn. Washington D.C.: American Psychiatric Publishing, 2021.

9. Nasser, A., Hull, J. T., Liranso, T., et al. The effect of viloxazine extended-release capsules on functional impairments associated with attention-deficit/hyperactivity disorder (ADHD) in children and adolescents in four phase 3 placebo-controlled trials. *Neuropsychiatric Dis Treat* 2021; 17: 1751–62. https://doi.org/10.2147/NDT.S312011

10. Rittig, S., Knudsen, U. B., Norgaard, J. P., Pedersen, E. B., Djurhuus, J. C. Abnormal diurnal rhythm of plasma vasopressin and urinary output in patients with enuresis. *Am J Physiol Renal Fluid Electrolyte Physiol* 1989; 256(4): F664–71. https://doi.org/10.1152/ajprenal.1989.256.4.f664

11. Shaffer, D., Costello, A. J., Hill, I. D. Control of enuresis with imipramine. *Arch Dis Childhood* 1968; 43(232): 665. https://doi.org/10.1136/adc.43.232.665

12. Yu, C., Garcia-Olivares, J., Candler, S., Schwabe, S., Maletic, V. New insights into the mechanism of action of viloxazine: serotonin and norepinephrine modulating properties. *J Exp Pharmacol* 2020; 12: 285–300. https://doi.org/10.2147/JEP.S256586

Case 15: Counting sheep and counting treatment trials: insomnia disorder in an adolescent

The Question: What is the evidence-based approach to addressing insomnia in adolescents?

The Psychopharmacological Dilemma: Managing sleep-related problems in adolescents – particularly in those with anxiety and/or depressive disorders – is complicated and requires an understanding of developmental and pharmacological principles

Pretest self-assessment question

Which of the following may be chronotropically dosed to re-entrain circadian rhythms?

A. Melatonin
B. Ramelteon
C. Suvorexant
D. Oxytocin (intranasal)

Answer: A (Melatonin)

Patient evaluation on intake

- 13-year-old adolescent with a history of persistent depressive disorder and generalized anxiety disorder who has been in remission for 18 months. However, she has significant difficulty falling asleep and typically lays in bed for 90–120 minutes prior to falling asleep
- She feels tired during the day and naps each afternoon for 30–45 minutes
- The patient and her parents are interested in a consultation for her insomnia
- She struggles to fall asleep on most nights and takes between 90 and 120 minutes to fall asleep. Clonidine 0.1 mg every night at bedtime was added by her primary care clinician and initially helped with her initial insomnia, but its effects dissipated within 1–2 weeks
- She falls asleep and stays in her own bed throughout the night
- She does not have any rocking movements at sleep onset
- Snoring does not usually occur
- Her mother does not report pauses in respiration during sleep nor hearing gasping or snorting sounds during sleep. The patient tends to breathe through her nose both while sleeping and awake. There is no history of adenotonsillectomy

- She denies hyperextending her neck, unusual sleep positions, bedwetting, sleepwalking, sleep talking, night terrors, nightmares, body pains prior to sleep onset, and teeth grinding
- She usually wakes up twice a night for about 10 minutes and cannot return to sleep easily. She will usually get out of bed and get a snack or something to drink
- She does not use her phone while in bed and occasionally reads while trying to fall asleep
- She takes naps 2–3 days per week and describes chronically feeling tired and having significant difficulty awakening in the morning
- She babysits for a neighbor on Saturday afternoons and finds it extremely difficult to awaken by 11 or 12 pm on those days
- On school days, she awakens at 6:45 am
- The clinician administers a five-item instrument known as the BEARS (B – Bedtime issues; E – Excessive daytime sleepiness; A – night Awakenings; R – Regularity and duration of sleep; and S – Snoring) and the Children's Sleep Habits Questionnaire (CSHQ) to explore sleep symptoms in detail
- The patient denies current depressive symptoms as well as anxiety
- She has no psychotic symptoms or illicit substance use
- There are no side effects associated with her fluoxetine

BEARS sleep screening tool

BEARS is divided into five major sleep domains (B = Bedtime Issues, E = Excessive Daytime Sleepiness, A = Night Awakenings, R = Regularity and Duration of Sleep, S = Snoring) and helps clinicians evaluate potential sleep problems in children 2–18 years old. Each sleep domain has a set of age-appropriate "trigger questions" for use in the clinical interview. The screen is free to use.

	Toddler/preschool (2–5 years)	School-aged (6–12 years)	Adolescent (13–18 years)
Bedtime problems	Does your child have any problems going to bed? Falling asleep?	Does your child have any problems at bedtime? (P) Do you have any problems going to bed? (C)	Do you have any problems falling asleep at bedtime? (C)
Excessive daytime sleepiness	Does your child seem overtired or sleepy a lot during the day? Does he/she still take naps?	Does your child have difficulty waking in the morning, seem sleepy during the day or take naps? (P) Do you feel tired a lot? (C)	Do you feel sleepy a lot during the day? In school? While driving? (C)
Awakenings during the night	Does your child wake up a lot at night?	Does your child seem to wake up a lot at night? Any sleepwalking or nightmares? (P) Do you wake up a lot at night? Have trouble getting back to sleep? (C)	Do you wake up a lot at night? Have trouble getting back to sleep? (C)

Regularity and duration of sleep	Does your child have a regular bedtime and wake time? What are they?	What time does your child go to bed and get up on school days? Weekends? Do you think he/she is getting enough sleep? (P)	What time do you usually go to bed on school nights? Weekends? How much sleep do you usually get? (C)
Snoring	Does your child snore a lot or have difficulty breathing at night?	Does your child have loud or nightly snoring or any breathing difficulties at night? (P)	Does your teenager snore loudly or nightly? (P)

(P) Parent-directed question (C) Child-directed question

Source: A Clinical Guide to Pediatric Sleep: Diagnosis and Management of Sleep Problems by Jodi A. Mindell and Judith A. Owens, Lippincott Williams & Wilkins

Psychiatric history

- Generalized anxiety disorder, onset 3 years ago
- Depressive symptoms began 2 years ago and have never met criteria for a major depressive episode
- No psychotic symptoms have been present, and there is no history of suicide attempts or self-injurious behavior
- There is no history of mania

Social and personal history

- She lives with her mother, father, and maternal grandmother, as well as her older and younger sisters
- She is in the eighth grade and earns Bs
- She has no Individualized Education Plan (IEP) or 504 Plan
- She babysits for a neighbor once weekly
- She plays volleyball on a recreational team and at her middle school
- There is no history of abuse or trauma

Medical history

- She was delivered at 36 weeks, 1 day, and has a twin sister
- She had in-utero growth restriction (IUGR) and a birthweight of 1400 g, and was hospitalized in the neonatal intensive care unit (NICU) for 10 days, but the only NICU interventions were 1 day of phototherapy for mild hyperbilirubinemia and supplemented breastmilk
- Her mother's pregnancy was further remarkable for cholestasis
- She has a peanut allergy and seasonal allergies and eczema
- She had normal developmental milestones

- She had COVID-19 at the age of 12½ and had mild upper-respiratory symptoms, including cough and congestion, and significant fatigue, as well as difficulties with concentration which resolved over 4–5 months

Family history

- Attention-deficit hyperactivity disorder (ADHD) in her father, maternal grandmother, and maternal aunt
- Anxiety in her mother and paternal grandmother
- Obsessive compulsive disorder (OCD), panic disorder, and depressive disorder in her maternal aunt
- There is no family history of completed suicide

Medication history

- Fluoxetine (Prozac) 60 mg daily
- Clonidine 0.1 mg every night at bedtime
- Melatonin 12 mg every night at bedtime

Current medications

- Fluoxetine (Prozac) 60 mg daily
- Clonidine 0.1 mg every night at bedtime
- Melatonin 12 mg every night at bedtime

Psychotherapy history

- The patient was seen in Cognitive Behavior Therapy (CBT) for her generalized anxiety disorder and persistent depressive disorder and did exceptionally well with this
- She completed psychotherapy and described using both skills that she learned in psychotherapy and also being able to still identify thinking patterns related to her anxiety (e.g. black-and-white thinking, fortune telling, discounting, overgeneralizing)

Further investigation

Is there anything else that you would like to know about the patient? What about caffeine use?

- She drinks an iced coffee each morning and two sodas per day, which each contain approximately 85 mg of caffeine

What about additional questionnaires to assess her daytime sleepiness?

Rating scales

EPWORTH SLEEPINESS SCALE QUESTIONNAIRE

Sitting and reading	High chance
Watching television	Slight chance
Sitting inactive in a public place (e.g. movie theater)	Slight chance
As a passenger in a car for an hour without a break	Slight chance
Lying down to rest in the afternoon when circumstances permit	High chance
Sitting and talking to someone	Slight chance
Sitting quietly after lunch	Slight chance
In a car, while stopped for a few minutes in traffic	Slight chance
Epworth Sleepiness Scale Score	12 (Excessive Daytime Sleepiness)

What about vitals?

- Her blood pressure is 120/72, heart rate is 89, weight is 67.6 kg, height is 166.5 cm and respiratory rate is 16

What about laboratory studies?

Testing: laboratory results, imaging, EKGs

CBC with Differential

	Value	Ref Range
WBC	4.0	4.5-13.0 K/mcL
RBC	4.67	4.50-5.30 M/mcL
HGB	13.2	13.0-16.0 gm/dL
HCT	39.0	37.0-49.0 %
MCV	82.8	78.0-94.0 fL
MCH	28.1	25.0-35.0 pg
MCHC	33.9	31.0-37.0 gm/dL
RDW	14.1	$\leq$14.6 %
PLATELET	199	135-466 K/mcL

Comp Metabolic Panel

	Value	Ref Range
SODIUM	140	136-145 mmol/L
POTASSIUM	4	3.3-4.7 mmol/L
CHLORIDE	108	100-112 mmol/L
CO2	24	17-31 mmol/L
ANION GAP	11	4-15 mmol/L
BUN	8	6-21 mg/dL
CREATININE	0.6	0.5-1.0 mg/dL
GLUCOSE	76	65-106 mg/dL
CALCIUM	9	8.3-10.6 mg/dL
PHOSPHORUS	3.6	2.8-5.1 mg/dL
ALBUMIN	4.1	3.3-4.8 gm/dL

TSH		
	Value	Ref Range
Thyroid Stimulating Hormone	3.1	0.43-4.0 mcIU/mL

Vitamin D		
	Value	Ref Range
25-OH-Vit-D	34 mg/dL	30-60 mg/dL

Iron Studies		
	Value	Ref Range
Total iron	35 mg/dL	Male: 59-158 µg/dL Female:37-145 µg/dL
TIBC	314	250-425 µg/dL
transferrin saturation	30	20-50% (male), 15-50% (female)
transferrin	308	200-360 mg/dL

Attending physician's mental notes: initial psychiatric evaluation

- This attending physician has paid particular attention to the patient's depressive and anxiety symptoms and was careful to assess whether they are in full remission. The attending physician is aware that up to three-quarters of depressed children and 90% of depressed adolescents report sleep disturbances, including initial, middle, and terminal insomnia, as well as hypersomnia
- Successful treatment of depression fails to relieve dyssomnia in 10% of children. Such sleep problems that persist after successfully treating the depressive episode may increase the risk of having another depressive episode (Skoch 2022)
- The attending physician is also aware that sleep problems are common among children and adolescents with anxiety disorders. Anxious children may fear sleeping alone, fear darkness/night-time, and experience separation worries (that are more pronounced at night). Having an anxiety disorder is also significantly associated with an increased risk of insomnia; however, anxiety symptoms precede a diagnosis of insomnia more than two-thirds of the time (Alfano et al. 2007). Moreover, sleep problems and anxiety symptoms may have a reciprocal influence on one another; tiredness that results from sleep problems can exacerbate anxiety, which further worsens sleep problems. In addition, many of the selective serotonin reuptake inhibitors (SSRIs) – which are the first-line pharmacotherapy for pediatric anxiety disorders – may influence sleep in anxious children and adolescents (Skoch et al. 2021)

- The attending physician has paid particular attention to snoring or her parents hearing gasping or snorting sounds, which could suggest obstructive airway pathology
- The attending physician has also assessed for parasomnias and associated symptoms
- The attending physician is aware that phase shifts in circadian rhythms are common in patients with depressive disorder (Figure 15.1)

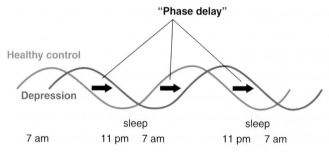

Figure 15.1 Depression can cause phase delay in circadian rhythms of sleep/wake cycles. Circadian rhythms describe events that occur on a 24-hour cycle. Many biological systems follow a circadian rhythm; in particular, circadian rhythms are key to the regulation of sleep/wake cycles. In patients with depression, the circadian rhythm is often "phase delayed," which means that because wakefulness is not promoted in the morning, such patients tend to sleep later. They also have trouble falling asleep at night, which further promotes feelings of sleepiness during the day. Reproduced from *Stahl's Essential Psychopharmacology*, 2021.

- The attending physician considers puberty-associated changes in chronotype. Adolescents and young adults are at high risk of "social jet lag," given their delayed circadian rhythms
- In adolescents, social jet lag results from a conflict between the biologically driven late phase of circadian entrainment (i.e. preference for later bedtimes) and the forced early awakening required by early start times for most schools. Additionally, on days when the adolescent doesn't have to awaken early (e.g. weekends) – as in our patient's case – the patient awakens later because of: (1) her later circadian phase and (2) her need to catch up to rectify sleep debt from the prior week
- The attending physician is also concerned about her caffeine intake, which may perpetuate her dyssomnia (Orbeta et al. 2006; Owens et al. 2014) and knows that caffeine, as an antagonist at purine

receptors, results in reduced adenosine from binding. Because these receptors are functionally coupled to post-synaptic dopamine receptors, this will enhance dopaminergic effects, and potentiate wakefulness (Figure 15.2)

Mechanism of action of caffeine: DA actions at D2 receptors

Adenosine and endogenous purines reduce DA binding

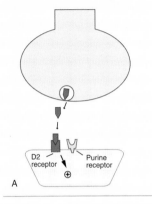
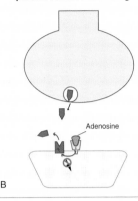

Caffeine antagonizes adenosine binding and enhances DA actions

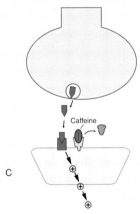

Figure 15.2 Caffeine and its effects on dopamine. Caffeine is an antagonist at purine receptors, and in particular adenosine receptors. (A) These receptors are functionally coupled with certain postsynaptic dopamine (DA) receptors, such as dopamine D_2 receptors, at which dopamine binds and has a stimulatory effect. (B) When adenosine binds to its receptors, this causes reduced sensitivity of D_2 receptors. (C) Antagonism of adenosine receptors by caffeine prevents adenosine from binding there, and thus can enhance dopaminergic actions. Adapted from *Stahl's Essential Psychopharmacology,* 2021.

- Finally, the attending physician has noted the dose of melatonin (12 mg), which is profoundly supraphysiologic. Given this, he is concerned that it is doing very little at this dose
- Regarding the patient's clonidine, it is commonly used to treat insomnia in children, although the evidence for clonidine is relatively limited

Question

Which of the following would be the most appropriate intervention after attempting to address the patient's insomnia through behavioral interventions?

- A trial of an antihistamine
- A trial of zolpidem (Ambien) 5 mg every night at bedtime
- Chloral hydrate 1 g orally every night at bedtime
- Discontinuation of fluoxetine (Prozac) and cross-titration to mirtazapine (Remeron) 7.5 mg every night at bedtime

Interim visit: week 4

- Since her last visit, cognitive behavioral therapy for insomnia (CBT-I) has been implemented, and she continues to report significant initial insomnia
- She has discontinued clonidine and a trial of diphenhydramine 50 mg every night at bedtime has been used, which initially produced some improvement, but its effect was no longer apparent after 2 weeks

Attending physician's mental notes: interim visit (week 4)

- Histamine antagonists such as diphenhydramine (Figure 15.3) – which promote sleep by blocking the wakefulness-promoting (Figure 15.4) and circadian-related effects of histamine – are the most commonly used medications to treat pediatric insomnia, despite a dearth of data from prospective trials (Owens et al. 2010)
- In one small study, diphenhydramine (1 mg/kg) at bedtime reduced sleep latency and night-time awakenings and increased sleep duration in 2–12-year-olds with similar effects observed in pediatric burn patients (Russo et al. 1976)
- Importantly, the attending physician is also aware that tachyphylaxis – a phenomenon that occurs when the body

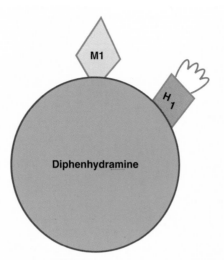

Figure 15.3 Diphenhydramine is a histamine 1 (H_1) receptor antagonist commonly used as a hypnotic. However, this agent is not selective for H_1 receptors and thus can also have additional effects. Specifically, diphenhydramine is also a muscarinic 1 (M_1) receptor antagonist and thus can have anticholinergic effects (blurred vision, constipation, memory problems, dry mouth). Adapted from *Stahl's Essential Psychopharmacology*, 2021.

becomes less responsive to the medication over time – results in a decreased hypnotic effect of diphenhydramine. This can be due to various pharmacologic and pharmacodynamic processes, such as a decrease in the number of H_1 receptors or the development of tolerance. Tachyphylaxis can occur with a variety of medications, including antihistamines, and may be more likely to occur with long-term use

PATIENT FILE

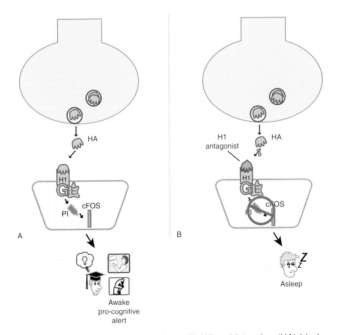

Figure 15.4 Histamine 1 antagonism. (A) When histamine (HA) binds to postsynaptic histamine 1 (H_1) receptors, it activates a G-protein-linked second-messenger system that activates phosphatidyl inositol (PI) and the transcription factor cFOS. This results in wakefulness and normal alertness. (B) H_1 antagonists prevent activation of this second messenger and thus can cause sleepiness. Adapted from *Stahl's Essential Psychopharmacology*, 2021.

Interim follow-up visit: week 8

- At her last visit, secondary to tachyphylaxis, diphenhydramine was discontinued
- She continues to take fluoxetine 60 mg daily, and her sleep complaints are unchanged
- She has good sleep hygiene but is increasingly frustrated by her insomnia and tiredness
- Between her last visit and today, her family practitioner, at her annual well-child check, prescribed trazodone to assist with her insomnia. She has been taking 50 mg every night at bedtime and notes that she has had some improvement in her insomnia but feels increasingly tired during the day and is now requiring naps of between 2 and 2½ hours daily. She has also noted worsening of her depressive symptoms, has been more irritable and more withdrawn, and has felt increased malaise since beginning trazodone

Attending physician's mental notes: interim follow-up visit (week 8)

- Her attending physician is very concerned about the potential interaction between trazodone and fluoxetine
- Fluoxetine is a potent inhibitor of CYP2D6 and in several large multicenter trials of children and adolescents with depressive disorders who received trazodone, outcomes for depressive symptoms were significantly worse (Shamseddeen et al. 2012). In the Treatment of SSRI-Resistant Depression in Adolescents (TORDIA) study (Brent et al. 2008), when trazodone was combined with antidepressants that inhibit CYP2D6 (e.g. fluoxetine, paroxetine), none of the trazodone-treated patients improved with regard to depressive symptoms. This finding – which was replicated in a separate cohort of depressed adolescents – may relate to CYP2D6 interactions and the accumulation of methylchloropiperazine (mCPP). This trazodone metabolite is associated with dysphoria, irritability, and depression. Thus, given the coadministration of fluoxetine and trazodone, she is largely unable to metabolize mCPP

Question

After discontinuing trazodone, which of the following represents a reasonable next-step intervention?

- A trial of melatonin (low dose)
- A trial of zolpidem 5 mg every night at bedtime
- A trial of suvorexant 10 mg every night at bedtime
- Discontinuation of fluoxetine and cross-titration to mirtazapine 7.5 mg every night at bedtime

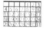

Interim follow-up visit: week 12

- Since beginning melatonin (1 mg) 4–6 hours before bedtime, she has noted improvements in sleep quality and daytime tiredness
- She continues to experience remission of her depressive and anxiety symptoms
- She reports no side effects associated with her fluoxetine
- She continues to abstain from caffeine

PATIENT FILE

Attending physician's mental notes: interim follow-up visit (week 12)

- Knowing that melatonin supplementation may be the preferred initial pharmacotherapy for sleep-onset insomnia due to its chronobiotic properties (Skoch 2022), the clinician has selected melatonin to address her insomnia
- The attending physician is aware of pediatric studies suggesting both immediate-release and extended-release melatonin improve sleep onset latency and total sleep duration (Schroder et al. 2019; van Geijlswijk et al. 2010). However, the increase in the total duration of sleep is greater with extended-release preparations (Schroder et al. 2019)
- The patient reports no side effects from the addition of melatonin, which is consistent with her attending physician's knowledge of tolerability data. Her attending physician is aware of 2-year randomized trials of prolonged-release melatonin for insomnia in pediatric patients that suggest no significant effects on growth, body mass index (BMI), and pubertal development (Malow et al. 2021; van Geijlswijk et al. 2011)

Interim follow-up visit: month 18

- She has done well in terms of school and in terms of friendships until approximately 6 months ago. However, she has experienced more daytime fatigue. She is now going to bed at 10–10:30 pm on weeknights and 11 pm to midnight on weekend nights
- She usually falls asleep within 30 minutes. She falls asleep and stays in her own bed throughout the night. She does not have any rocking movements at sleep onset
- The family continues to deny snoring, and there are no additional changes in her medical history. The family and patient report some sleep talking, leg discomfort, and leg jerking
- She awakens three to four times a night for about 15 minutes and cannot return to sleep without help. She will usually get out of bed and get a snack or something to drink
- In the morning, she awakens at 6:30 am on weekdays and 10–11 am on weekends. She wakes with difficulty and reports feeling irritable in the morning
- She denies morning headaches
- She continues to take fluoxetine 60 mg daily and melatonin

Question

Which of the following is the next best intervention?

- Discontinue melatonin
- A trial of zolpidem 5 mg every night at bedtime
- A trial of suvorexant 10 mg every night at bedtime
- Refer to sleep medicine for evaluation for sleep study

Attending physician's mental notes: interim follow-up visit (month 18)

- Her attending physician is concerned about the possibility of periodic limb movement disorder. He orders repeat iron studies and refers her for consultation with a sleep medicine specialist

Testing: laboratory results, imaging, EKGs

SLEEP STUDY

There were 464.5 minutes of total study time analyzed, of which 384.0 minutes were spent in sleep for a sleep efficiency of 82.7%.

Sleep latency was 31 minutes.

REM latency was 200.5 minutes.

There was 22.9% of the sleep time spent in REM sleep, 7.0% in NREM1, 58.6% in NREM2, and 11.5% in NREM3. There were 3 REM cycles identified during the sleep study.

There were 109 episodes of arousal for an arousal index of 17.0.

The patient spent 29.8% of the total sleep time in the supine position, with 5.2% in supine REM, 0.0% in the prone position, 0.0% on the right side, and 70.2% on the left side.

There were 195 PLMs noted during sleep, making the PLM index 30.5.

IMPRESSION

This diagnostic polysomnogram was notable for the presence of periodic limb movements of sleep. Given the associated sleep continuity disruption, this is supportive of a diagnosis of periodic limb movement disorder. The remainder of the study was generally reassuring without evidence of clinically significant central or obstructive sleep apnea (rare obstructive events followed arousals). Hypoventilation was not

present based upon end-tidal pCO2 monitoring. The
arousal index was elevated, and the proportion of
NREM 3 was lower than typically seen.

Additionally, in the sleep medicine clinic, repeat iron studies were
obtained and revealed:

Iron Studies

	Value	Ref Range
Ferritin	L 7.4	8-100 ng/mL
TIBC	H 407	280-370 mcg/dL
Percent saturation	36	15-50%
Iron level	145	19-121 mg/dL

An electrocardiogram (EKG) was also obtained:

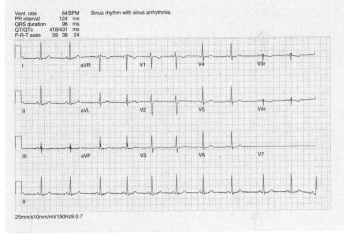

Vent. rate 64 BPM Sinus rhythm with sinus arrhythmia.
PR interval 124 ms
QRS duration 96 ms
QT/QTc 418/431 ms
P-R-T axes 59 38 24

25mm/s10mm/mV150Hz9.0.7

Interim follow-up visit: month 22

- The patient has been diagnosed with periodic limb movement
  (PLM) disorder based on the recent sleep study, which revealed a
  Periodic Limb Movement Index (PLMi) of 30.5 and associated sleep
  fragmentation
- Iron supplementation has been initiated, and the patient notes
  significant improvements in terms of sleep quality and daytime
  fatigue
- She no longer awakens overnight and continues to no longer need
  naps during the day

Take-home points

- Clinicians should consider several structured assessments for evaluating insomnia and sleep disorders in children and adolescents:
  - BEARS, a five-item instrument that evaluates the following: B – Bedtime issues; E – Excessive daytime sleepiness; A – night Awakenings; R – Regularity and duration of sleep; S – Snoring
  - The CSHQ, which explores sleep symptoms in detail
  - Two-week sleep diaries to assess sleep–wake patterns
  - A graphic sleep diary is available from http://www.sleepfoundation.org/
- When assessing sleep disorders, in addition to *DSM-5*, clinicians may consider formal criteria, such as those of the International Classification of Sleep Disorders (ICSD)
- When there are concerns related to sleep apnea or PLM disorder, consider a consultation with a sleep medicine specialist and polysomnography (PSG) (Skoch, 2022). Additionally, the Multiple Sleep Latency Test can be used to provide an objective measure of daytime sleepiness and is typically used to diagnose narcolepsy or other hypersomnias
- Regarding pharmacotherapy for insomnia disorder in children and adolescents, melatonin may have a particularly important role in circadian rhythm sleep disorders. In this regard, low-dose melatonin (0.5 mg), when timed relative to the endogenous dim light melatonin onset, is more effective in shifting sleep phase than higher doses, suggesting that timing may have a greater impact than dosage
- Variation across studies has contributed to a lack of consensus regarding pediatric melatonin dosing. For example, 0.05 mg/kg may be a minimal effective dose when given 1–2 hours prior to bedtime; however, in surveys, doses vary considerably, with typical doses of 2.5–3 mg for prepubertal children and 5 mg for adolescents
- In patients with decreased CYP1A2 activity, a lack of diurnal variation in melatonin serum concentration may decrease the effectiveness of exogenous melatonin
- In patients with depressive disorders who are treated with SSRIs that inhibit CYP2D6 or who are CYP2D6 poor metabolizers, several studies suggest that trazodone should be avoided
- Antihistamines can be helpful, but may be best used on an as-needed basis secondary to tachyphylaxis

- Zolpidem and other Z-drugs may be helpful, but their evidence is limited in pediatric patients (de Zambotti et al. 2018; Weiss and Garbutt 2010). Additionally, orexin modulators may be beneficial, although results from prospective, randomized controlled trials are not currently available in pediatric patients

Two-minute tutorial: sleep in pediatric patients

- *Sleep architecture in healthy children: middle childhood*
  - School-aged children (ages 6–12 years) typically need 9 to 10 hours of sleep over 24 hours
  - This developmental period is critical for children to develop healthy sleep habits; however, developmentally appropriate cognitive and social/emotional factors may interfere with the quality and quantity of sleep in this age group
  - Middle childhood is a time when children can understand the dangers of the outside world (i.e. violence, health problems), and this resulting anxiety can disrupt sleep. Parents are usually less involved in bedtime as children approach adolescence, leading to later bedtimes
  - At this stage, many children begin to take on more serious roles in their academic and extracurricular activities, peer relationships become more important, and electronic use (e.g. television, video games, internet, and handheld devices) increases – all of which compete with sleep
  - Frequent sleep issues during middle childhood (ages 4–12 years) include: (1) irregular sleep–wake schedules, (2) later bedtimes, (3) decreased night-time sleep, (4) increased caffeine intake, (5) parental presence at bedtime, and (6) daytime sleepiness

- *Sleep architecture in healthy adolescents:*
  - The National Sleep Foundation (NSF) recommends adolescents obtain at least 9 hours of sleep per night, with 8–10 hours being "recommended," and noting that for some adolescents, as much as 11 hours of sleep a night "may be appropriate." However, this contrasts with NSF findings from their Sleep in America Poll, which revealed that 75% of twelfth graders report <8 hours of sleep nightly
  - Many adolescents experience delayed sleep phase syndrome or delayed sleep–wake phase disorder, which involves a persistent phase shift of more than 2 hours in the sleep–wake schedule that conflicts with the adolescent's school, work, or lifestyle demands. Such circadian rhythm disorders typically result

from the poor match between the sleep–wake schedule and the demands of the adolescent's life or a failure to synchronize their internal clock with a 24-hour circadian clock

- ○ Children typically become tired after sunset, but puberty is associated with reduced slow-wave sleep and changes in circadian rhythms. As a result, a 3-hour delay (delayed phase preference) is common in adolescents
- ○ Around age 20, people become tired again after sunset and awaken earlier in the morning – a pattern driven by sunlight and the timing of melatonin release that will remain stable until the sixth decade of life

Tips and pearls

- Diagnosing and treating sleep-related problems in children and adolescents is critical, as children and teens require sufficient sleep to engage in their activities of daily living, such as academics, social relationships, and after-school commitments
- Screening questionnaires such as the CSHQ (Owens et al. 2000) and BEARS (Owens and Dalzell 2005) can be helpful in terms of addressing factors and behaviors that may contribute to sleep difficulties
- Unstructured questions related to sleep timing (bedtime, sleep onset time, variable or fixed bedtime, sleep onset latency, weekend catch-up sleep, napping during the daytime, sleeping through, wake-up time, sleep duration, sleep quality, sleepiness during daytime) can be helpful
- Techniques to promote healthy sleep in pediatric populations include setting a developmentally appropriate bedtime, a consistent wake time (weekdays and weekends), avoiding naps, avoiding caffeine, creating an environment that is soothing for sleep (dark, cool, safe, comfortable), removing of electronics from the bedroom, establishing bedtime routines and encouraging a relaxation/wind-down period before bed
- CBT-I is the recommended first-line treatment for pediatric insomnia and includes cognitive restructuring of anxious thoughts, relaxation training, stimulus control, and sleep restriction
- In certain circumstances, medication is warranted. Data regarding melatonin administration suggest that the optimal timing for melatonin administration is 4–6 hours prior to a child's preferred bedtime, and doses of 0.5–1 mg have been effective
- The use of medications such as clonidine, trazodone, diphenhydramine, and mirtazapine may be indicated for children and teens who have not responded to CBT-I or melatonin

Mechanism of action moment: melatonin

- Melatonin is secreted by the pineal gland and acts especially in the suprachiasmatic nucleus to regulate circadian rhythms. In normal physiologic settings, light is the most powerful synchronizer of circadian rhythms. When light enters through the eye it is translated via the retinohypothalamic tract to the suprachiasmatic nucleus (SCN) within the hypothalamus. The SCN, in turn, signals the pineal gland to turn off melatonin production. During darkness, there is no input from the retinohypothalamic tract to the SCN within the hypothalamus (Figure 15.5). However, it is important to remember that light, and in particular blue light (e.g. light from many digital devices), can counteract the effects of darkness at the SCN

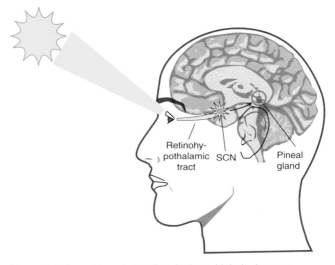

Figure 15.5 The setting of circadian rhythms. Light is the most powerful synchronizer of circadian rhythms. When light enters through the eye it is translated via the retinohypothalamic tract to the suprachiasmatic nucleus (SCN) within the hypothalamus. The SCN, in turn, signals the pineal gland to turn off melatonin production. During darkness, there is no input from the retinohypothalamic tract to the SCN within the hypothalamus. Thus, darkness signals the pineal gland to produce melatonin. Melatonin, in turn, can act on the SCN to reset circadian rhythms. Adapted from *Stahl's Essential Psychopharmacology,* 2021.

- Melatonin shifts circadian rhythms, especially in those with phase delay, when taken at the desired bedtime, particularly in adolescents
- Melatonin acts at three different sites: MT_1 and MT_2 receptors as well as MT_3 receptors

- MT$_1$-mediated inhibition of neurons in the SCN is thought to promote sleep by decreasing the wake-promoting actions of the circadian "clock" that functions there, perhaps by attenuating the SCN's alerting signals and allowing sleep signals to predominate, thus inducing sleep
- Phase shifting and circadian rhythm effects of the normal sleep–wake cycle are thought to be primarily mediated by MT$_2$ receptors, which entrain these signals in the SCN

Mechanism of action moment: clonidine

- Clonidine is often used as an initial psychopharmacologic treatment for insomnia in pediatric patients. That norepinephrine (NE) is targeted by these soporifics relates to the normal role of norepinephrine in promoting wakefulness and arousal. Thus, turning down the noradrenergic volume can produce sedation
- Understanding the effects of this α_2 agonist requires a review of the physiology of noradrenergic neurons, including the role of the α_2 receptor in modulating NE release and the firing of NE neurons
- The noradrenergic neuron is regulated by a multiplicity of receptors for NE (Figure 15.6). NE receptors are classified as α_1, α_{2A}, α_{2B}, or α_{2C}, or as β_1, β_2, or β_3. All can be postsynaptic, but only α_2 receptors can act as presynaptic autoreceptors. Importantly, α_2 receptors are found densely in the pontine locus coeruleus and clonidine's sedating properties likely are related to the inhibition of this nucleus
- Presynaptic α_2 receptors regulate NE release, so they are called "autoreceptors." Presynaptic α_2 autoreceptors are located both on the axon terminal (i.e. terminal α_2 receptors) (Figure 15.7) and at the cell body (soma) and nearby dendrites; thus, these latter α_2 presynaptic receptors are called somatodendritic α_2 receptors (Figure 15.8)
- Presynaptic α_2 receptors are important because both the terminal and the somatodendritic α_2 receptors are autoreceptors. That is, when presynaptic α_2 receptors recognize NE, they turn off further release of NE (Figure 15.7 and 15.8). Thus, presynaptic α_2 autoreceptors act as a brake for the NE neuron and also cause what is known as a negative feedback regulatory signal. Using an α_2 agonist, like clonidine, stimulates this receptor (i.e. stepping on the brake) and stops the neuron from firing. This probably occurs physiologically to prevent overfiring of the NE neuron since it can shut itself off once the firing rate gets too high and the autoreceptor becomes stimulated

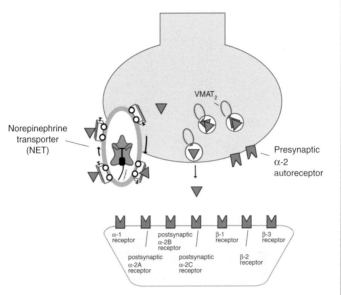

Figure 15.6 Norepinephrine receptors. The norepinephrine transporter (NET) exists presynaptically and is responsible for clearing excess norepinephrine out of the synapse. The vesicular monoamine transporter-2 (VMAT2) takes norepinephrine up into synaptic vesicles and stores it for neurotransmission. The presynaptic α_2 autoreceptor regulates release of norepinephrine from the presynaptic neuron. In addition, there are several postsynaptic receptors, including α_1, α_{2A}, α_{2B}, α_{2C}, β_1, β_2, and β_3 receptors. Reproduced from *Stahl's Essential Psychopharmacology*, 2021.

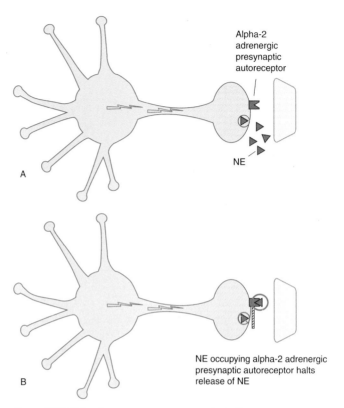

Figure 15.7 Alpha-2 receptors on axon terminal. Shown here are presynaptic α_2-adrenergic autoreceptors located on the axon terminal of the norepinephrine (NE) neuron. These autoreceptors are "gatekeepers" for norepinephrine. (A) When they are not bound by norepinephrine, they are open, allowing norepinephrine release. (B) When norepinephrine binds to the gatekeeping receptors, they close the molecular gate and prevent norepinephrine from being released. Reproduced from *Stahl's Essential Psychopharmacology*, 2021.

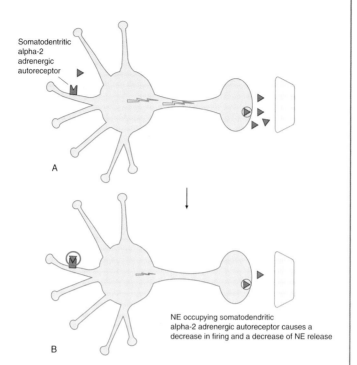

Figure 15.8 Somatodendritic α_2 receptors. Shown here
are presynaptic α_2-adrenergic autoreceptors located in the
somatodendritic area of the norepinephrine neuron. (A) When
they are not bound by norepinephrine, there is normal neuronal
impulse flow, with resultant release of norepinephrine. (B) When
norepinephrine binds to these α_2 receptors, it shuts off neuronal
impulse flow (see loss of lightning bolts in the neuron), and this
stops further norepinephrine release. Reproduced from *Stahl's
Essential Psychopharmacology*, 2021.

Post test question

Which of the following may be chronotropically dosed to re-entrain circadian rhythms?

A. Melatonin
B. Ramelteon
C. Suvorexant
D. Oxytocin (intranasal)

Answer: A (Melatonin)

Regarding pharmacotherapy for insomnia disorder in children and adolescents, low-dose melatonin (0.5 mg) (A), when timed relative to the endogenous dim light melatonin onset, is considered a first-line intervention. However, melatonin (0.05 mg/kg) may be effective. Ramelteon (B) and suvorexant (C) have not been systematically evaluated in pediatric patients with insomnia disorder. Finally, intranasal oxytocin (D) has been evaluated in autism spectrum disorder but has not been evaluated in pediatric patients with insomnia.

References

1. Alfano, C. A., Ginsburg, G. S., Kingery, J. N. Sleep-related problems among children and adolescents with anxiety disorders. *J Am Acad Child Adolesc Psychiatry* 2007; 46: 224–32. https://doi.org/10.1097/01.chi.0000242233.06011.8e

2. Brent, D., Emslie, G., Clarke, G., et al. Switching to another SSRI or to venlafaxine with or without cognitive behavioral therapy for adolescents with SSRI-resistant depression: the TORDIA randomized controlled trial. *JAMA* 2008; 299(8): 901–13. https://doi.org/10.1001/jama.299.8.901

3. de Zambotti, M., Goldstone, A., Colrain, I. M., Baker, F. C. Insomnia disorder in adolescence: diagnosis, impact, and treatment. *Sleep Med Rev* 2018; 39: 12–24. https://doi.org/10.1016/j.smrv.2017.06.009

4. Skoch, S. H., Mills, J. A., Ramsey, L., Strawn, J. R. Letter to the editor: sleep disturbances in selective serotonin reuptake inhibitor-treated youth with anxiety disorders and obsessive compulsive disorder: a Bayesian hierarchical modeling meta-analysis. *J Child Adolesc Psychopharmacol* 2021; 31(5): 387–88. https://doi.org/10.1089/cap.2020.0169

5. Malow, B. A., Findling, R. L., Schroder, C. M., et al. Sleep, growth, and puberty after 2 years of prolonged-release melatonin in children with autism spectrum disorder. *J Am Acad Child Adolescent Psychiatry* 2021; 60(2): 252–61.e3. https://doi.org/10.1016/j.jaac.2019.12.007

6. Orbeta, R. L., Overpeck, M. D., Ramcharran, D., Kogan, M. D., Ledsky, R. High caffeine intake in adolescents: associations with difficulty sleeping and feeling tired in the morning. *J Adolesc Health* 2006; 38(4): 451–53. https://doi.org/10.1016/j.jadohealth.2005.05.014

7. Owens, J. A., Dalzell, V. Use of the "BEARS" sleep screening tool in a pediatric residents' continuity clinic: a pilot study. *Sleep Med* 2005; 6(1): 63–69. https://doi.org/10.1016/j.sleep.2004.07.015

8. Owens, J. A., Mindell, J., Baylor, A. Effect of energy drink and caffeinated beverage consumption on sleep, mood, and performance in children and adolescents. *Nutrition Reviews* 2014; 72(S1): 75–61. https://doi.org/10.1111/nure.12150

9. Owens, J. A., Rosen, C. L., Mindell, J. A., Kirchner, H. L. Use of pharmacotherapy for insomnia in child psychiatry practice: a national survey. *Sleep Med* 2010; 11(7): 692–700. https://doi.org/10.1016/j.sleep.2009.11.015

10. Owens, J. A., Spirito, A., McGuinn, M. The Children's Sleep Habits Questionnaire (CSHQ): psychometric properties of a survey instrument for school-aged children. *Sleep* 2000; 23(8): 1–9. https://doi.org/10.1093/sleep/23.8.1d

11. Russo, R. M., Gururaj, V. J., Allen, J. E. The effectiveness of diphenhydramine HCl in pediatric sleep disorders. *J Clin Pharmacol* 1976; 16(5–6): 284–88. https://doi.org/10.1002/j.1552-4604.1976.tb02406.x

12. Schroder, C. M., Malow, B. A., Maras, A., et al. Pediatric prolonged-release melatonin for sleep in children with autism spectrum disorder: impact on child behavior and caregiver's quality of life. *J Autism Develop Disord* 2019; 49(8): 3218–30. https://doi.org/10.1007/s10803-019-04046-5

13. Shamseddeen, W., Clarke, G., Keller, M. B., et al. Adjunctive sleep medications and depression outcome in the treatment of serotonin-selective reuptake inhibitor resistant depression in adolescents study. *J Child Adolesc Psychopharmacol* 2012; 22(1): 29–36. https://doi.org/10.1089/cap.2011.0027

14. Skoch, S. H. Pediatric insomnia: treatment. *Curr Psychiatry* 2022; 21(1): 15–21. https://doi.org/10.12788/cp.0200

15. van Geijlswijk, I. M., Mol, R. H., Egberts, T. C. G., Smits, M. G. Evaluation of sleep, puberty and mental health in children with long-term melatonin treatment for chronic idiopathic childhood sleep onset insomnia. *Psychopharmacology* 2011; 216(1): 111–20. https://doi.org/10.1007/s00213-011-2202-y

16. van Geijlswijk, I. M., van der Heijden, K. B., Egberts, A. C. G., Korzilius, H. P. L. M., Smits, M. G. Dose finding of melatonin

for chronic idiopathic childhood sleep onset insomnia: an RCT. *Psychopharmacology* 2010; 212(3): 379–91. https://doi.org/10.1007/s00213-010-1962-0

17. Weiss, S. K., Garbutt, A. Pharmacotherapy in pediatric sleep disorders. In Sass, A. E., Kaplan, D. W. (eds.), *Adolescent Medicine: State of the Art Reviews*. Itasca, IL: American Academy of Pediatrics, 2005. https://doi.org/10.1542/9781581105803-pharmacotherapy

Case 16: Second-generation antipsychotics/mixed dopamine–serotonin receptor agonists (SGAs), side effects, and the autism spectrum: SGA-related side effects in a boy with autism spectrum disorder (ASD)

The Questions: What is the evidence-based workup for a child with ASD? Which SGAs have evidence for specific symptoms in children and adolescents with ASD and how should they be diagnosed? How should tolerability of SGAs be monitored in children and adolescents with ASD?

The Psychopharmacological Dilemma: Managing SGAs in children and adolescents with ASD can be complicated, but awareness of pharmacological/pharmacogenetic principles can help to predict specific tolerability concerns

Pretest self-assessment question

Which of the following is associated with the greatest incidence of hyperprolactinemia?

A. Aripiprazole (Abilify)

B. Risperidone (Risperdal)

C. Paliperidone (Invega)

D. Vortioxetine (Trintillix)

E. All of the above

Answer: C (Paliperidone, Invega)

Patient evaluation on intake

- 11-year-old boy with fragile X syndrome, ASD with accompanying intellectual impairment, associated with known genetic condition (fragile X syndrome), requiring substantial support and attention-deficit/hyperactivity disorder (ADHD), combined presentation
- The patient struggles with chronic irritability and aggression, which have not been responsive to several environmental changes and adaptations, including a home-based consultation from an applied behavioral analysis (ABA) therapist
- His difficulties are present at school and home
- He denies depressed mood, and there is no evidence of anhedonia
- There is no evidence of psychosis
- There are no obsessive-compulsive symptoms, although he likes to order and count medieval knight figurines he collects. Additionally, he struggles with rigidity and transitions and is upset when routines are disrupted. Often, this is a precipitant of aggressive outbursts, which have resulted in minor injuries to himself and to his family members

- The family denies any history of tics
- His ADHD symptoms are well controlled

Psychiatric history

- History of global developmental delay and was diagnosed with intellectual disability disorder at age 7
- He was diagnosed with ASD based on the Autism Diagnostic Observation Scale (ADOS) (Gotham et al. 2007, 2009) administered at an autism center in a large academic center
- He is prescribed clonidine extended-release formulation 0.1 mg twice daily, and his parents have given low-dose melatonin every night at bedtime (1.5 mg) on an as-needed basis to help with insomnia

Social and personal history

- He lives with his mother and father
- His mother stays at home, and his father is a software engineer who travels monthly for his job
- An Individualized Education Plan (IEP) is in place at school, and he learns in a self-contained classroom with a teacher:student ratio of 1:4
- There is no history of abuse or neglect
- He has limited peer relationships but an older cousin who lives near the family will spend time with him several times each month. He does not participate in any organized sports or other activities

Medical history

- He was delivered at 40 weeks to a 40-year-old mother and 40-year-old father
- At birth, there was mild hypotonia which decreased over the first 6 months of life
- Developmental milestones were delayed for gross motor and fine motor. He began making sounds at approximately 5–6 months of age and had an expressive language delay. Specifically, he did not use words until age 3 years
- He received speech and language therapy and occupational therapy in the past and continues to receive occupational therapy at school
- He has a history of recurrent otitis media
- He has no history of seizure disorder

Family history

- Mother with obsessive compulsive disorder (OCD)

Medication history

- Clonidine 0.1 mg twice daily
- History of methylphenidate OROS titrated to 18 mg daily, which was associated with disinhibition
- Melatonin 1.5 mg every night at bedtime as needed – insomnia

Current medications

- Clonidine 0.1 mg twice daily
- Melatonin 1.5 mg every night at bedtime as needed – insomnia

Psychotherapy history

- He previously participated in a social communication group for 6 months and has worked with a therapist who used applied behavioral analysis-based approaches to assist with managing impulsive aggression and "anger" at home
- He also received occupational therapy to address "sensory problems"

Further investigation

Is there anything else that you would like to know about the patient? What about additional physical symptoms?

What about prior psychological testing?

- His complete neuropsychological evaluation is unavailable. However, his parents provided a copy of the Weschler Intelligence Scale for Children 5th edition (WISC-V) in addition to an assessment of adaptive functioning (Table 16.1)

Testing: laboratory results, imaging, EKGs
Table 6.1 Weschler Intelligence Scale for Children (WISC-V)

Scales	Scaled Score	Standard Score	Percentile Rank
Full Scale IQ		59	0.3
Verbal Comprehension Index		84	14
Similarities	5		
Vocabulary	9		*
Visual Spatial Index		69	2
Block Design	2		
Visual Puzzles	7		

Scales	Scaled Score	Standard Score	Percentile Rank
Fluid Reasoning Index		67	1
Matrix Reasoning	2		
Figure Weights	6		
Working Memory Index		51	0.1
Digit Span	2		
Picture Span	1		
Processing Speed Index		45	<0.1
Coding	1		
Symbol Search	1		

The WISC-V yields a Full-Scale Intelligence Quotient (FSIQ), which provides an estimate of current overall cognitive functioning. The WISC-V has a mean of 100 and a standard deviation of 15, indicating that normal limits fall within the range of 85–115. The patient's FSIQ is classified as very low.

In addition to the full-scale score, the WISC-V provides five index scores, each of which is comprised of selected subtests. The patient's verbal abilities are a notable strength; whereas his short-term memory, concentration, attention and motor speed, and speed of visual processing mental reasoning are a notable weakness, a finding that should play an essential role for developing education interventions.

Scales of Independent Behavior-Revised (SIB-R)

Domain/Composite Area	Standard Score	Age Equivalent	Percentile Rank
Broad Independence Composite	52	5–8	0.1
Motor Skills	60	5–8	0.4
Gross Motor Skills		6–1	
Fine Motor Skills		5–5	
Social/Communication Skills	68	5–11	2
Social Interactions		5–9	
Language Comprehension		4–9	
Language Expression		6–5	
Personal Living	63	5–1	1
Eating		6–5	
Toileting		5–3	
Dressing		4–1	
Self-care		5–10	
Domestic Skills		6–10	
Community Living Skills	44	5–9	0.1
Time and Punctuality		6–7	

Domain/Composite Area	Standard Score	Age Equivalent	Percentile Rank
Money and Value		5-6	
Work Skills		5-2	
Home-Community		4-6	

The patient's Broad Independence, an overall measure of adaptive behavior, is comparable to that of the average individual at age 5 years 8 months. His functional independence is limited. When presented with age-level tasks, his motor skills, social interaction and communication skills, and personal living skills are limited. His community living skills are limited to very limited. The patient has limitations in 12 adaptive skill areas: gross motor skills, fine motor skills, social interaction, language comprehension, eating and meal preparation, toileting, dressing, personal self-care, time and punctuality, money and value, work skills, and home/community orientation.

The patient's greatest strengths include his social interaction and communication skills. His lowest scores include his community living skills.

What about a physical examination and vital signs?

- His vital signs are within normal limits, although his height is 90th percentile for age and sex
- He denies cardiac symptoms, including palpitations
- Physical examination is remarkable for a prominent forehead, a long, narrow face, a prominent jaw, and protuberant ears. Additionally, he has dental crowding and a history of malocclusion. The remainder of the physical examination is unremarkable, and his neurologic examination is summarized as:
  - On the mental status exam, he was alert, and his speech was mildly dysarthric with poor articulation and difficulty with /th/ and /s/ but he was fluent
  - On cranial nerve exam, pupils were equal, round, and reactive to light bilaterally. He had no afferent pupillary defect. Extraocular movements were intact. There was no nystagmus. Smile, eye closure, and palatal elevation were symmetric. Facial sensation and hearing were intact. Shoulder shrug was normal bilaterally. Tongue protrusion was in the midline
  - On motor exam, he had decreased muscle tone. Motor strength was 5/5 bilaterally. Deep tendon reflexes were 2/4 throughout. No Babinski sign
  - Sensation was intact to light touch
  - There was no tremor, dysdiadochokinesia, dysmetria, chorea, dystonia, or myoclonus
  - Gait was narrow-based. He was able to toe-walk, heel-walk, and tandem walk. No Romberg sign

Attending physician's mental notes: initial psychiatric evaluation

- The attending physician notes that the prior diagnosis of autism spectrum disorder was based on the "gold standard" ADOS (Gotham et al. 2007, 2009); however, he considers the contribution of medical comorbidity related to his fragile X syndrome and his deficits in communication. His attending has obtained old medical records, including the genetic testing results (Muhle et al. 2017; Savatt and Myers 2021)

- The attending physician has asked about several additional physical symptoms (e.g. gastroesophageal reflux, dental problems, hypermobility), given that medical comorbidity is common in patients with fragile X syndrome (Hersh and Saul 2021)

- The patient's phenotype is consistent with fragile X syndrome, although some features are difficult to detect in prepubertal patients. His history of developmental delay and intellectual disability disorder are consistent with fragile X syndrome

- Additionally, the attending physician notes a prominent forehead, a long, narrow face, a prominent jaw, and protuberant ears, which is a common phenotype in fragile X syndrome. Additionally, his attending physician is aware that other features are also common, including macroorchidism (present in 80% of adolescent males) as well as connective tissue dysplasia, soft velvet-like skin, and joint hypermobility (especially in the fingers) (Hersh and Saul 2021)

- His attending physician will also ask about seizures, as these are present in approximately 15% of males with fragile X syndrome (Hersh and Saul 2021)

- In reviewing his developmental history, his attending physician notes a history of accelerated linear growth with tall stature, although this tends to be less common postpubertally (Hersh and Saul 2021)

- From a cognitive standpoint, the attending physician is aware that his deficits may complicate reporting of symptoms in expressive language

Question

Given his prior psychotherapy and current pharmacologic treatment, which of the following would be your next step?

- Trial of a mixed amphetamine salt (Adderall)
- Adjunctive guanfacine extended release formulation (Intuniv)
- Trial of risperidone (Risperdal)
- Conversion of immediate-release melatonin to extended-release melatonin

Case outcome: first interim follow-up (week 1)

- At his last appointment, risperidone 0.25 mg twice daily was added and titrated to 0.5 mg twice daily approximately 4 days later
- His parents have noted a significant decrease in his repetitive behaviors, and he has been able to engage more with his family and can sit through meals
- There is no excessive tiredness, and his teachers have commented on his ability to tolerate frustration and his improved ability to transition from one activity to another
- His parents have observed improvements in his flexibility, and his episodes of aggression have significantly improved in frequency and severity. However, episodes of aggressive outbursts occur every other day at home and last for approximately 25 to 45 minutes

Attending physician's mental notes: first interim follow-up (week 1)

- The attending physician selected risperidone based on its U.S. Food and Drug Administration (FDA) indication for "treatment of irritability associated with autistic disorder in children and adolescents aged 5–16 years" and prior studies suggesting its efficacy (Aman et al. 2015; McCracken et al. 2002), including in patients with fragile X syndrome (Dominick et al. 2018; Erickson et al. 2011). Based on registration studies, his attending physician is aware that improvement emerges early during treatment and then plateaus (Figure 16.1)

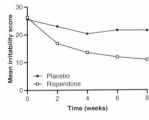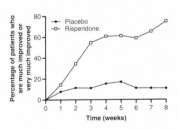

Figure 16.1 Improvement in pediatric patients with ASD during acute treatment with risperidone. Mean scores for irritability in patients receiving risperidone or placebo are shown (left), while the percentage of children who were responders (defined based on Clinical Global Impression – Improvement Scale) are shown (right). Adapted from McCracken et al. Risperidone in children with autism and serious behavioral problems. *N Engl J Med* 2002; 347: 314–21.

- His attending physician is encouraged by the improvement in irritability and outbursts, as well as episodes of aggression
- His attending physician recalls the dosing used in the pediatric studies of risperidone in ASD. In these studies, patients weighing between 20 and 45 kg received an initial dose of 0.5 mg every night at bedtime and this was increased to 0.5 mg twice daily on the fourth day of treatment. Thereafter, doses were increased in 0.5-mg increments to a maximum dose of 2.5 mg daily (1 mg every morning and 1.5 mg at bedtime). Children who weighed more than 45 kg were titrated more quickly and to a maximum dose of 1.5 mg every morning and 2 mg every night at bedtime (McCracken et al. 2002). With this information in hand, his attending physician considers his options with regard to titration of risperidone and would like to see more reductions in the frequency and severity of his aggressive episodes
- In thinking about his prognosis based on studies of children and adolescents with ASD who were treated with risperidone, baseline symptom severity and adherence significantly predicted improvement

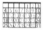

Case outcome: second interim follow-up (week 5)

- During two brief telehealth visits over the past 2 weeks, risperidone has been titrated to 1.5 mg every morning and 2 mg every night at bedtime. The patient's aggressive outbursts are profoundly less frequent, and he has had no episodes over the prior week
- His teachers and intervention specialist at school have noted continued improvements
- There are continued improvements in his frustration tolerance, and his parents note that previously reported bedtime difficulties are markedly better
- His blood pressure and heart rate remain within the normal range, and he denies any additional physical symptoms. However, his parents have noted significant weight gain over the past 2 weeks

Attending physician's mental notes: second interim follow-up (week 5)

- The attending physician is very happy with the patient's current symptoms and the parents' and teachers' reports of improvement
- The attending physician is concerned by the weight gain and knows that risperidone-treated patients with ASD may experience more weight gain (Figure 16.2) in addition to more sedation and higher prolactin concentrations (Kloosterboer et al. 2021)

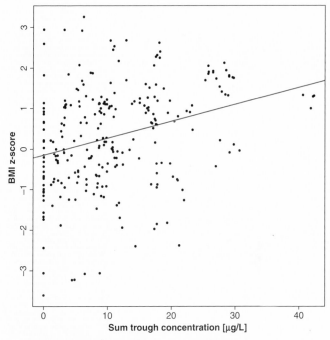

Figure 16.2 Higher concentrations of risperidone +
9-OH-risperidone predict increases in body mass index (BMI)
z-scores in children and adolescents treated with risperidone.
Adapted from Kloosterboer et al. Risperidone plasma concentrations are associated with side effects and effectiveness in children and adolescents with autism spectrum disorder. *Br J Clin
Pharmacol* 2021; 87: 1069–81.

Case outcome: third interim follow-up (week 12)

- The patient has continued to gain weight over the past 4 weeks,
  although his behavioral symptoms remain well-controlled on his
  current regimen
- In addition, he notes more frequent headaches and his parents have
  been concerned about breast enlargement and possible breast pain.
  Also, last week, his mother noted galactorrhea

Testing: laboratory results, imaging, EKGs (week 12)

- The attending physician has ordered several laboratory studies, in
  addition to the routine studies recommended for the monitoring
  of patients treated with mixed dopamine–serotonin receptor
  antagonists (formerly second-generation antipsychotics, SGAs)

Pharmacogenetic testing		
	Genotype	Phenotype
CYP2D6	*1/*2x2	Ultrarapid metabolizer
CYP2C19	*17/*17	Ultrarapid metabolizer

Hemoglobin A1 C		
	Value	Ref Range
Hemoglobin A1 C	5.5	<5.6%

Lipid Profile W/ HDL		
	Value	Ref Range
HDL CHOLESTEROL	40	>=40 mg/dL
CHOLESTEROL LEVEL	129	<=199 mg/dL
TRIGLYCERIDES	129	<=129 mg/dL
LDL CHOLESTEROL	75	<=129 mg/dL

Insulin		
	Value	Ref Range
INSULIN	**(H) 9.4**	**3-8 mcIU/mL**

CBC with Differential		
	Value	Ref Range
WBC	8.8	4.5 - 13.0 K/mcL
RBC	5.09	4.50 - 5.30 M/mcL
HGB	15.8	13.0 - 16.0 gm/dL
HCT	44.7	37.0 - 49.0 %
MCV	87.8	78.0 - 94.0 fL
MCH	30.9	25.0 - 35.0 pg
MCHC	35.2	31.0 - 37.0 gm/dL
RDW	11.5	≤14.6 %
PLATELET	204	135 - 466 K/mcL

Comp Metabolic Panel		
	Value	Ref Range
SODIUM	141	136 - 145 mmol/L
POTASSIUM	4.1	3.3 - 4.7 mmol/L
CHLORIDE	105	100 - 112 mmol/L
CO2	26	17 - 31 mmol/L
ANION GAP	10	4 - 15 mmol/L
BUN	12	6 - 21 mg/dL
CREATININE	0.96	0.46 - 1.00 mg/dL
B/C RATIO	12	≤25
GLUCOSE	93	65 - 106 mg/dL
CALCIUM	9.4	8.3 - 10.6 mg/dL
ALBUMIN	4.6	3.3 - 4.8 gm/dL
TOTAL PROTEIN	7.4	6.2 - 8.1 gm/dL
ALKALINE PHOS	136	48 - 138 unit/L
ALT	34	<=49 unit/L
AST	**37**	**10 - 36 unit/L**
BILIRUBIN	1.2	0.1-1.2 mg/dL

| GLOBULIN | 3.0 | gm/dL |
| A/G RATIO | 2 | 1 - 2 |

GGT		
	Value	Ref Range
GGT	17	9 - 49 unit/L

TSH with Reflex to T4 Free, Rapid		
	Value	Ref Range
TSH	1.92	0.43 - 4.0 mcIU/mL

Prolactin		
	Value	Ref Range
Prolactin	(H) 56	3-18 ng/mL

Risperidone + 9-OH-risperidone		
	Value	Ref Range
RISPERIDONE + 9-OH RISPERIDONE	(H) 40	15-25 ug/L*

* Kloosterboer et al., 2021 in youth with autism spectrum disorder

Attending physician's mental notes: third interim follow-up (week 12)

- The attending physician notes that the patient has hyperprolactinemia and that this is likely related to his increased risperidone + 9-OH-risperidone exposure (i.e. blood levels) and that this may be related to his higher dose of risperidone and by the increased conversion of risperidone to 9-OH-risperidone (Figure 16.3) given that he is an ultrarapid metabolizer of CYP2D6 and that he has a duplication
- Importantly, 9-OH-risperidone is associated with a higher risk of hyperprolactinemia compared to risperidone
- The attending physician notes that his HbA1C is near the upper limit of normal and that his fasting insulin concentration is mildly increased. As such, his physician is concerned about the potential for later risperidone-related adverse metabolic effects

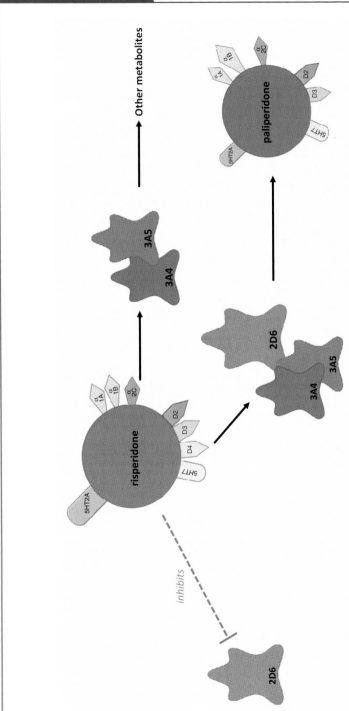

Figure 16.3 Risperidone and paliperidone (9-OH-risperidone) pharmacological and binding profiles. This figure portrays a qualitative consensus of current thinking about the binding properties of risperidone and paliperidone. Note that this conversion is dependent on CYP2D6. Adapted from *Stahl's Essential Psychopharmacology*, 2021.

Question

Given the patient's prior psychotherapy and current pharmacologic treatment, which of the following would be your next step?

- Discontinue risperidone (Risperdal) and begin escitalopram (Lexapro)
- Discontinue risperidone (Risperdal) and begin aripiprazole (Abilify)
- Cross-titrate risperidone (Risperdal) to aripiprazole (Abilify)
- Add bromocriptine

Case outcome: fourth, fifth and sixth interim follow-up (week 14–24)

- Two weeks after beginning aripiprazole (2 mg every night at bedtime), the patient continues to do well
- Over the subsequent several weeks, risperidone has been slowly decreased, while aripiprazole has been titrated to 2.5 mg every night at bedtime and then 5 mg every night at bedtime
- His hyperprolactinemia has resolved and weight gain normalized

Performance in practice: confessions of a psychopharmacologist

- The patient had extensive behavioral interventions prior to treatment with a mixed dopamine–serotonin receptor antagonist; however, he experienced significant adverse effects. Whether titration of his clonidine extended-release formulation could have produced additional improvement or resulted in the patient needing less risperidone is unclear
- Pharmacogenetic testing was not obtained until the patient began treatment with risperidone. The decision of when to begin pharmacogenetic testing remains a debated question in pediatric psychopharmacology (Figure 16.4). However, current guidance suggests that if a medication with actionable pharmacogenetic dosing guidance is available, pharmacogenetic testing should be obtained prior to treatment. In this case, recommendations related to CYP2D6 dosing are mixed
- The pediatric psychopharmacologist regrets not having obtained this information in advance as knowing that the patient is an ultrarapid metabolizer for CYP2D6 would have led him to choose an alternative agent such as aripiprazole which also has an FDA indication for irritability associated with ASD in children and adolescents but – because of its partial D_2 agonism – might have produced less hyperprolactinemia

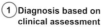
① Diagnosis based on clinical assessment

② Determine whether pharmacotherapy is warranted

③ Choose medication based on evidence, FDA, or guidelines

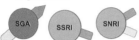

④ Review PGx results (PK & hypersensitivity genes) relevant to the medication selected if they are available

⑤ Review FDA package insert and CPIC guidelines

⑥ Determine dosing strategy or alternative medication

Figure 16.4 Approach to pharmacogenetic testing in children and adolescents. Adapted from Ramsey et al. *J Am Acad Child Adolesc Psychiatry* 2021; 60(6): 660–64.

Take-home points

- Several mixed dopamine–serotonin receptor antagonists are FDA approved for the treatment of irritability in pediatric patients with ASD
- Fragile X syndrome is the most common inherited form of developmental disability and is the most common single-gene cause of ASD. Additionally, in individuals with fragile X syndrome, irritable behavior, aggression, self-injury, and severe tantrums may be targets of treatment. However, there are few randomized controlled trials in fragile X syndrome, and therefore, most evidence for psychopharmacologic interventions comes from studies of patients with idiopathic autism. Both risperidone and aripiprazole have been studied in open-label trials of children and adolescents with fragile X syndrome (Erikson et al. 2010; Dominick et al. 2018)
- In cross-titrating from risperidone (a full D_2 antagonist) to aripiprazole (a partial D_2 antagonist), psychopharmacologists should consider beginning aripiprazole prior to reducing the dose of risperidone, given the D_2 partial antagonism and the risk of displacing some risperidone (Figure 16.5)

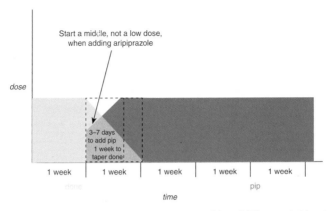

Figure 16.5 Switching to aripiprazole from a "done." When switching to aripiprazole ("pip") from a "done" (risperidone, paliperidone, ziprasidone, iloperidone, lurasidone), it is recommended to start aripiprazole at a middle dose, rather than a low dose, while down-titrating the done over 1 week. Adapted from *Stahl's Essential Psychopharmacology*, 2021.

Tips and pearls

- Mixed dopamine–serotonin receptor antagonists can effectively reduce irritability and aggressive outbursts in children and adolescents with ASD; however, clinicians should always consider the underlying etiology of these episodes and should consider behavioral interventions first
- When considering mixed dopamine–serotonin receptor antagonists consider the side-effect profile and the relationship between pharmacokinetic and pharmacodynamic factors:
  - Risperidone and 9-OH-risperidone are associated with hyperprolactinemia (Kloosterboer et al. 2021), although the latter is associated with greater hyperprolactinemia
  - D_2 antagonism vs. D_2 partial antagonism has different effects in terms of the risk of hyperprolactinemia, with some partial D_2 antagonists potentially ameliorating hyperprolactinemia associated with other mixed dopamine–serotonin receptor antagonists
- For risperidone-treated patients, side effects (and potential efficacy) are related to plasma concentrations of risperidone and 9-OH-risperidone. Recent studies suggest a therapeutic trough level of 15–25 µg/L in pediatric patients with an ASD (Kloosterboer et al. 2021)

Mechanism of action moment

- For decades it has been known that D_2 antagonists markedly increase pituitary prolactin secretion in proportion to their individual abilities to block pituitary dopamine D_2

- Pituitary prolactin secretion is negatively regulated by dopamine, such that decreasing dopamine unleashes pituitary lactotrophs, which secrete prolactin, from tonic dopaminergic inhibition (Strawn and Geracioti 2023). Further, serotonin and dopamine have reciprocal roles in the regulation of prolactin secretion, with dopamine inhibiting prolactin release via stimulation of D_2 receptors and serotonin promoting prolactin release via stimulation of 5-HT$_{2A}$ receptors (Figure 16.6)

- Thus, when D_2 receptors alone are blocked by D_2 antagonism, dopamine can no longer inhibit prolactin release, so prolactin levels rise (Figure 16.6). However, in the case of a drug that has both D_2 antagonism and 5-HT$_{2A}$ antagonism, there is simultaneous inhibition of 5-HT$_{2A}$ receptors, so serotonin can no longer stimulate prolactin release (Figure 16.6). This mitigates the hyperprolactinemia of D_2 receptor blockade

- The brain-pituitary hormone prolactin is well known to promote galactorrhea and lactation, as the name of the polypeptide implies ("pro-lactin")

- A clinically important, major adverse effect of hyperprolactinemia is hypogonadism, with suppression of sex hormone release. Hyperprolactinemia-generated hypogonadism can be of greater or lesser severity depending on the degree of suppression of brain gonadotropic releasing hormone (GnRH) and, in turn, pituitary luteinizing hormone and follicular-stimulating hormone activity – but it is sometimes profound

- In adults and in children and adolescents, hyperprolactinemia-induced hypothalamic–pituitary–gonadal (HPG) suppression results in reductions in circulating androgens and estrogens. However, our understanding of the long-term effects of suppressed HPG axis functioning in children and adolescents is underdeveloped

- Clinical signs and symptoms of hyperprolactinemia and hypogonadism may be difficult to appreciate in prepubertal children. Typically, it is not until puberty is delayed or arrested, secondary sexual characteristics fail to develop, menarche does not occur, menses cease, or irregular menstruation is reported that clinicians suspect hypogonadism (Strawn and Geracioti 2023)

- In children and adolescents, prolactin increases rapidly after exposure to some dopamine–serotonin receptor antagonists and peaks within

4–5 weeks, but may linger indefinitely, especially for the "prolactin-raising" dopamine–serotonin receptor antagonists (risperidone and olanzapine). However, while prolactin concentrations increase quickly and peak within 4–5 weeks for many, they may subsequently decline over time in some children and adolescents (Koch et al. 2023)

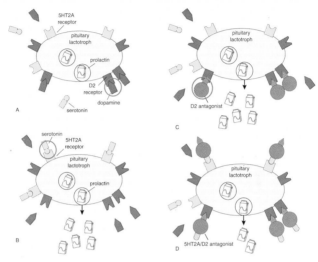

Figure 16.6 Dopamine and serotonin regulate prolactin release. (A) Dopamine binding at inhibitory D_2 receptors (red circle) prevents prolactin release from pituitary lactotroph cells in the pituitary gland. (B) Serotonin (5-HT) binding at excitatory 5-HT$_{2A}$ receptors (red circle) stimulates prolactin release from pituitary lactotroph cells in the pituitary gland. Thus, dopamine and serotonin have a reciprocal regulatory action on prolactin release. (C) D_2 antagonism (red circle) blocks dopamine's inhibitory effect on prolactin secretion from pituitary lactotrophs. Thus, these drugs increase prolactin levels. (D) As dopamine and serotonin have reciprocal regulatory roles in the control of prolactin secretion, one cancels the other. Thus, 5-HT$_{2A}$ antagonism reverses the ability of D_2 antagonism to increase prolactin secretion. Adapted from *Stahl's Essential Psychopharmacology*, 2021.

Two-minute tutorial

- The genetic work-up in patients first presenting with developmental disabilities (DD) is important. Diagnostic genetic testing aimed at establishing the molecular diagnosis is now standard-of-care for all individuals with unexplained (idiopathic) DD. This work-up is recommended by multiple professional organizations, including the American Academy of Child and Adolescent Psychiatry (AACAP), the American College of Medical Genetics (ACMG), and the American Academy of Pediatrics (AAP) (Muhle et al. 2017)

- Current recommendations for standard-of-care genetic testing patients with ASD, intellectual disability, or global developmental delay include:
  - Chromosomal microarray in all individuals (regardless of sex, IQ, or co-occurring medical conditions) to identify microdeletions and microduplications in the genome (copy number variants)
  - Fragile X gene testing in all boys and in girls with intellectual disability
- Also, based on the history and physical examination, additional testing may be indicated as described below. However, in these situations, consultation with a developmental pediatrician, medical geneticist, or child and adolescent psychiatrist who works with these populations can be helpful in guiding workup. Some specific examples of targeted testing include:
  - *PTEN* (phosphatase and tensin homolog) gene testing if the patient's head circumference is more than 2.5 standard deviations above the mean for age
  - *MECP2* (methyl CpG binding protein 2) gene testing for Rett syndrome in girls with severe intellectual disability
  - Karyotype analysis if a chromosomal syndrome is suspected
- Finally, some suggest that whole-exome sequencing may become an additional standard-of-care evaluation as this becomes more affordable, given that it may detect small changes in the DNA sequence that chromosomal microarray cannot detect

Post test question

Which of the following is associated with the greatest incidence of hyperprolactinemia?

A. Aripiprazole (Abilify)
B. Risperidone (Risperdal)
C. Paliperidone (Invega)
D. Vortioxetine (Trintillix)
E. All of the above

Answer: C (Paliperidone, Invega)

While both risperidone (B) and paliperidone (C) are associated with hyperprolactinemia, paliperidone, or 9-OH-risperidone, the primary metabolite of risperidone (C) is associated with a greater risk of hyperprolactinemia. Aripiprazole (A) is a partial D_2 antagonist and may help ameliorate mixed dopamine–serotonin receptor antagonist-related hyperprolactinemia. Vortioxetine (D) is not associated with hyperprolactinemia in pediatric studies.

References

1. Aman, M., Rettiganti, M., Nagaraja, H. N., et al. Tolerability, safety, and benefits of risperidone in children and adolescents with autism: 21-month follow-up after 8-week placebo-controlled trial. *J Child Adolesc Psychopharmacol* 2015; 25(6): 482–93. https://doi.org/10.1089/cap.2015.0005

2. Dominick, K. C., Wink, L. K., Pedapati, E. V., et al. Risperidone treatment for irritability in fragile X syndrome. *J Child Adolesc Psychopharmacol* 2018, 28(4): 274–78. https://doi.org/10.1089/cap.2017.0057

3. Erickson, C. A., Stigler, K. A., Wink, L. K., et al. A prospective open-label study of aripiprazole in fragile X syndrome. *Psychopharmacology* 2011; 216(1): 85–90. https://doi.org/10.1007/s00213-011-2194-7

4. Gotham, K., Pickles, A., Lord, C. Standardizing ADOS scores for a measure of severity in autism spectrum disorders. *J Autism Develop Disord* 2009; 39(5): 693–705. https://doi.org/10.1007/s10803-008-0674-3

5. Gotham, K., Risi, S., Pickles, A., Lord, C. The autism diagnostic observation schedule: revised algorithms for improved diagnostic validity. *J Autism Develop Disord* 2007; 37(4): 613–27. https://doi.org/10.1007/s10803-006-0280-1

6. Hersh, J. H., Saul, R. A. Health supervision for children with fragile X syndrome (clinical report). In *Pediatric Clinical Practice Guidelines & Policies*. Itasca, IL: American Academy of Pediatrics, 2021. https://doi.org/10.1542/9781581108224-health8_sub01

7. Kloosterboer, S. M., de Winter, B. C. M., Reichart, C. G., et al. Risperidone plasma concentrations are associated with side effects and effectiveness in children and adolescents with autism spectrum disorder. *Br J Clin Pharmacol* 2021; 87(3): 1069–81. https://doi.org/10.1111/bcp.14465

8. Koch, M. T., Carlson, H. E., Kazimi, M. M., Correll, C. U. Antipsychotic-related prolactin levels and sexual dysfunction in mentally ill youth: a 3-month cohort study. *J Am Acad Child Adolesc Psychiatry* 2023; 15: S08908567(23)00125-9. doi: 10.1016/j.jaac.2023.03.007. Epub ahead of print. PMID: 36931560.

9. McCracken, J. T., McGough, J., Shah, B., et al. Risperidone in children with autism and serious behavioral problems. *N Engl J Med* 2002; 347(5): 314–21. https://doi.org/10.1056/nejmoa013171

10. Muhle, R. A., Reed, H. E., Vo, L. C., et al. Clinical diagnostic genetic testing for individuals with developmental disorders. *J Am*

Acad Child Adolesc Psychiatry 2017; 56(11): 910–13. https://doi.org/10.1016/j.jaac.2017.09.418

11. Savatt, J. M., Myers, S. M. Genetic testing in neurodevelopmental disorders. *Front Pediatr* 2021; 9. https://doi.org/10.3389/fped.2021.526779

12. Strawn, J. R., Geracioti, T. D. Editorial: a better perspective on antipsychotic-related hyperprolactinemia in children and adolescents. *J Am Acad Child Adolesc Psychiatry* 2023: S0890-8567(23)00240-X. doi: 10.1016/j.jaac.2023.05.003. Epub ahead of print. PMID: 37172820.

Case 17: The "standard treatment" is earning a "D": treatment-resistant schizophrenia

The Question: When and how should clozapine be used in older adolescents with treatment-resistant schizophrenia?

The Psychopharmacological Dilemma: When to use clozapine and how to dose and monitor its use is a source of debate and uncertainty for many clinicians, yet the evidence – largely based on decades of studies in adults – suggests that this agent has response rates substantially higher than those for other second-generation antipsychotics (SGAs) in patients with treatment-resistant schizophrenia

Pretest self-assessment question

In addition to D_2 antagonism, clozapine's effect at which of the following receptors may contribute to its antipsychotic efficacy?

A. H_1
B. D_3
C. 5-HT_{2A}
D. 5-HT_{2C}
E. α_1

Answer: C (5-HT_{2A})

Patient evaluation on intake

- A 17-year-old adolescent who developed psychotic symptoms approximately 2 years ago has been more withdrawn, no longer spending time with friends, and, at home, has been responding to internal stimuli
- The patient reports ongoing psychotic symptoms, including auditory hallucinations and persecutory delusions
- She experiences constant worry and an inability to trust others and thinks poorly of her abilities; however, she is reluctant to admit this to others
- She denies obsessions, including hearing songs or sentences in her head over and over, having thoughts of hurting herself or hurting someone else, or that bad things might happen to someone or that she might get contaminated by germs or dirt. Similarly, she denies compulsions
- In social situations, she describes some fear related to embarrassment or humiliation but notes that most of her "social problems" stem from her distrust of others

- Despite her withdrawal and decreased motivation, she denies depressed mood, feelings of guilt or worthlessness, changes in appetite, anergia, and suicidal ideation, intent, or plan
- She denies manic symptoms, including persistently elevated, expansive mood as well as inflated self-esteem, decreased need for sleep, pressured speech, flight of ideas/racing thoughts, and distractibility
- There is no history of attention-deficit hyperactivity disorder (ADHD)
- In terms of medication, she reports taking her risperidone every day
- She denies any side effects, including akathisia/extrapyramidal symptoms

Psychiatric history

- Prodromal symptoms emerged 12 months before the onset of auditory hallucinations
- During her initial psychotic episode, she was withdrawn and expressed persecutory delusions related to foods having been poisoned and that people are listening to her thoughts. She experienced significant anxiety related to her psychosis, and several of her longer-term friendships were ruptured at this time
- She had one prior psychiatric hospitalization, which was 10 days and related to her "psychotic break." During this hospitalization, an encephalitis panel was negative, and reversible causes of psychosis were eliminated
- There is no family history of substance-use disorders

Social and personal history

- The patient lives with her mother, who divorced her father when the patient was 12 years of age
- She has a younger brother, age 14, with whom she has a close relationship
- She attends a private high school and has been accepted to a local university where she plans on majoring in clinical laboratory science
- Academically, she earns As and excels in math-based coursework
- She has few close friends, although she is close with an 18-year-old girl online, who lives 5 hours away and with whom she chats nightly
- There is no history of abuse

Medical history

- She was delivered by planned cesarian section at 39 weeks to a 32-year-old mother and 32-year-old father. She had no pre- or perinatal complications
- Her mother had prenatal care throughout the pregnancy and took a multivitamin
- She had normal developmental milestones

Family history

- The patient's paternal grandfather has schizophrenia, coronary artery disease, type II diabetes, obstructive sleep apnea, and obesity
- Her paternal uncle has had multiple psychiatric hospitalizations and has been treated with multiple dopamine receptor antagonists as well as serotonin-dopamine receptor antagonists. He has diabetes, stage 3 chronic kidney disease, obesity, hyperlipidemia, and chronic obstructive pulmonary disease (COPD). He is treated with clozapine (Clozaril) 600 mg daily, extended-release metformin (Glucophage XR) 1500 mg daily, losartan (Cozaar) 100 mg daily, rosuvastatin (Crestor) 5 mg daily, tiotropium 18 mcg daily, and albuterol (metered dose inhaler) as needed

Medication history

- Her initial antipsychotic treatment was aripiprazole (Abilify) monotherapy (titrated to 15 mg every night at bedtime) with partial response (total of 3 months of treatment)
- Thereafter, aripiprazole was cross-titrated to extended-release quetiapine (Seroquel XR, 600 mg every night at bedtime). However, over 2 months, positive and negative symptoms not only persisted, but she had recrudescence of some of her auditory hallucinations
- Following her trial of extended-release quetiapine (Seroquel XR), risperidone was begun and titrated to 3 mg twice daily. And, over the first month of treatment with risperidone, quetiapine was discontinued
- She has been treated with risperidone (Risperdal) 3 mg twice daily for 6 months; however, she continues to experience significant functional impairment and auditory hallucinations

Current medications

- Risperidone (Risperdal) 3 mg twice daily

Psychotherapy history

- She is working intermittently in supportive psychotherapy
- Her family has also participated in the Family-to-Family Program through the National Alliance on Mental Illness (NAMI)

Further investigation

Is there anything else that you would like to know about the patient? What about possible safety concerns?

- She denies suicidal ideation, intent, and plan
- There have been no recent exposures to suicide attempts or completed suicides
- She does not possess any firearms

Attending physician's mental notes: initial psychiatric evaluation

- In reflecting on her prior psychopharmacologic treatment, her attending physician notes that her current dose of risperidone, assuming that she is not a CYP2D6 ultrarapid metabolizer, would likely produce 80% D_2 receptor blockade (Kapur et al. 1995). Eighty percent occupancy thresholds are generally considered sufficient thresholds for antipsychotic efficacy for many patients when using first- and second-generation antipsychotics and this threshold is achieved at higher doses than for 5-HT$_2$ occupancy (Figure 17.1) (Meyer and Stahl 2019)

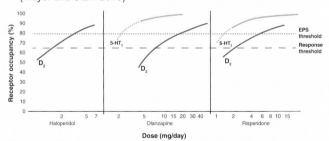

Figure 17.1 Response and adverse effects based on fitted D_2 occupancy curves for D_2 antagonist antipsychotics. Adapted from: Kapur, S. and Seeman, P. Does fast dissociation from the dopamine (D2) receptor explain the action of atypical antipsychotics? A new hypothesis. *Am J Psychiatry* 2021; 158: 360–69.

- However, her attending physician is aware that D_2 occupancy thresholds do not apply to medications whose mechanism is not highly dependent on D_2 antagonism (Meyer and Stahl 2021) and that the relationship between D_2 blockade is complex for quetiapine because of its rapid dissociation from the D$_2$ receptor (Kapur et al. 2000)

- Psychologically, the attending physician is concerned by her disconnection from others and her tendency to feel alone. He is concerned that this tendency relates both to her psychotic disorder and her low self-esteem and limits her ability to experience positive social interactions

- The attending physician is aware that while she reports her adherence to be high, this varies substantially even in "stable" patients with schizophrenia (MacEwan et al. 2016; Yaegashi et al. 2020). He recalls that various thresholds for "adherence" are common in the literature and range from 70–80% of doses being taken. Nonadherence can clearly be seen in most patients (Figure 17.2) and an 80% threshold for adherence is generally suggested as a goal in meta-analyses and individual monitoring studies (Yaegashi et al. 2020). Painfully, however, the attending physician knows that clinicians and patients generally perceive adherence to be higher than reality (Lopez et al. 2017; Velligan et al. 2006) and that adherence is dynamic (Meyer and Stahl 2021)

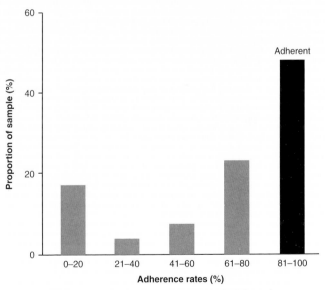

Figure 17.2 Rates of adherence in stable schizophrenia patients monitored over 4 weeks. Adapted from Remington et al. Examining levels of antipsychotic adherence to better understand nonadherence. *J Clin Psychopharmacol* 2013; 33: 261–63.

Question

Given her current symptoms and presentation, what would be your next step?

- Obtain risperidone and 9-OH risperidone trough concentrations
- Obtain pharmacogenetic testing to determine her genotype for the *methyl tetrahydrofolate reductase (MTHFR)* gene
- Referral for psychological testing

Testing: laboratory results, imaging, EKGs

Neither pharmacogenetic testing nor psychological testing were obtained as these would not change acute management. However, routine laboratory studies, as well as a trough risperidone level, were obtained.

RISPERIDONE	Value	Ref Range
RISPERIDONE	26 ng/dL	Not established
9-HYDROXYRISPERIDONE	20 ng/dL	Not established
TOTAL (RISP+9-HYDROXY)	46 ng/dL	20-60 ng/mL

Hemoglobin A1 C		
	Value	Ref Range
Hemoglobin A1C	5.0	<5.6%

Lipid Profile W/ HDL		
	Value	Ref Range
HDL CHOLESTEROL	**39**	**>=40 mg/dL**
CHOLESTEROL LEVEL	128	<=199 mg/dL
TRIGLYCERIDES	125	<=129 mg/dL
LDL CHOLESTEROL	75	<=129 mg/dL

Insulin		
	Value	Ref Range
INSULIN	7.4	2-8 mcIU/mL

CBC with Differential		
	Value	Ref Range
WBC	8.8	4.5 - 13.0 K/mcL
RBC	5.09	4.50 - 5.30 M/mcL
HGB	15.8	13.0 - 16.0 gm/dL
HCT	44.7	37.0 - 49.0 %
MCV	87.8	78.0 - 94.0 fL
MCH	30.9	25.0 - 35.0 pg
MCHC	35.2	31.0 - 37.0 gm/dL
RDW	11.5	<14.6 %
PLATELET	204	135 - 466 K/mcL

Comp Metabolic Panel		
	Value	Ref Range
SODIUM	141	136 - 145 mmol/L
POTASSIUM	4.1	3.3 - 4.7 mmol/L
CHLORIDE	105	100 - 112 mmol/L
CO2	26	17 - 31 mmol/L
ANION GAP	10	4 - 15 mmol/L
BUN	12	6 - 21 mg/dL

CREATININE	0.96	0.46 – 1.00 mg/dL
B/C RATIO	12	<25
GLUCOSE	93	65 – 106 mg/dL
CALCIUM	9.4	8.3 – 10.6 mg/dL
ALBUMIN	4.6	3.3 – 4.8 gm/dL
TOTAL PROTEIN	7.6	6.2 – 8.1 gm/dL
ALKALINE PHOS	130	48 – 138 unit/L
ALT	34	<=49 unit/L
AST	35	10 – 36 unit/L
BILIRUBIN	1.2	0.1–1.2 mg/dL
GLOBULIN	3.0	gm/dL
A/G RATIO	2	1 – 2

GGT

	Value	Ref Range
GGT	17	9 – 49 unit/L

TSH with Reflex to T4 Free, Rapid

	Value	Ref Range
TSH WITH REFLEX TO T4 FREE, RAPID	1.861	0.430 – 4.000 mcIU/mL

TOXICOLOGY – MASS SPEC

	Value	Ref Range
AMPHETAMINES	Not Detected	Not Applicable
BARBITURATES	Not Detected	Not Applicable
BENZODIAZEPINES	Not Detected	Not Applicable
CANNABINOIDS	Not Detected	Not Applicable
COCAINE	Not Detected	Not Applicable
OPIOID	Not Detected	Not Applicable
METHADONE INTERP	Not Detected	Not Applicable
BUPRENORPHINE INTERP	Not Detected	Not Applicable
MUSCLE RELAXANTS INTERP	Not Detected	Not Applicable
PHENCYCLIDINE	Not Detected	Not Applicable
NICOTINE INTERP	Not Detected	Not Applicable

Question

Given her current symptoms and the results of the work-up, what would be your next step?

- Convert risperidone (Risperdal) 6 mg daily to paliperidone (Invega) 3 mg every night at bedtime
- Cross-titrate risperidone (Risperdal) to asenapine (Saphris)
- Cross-titrate risperidone (Risperdal) to clozapine (Clozaril)
- Begin fluoxetine (Prozac) 20 mg daily to address her negative symptoms

Case outcome: first interim visit (week 1)

- At her last visit, her clinician began cross-titrating risperidone (Risperdal) to clozapine (Clozaril)
- The physician had a thorough discussion of risks and benefits of clozapine using the discussion points described in Jonathan

Meyer's and Stephen Stahl's *Clozapine Handbook* (Meyer and Stahl 2019) (Table 17.1). The attending physician uses the checklist to document these discussions and provide a scaffold for the informed consent discussion

- The attending physician will meet regularly with the patient as clozapine is titrated and will follow the titration schedule shown in Table 17.2

Table 17.1

Checklist of patient and caregiver information prior to initiating clozapine.

Item	Date
1. The indication for clozapine has been explained.	
2. The reasons for clozapine monitoring have been explained.	
3. Clozapine's common side effects have been explained and actions to take should they occur.	
4. Signs and symptoms of infection have been explained and what to do should they occur.	
5. The importance of regular blood tests has been discussed and what may happen if they miss their blood test.	
6. Discuss the importance of continuing clozapine.	
7. Document that dietary and lifestyle advice has been given to the patient.	
8. What to do if they miss a dose, especially if more than 48 hours has elapsed.	
9. Explain how smoking can affect clozapine levels and the importance of letting the prescriber know if they intend to stop or cut down smoking, or start smoking.	
10. Whom to contact in an emergency both during and after office hours.	

Reproduced from Meyer and Stahl, *Clozapine Handbook*, 2019.

Table 17.2

Example outpatient titration for clozapine

Day	Adult dose (smoker) (mg every night at bedtime)	Adult dose (nonsmoker) (mg every night at bedtime)
1	25	12.5
3	50	25
6	100	50
9	150	75
12	200	100
15	250	125
18	300	150
21	350	175
24	400	200

Reproduced from Meyer and Stahl, *Clozapine Handbook*, 2019.

- Since beginning clozapine, the patient notes no current orthostatic symptoms; she denies fever and constipation and denies any significant change in her psychotic symptoms

- She describes excellent adherence, and her parents have helped her to monitor her medication adherence
- An Abnormal Involuntary Movement Scale (AIMS) has been administered and reveals a score of 1

Current medications

- Risperidone (Risperdal) 1 mg every morning and 2 mg every night at bedtime
- Clozapine (Clozaril) 50 mg every night at bedtime

Attending physician's mental notes: first interim visit (week 1)

- The attending physician has selected clozapine based on the failure of three other dopamine-serotonin receptor agonists and has obtained trough risperidone concentrations to determine that she has an exposure that would be expected based on her current dose. Additionally, the attending physician notes roughly a 1:1 ratio of risperidone to its primary metabolite, 9-OH-risperidone
- He has chosen a slower cross-titration from risperidone to clozapine and enquired about her smoking status, given that smoking significantly increases clozapine exposure
- Additionally, the attending physician has confirmed that she is not treated with any CYP1A2 inhibitors, which could increase clozapine exposure (i.e. blood levels)

Case outcome: second, third, and fourth interim follow-up visits (weeks 2–5)

- The patient is seen weekly and has several "nurse visits" over the first month of treatment
- By the fifth week of treatment, she is taking clozapine 100 mg twice daily, and risperidone has been decreased to 0.5 mg twice daily
- She notes improvement in auditory hallucinations, and her parents report that she is more engaged, particularly at several recent family events. She is more animated in discussing her longer-term career goals and has joined a preprofessional society at her school
- Her weekly absolute neutrophil counts (ANCs) are stable, and her vital signs are remarkable for mild tachycardia (heart rate 100–112). However, she denies any palpitations or orthostatic intolerance. Additionally, she denies chest pain, constipation, fever, chills, nausea, and vomiting

Current medications

- Risperidone (Risperdal) 0.5 mg twice daily
- Clozapine (Clozaril) 100 mg twice daily

Attending physician's mental notes: second, third, and fourth interim follow-up visits (weeks 2–5)

- Her attending physician is encouraged by her progress and her reported adherence
- He consults the monitoring guidelines for ANC and adheres to the clozapine Risk Evaluation and Mitigation Strategy (REMS) requirement to send the results of her ANC to the central REMS program and discusses the importance of monitoring with the patient

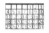

Case outcome: fifth interim follow-up visit (week 8)

- At her last visit, risperidone was discontinued, and the patient continues to do very well
- ANCs remain stable
- Her vital signs are remarkable for mild tachycardia (heart rate 100–106 bpm), and she denies any palpitations or orthostatic intolerance. Additionally, she denies chest pain, constipation, fever, chills, nausea, and vomiting
- She describes excellent adherence to her medication regimen and uses a "pill tracker" app to ensure that she does not miss any doses. She has noted that she "almost misses" her morning dose if she runs late for classes in the morning and asks about the possibility of taking her clozapine dose in the evening. Following a discussion, she and her physician agree to try this approach
- Finally, she confirms no new concomitant medications

Current medications

- Clozapine (Clozaril) 200 mg every night at bedtime

Attending physician's mental notes: fifth interim follow-up visit (week 8)

- Her attending physician continues to be encouraged by her progress and reported adherence
- Regarding the discussion of twice-daily vs. once-daily administration, clozapine has a mean peripheral half-life of only 12 hours; however, its active metabolite, norclozapine, has a half-life of nearly 24 hours. As in this case, initial titration often uses twice

daily dosing, given that the medication may be sedating initially (Meyer and Stahl 2019).

- Her attending physician is aware that the use of once-daily dosing may be possible given that clozapine's primary mechanism is not solely dependent on D_2 antagonism. Interestingly, clozapine only transiently reaches 60% D_2 receptor occupancy (Figure 17.3) and some of its efficacy may relate to 5-HT_{2A} antagonism, which – unlike D_2 occupancy – remains high throughout the day

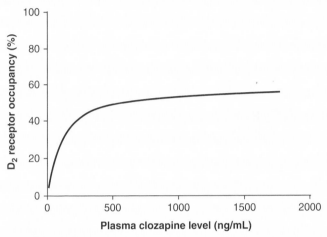

Figure 17.3 Relationship between the daily dose of clozapine and the steady-state trough serum concentration of clozapine for N = 68 patients. The recommended therapeutic reference range of clozapine (350–600 ng/mL) in adults is highlighted. Reproduced from Wohkittel, C., et al. Relationship between clozapine dose, serum concentration, and clinical outcome in children and adolescents in clinical practice. *J Neural Transm (Vienna)* 2016; 123(8): 1021–31.

Question

Given her current stable symptoms, would you consider obtaining plasma clozapine and norclozapine concentration prior to her next visit?

- No
- Yes

Case outcome: sixth interim follow-up visit (week 12)

- She continues to do well in terms of her psychotic symptoms and reports no auditory hallucinations over the past 4 weeks. She continues to be increasingly engaged at school, and with friends and family

- There are no significant depressive or anxiety symptoms
- ANCs remain stable
- Her vital signs remain remarkable for mild tachycardia (heart rate 100–106), and she continues to deny any palpitations or orthostatic intolerance. Additionally, she denies chest pain, constipation, fever, chills, nausea, and vomiting

Testing: laboratory results, imaging, EKGs

CLOZAPINE (Clozaril)*	Value	Ref Range
CLOZAPINE	430 ng/mL	350-650 ng/mL
NORCLOZAPINE	250 ng/mL	Not established
TOTAL (Cloz+Norcloz)	680 ng/mL	Not established

*Patients dosed with 400 mg clozapine daily for 4 weeks were most likely to exhibit a therapeutic effect when the sum of clozapine and norclozapine concentrations was at least 450 ng/mL. Toxic ranges are not well established. Serum/plasma concentrations >1500 ng/mL (clozapine, norclozapine, and clozapine-N-oxide combined) may cause drug-induced agranulocytosis, Stevens-Johnson syndrome, seizures, hypotension, cardiovascular abnormalities, drowsiness, and death REFERENCE: Hiemke, C., Baumann, P., Bergemann, N., et al. AGNP Consensus Guidelines for Therapeutic Drug Monitoring in Psychiatry: Update 2011, Pharmacopsychiatry Sep 2011; 44(6):195-235.

Hemoglobin A1C		
	Value	Ref Range
Hemoglobin A1C	4.9	<5.6%

CBC		
	Value	Ref Range
WBC	8.5	4.5 - 13.0 K/mcL
RBC	5.09	4.50 - 5.30 M/mcL
HGB	15.8	13.0 - 16.0 gm/dL
HCT	44.7	37.0 - 49.0 %
MCV	87.8	78.0 - 94.0 fL
MCH	30.9	25.0 - 35.0 pg
MCHC	35.2	31.0 - 37.0 gm/dL
RDW	11.5	<14.6 %
PLATELET	204	135 - 466 K/mcL

ANC		
	Value	Ref Range
4.8	1.5-7.5 x 10^3/µL	

Attending physician's mental notes: sixth interim follow-up visit (week 12)

- Her attending physician continues to be encouraged by her progress and reported adherence and has elected to obtain a clozapine/norclozapine level for several reasons
- Her attending physician is aware that the likelihood of response (which this patient has already met) is uncommon at levels >1000 ng/mL ("point of futility") (Meyer and Stahl 2019), but that

the likelihood of response is greatest at levels >350 ng/mL and that >350 ng/mL, >600 ng/mL, and >700 ng/mL identify intervals with a marked reduction in the proportion of nonresponders (Figure 17.4)

- In reviewing the laboratory results, her attending physician is aware that many laboratories report an "upper limit" for clozapine levels, but there are patients who benefit from and tolerate these high plasma levels
- Regarding the decision to obtain a clozapine level, her attending physician hopes that this will be a baseline reference for her concentration at a time when she was doing well with regard to psychotic symptoms. Additionally, should concomitant medications be added or her adherence change, her attending physician can compare future concentrations to her current level

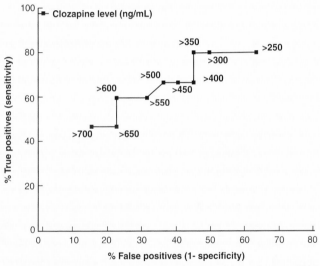

Figure 17.4. Receiver operating characteristic (ROC) curve from 1995 data on the proportion of clozapine responders and nonresponders for plasma clozapine concentrations in 50 ng/mL increments. Adapted from Kronig, M. H., et al. Plasma clozapine levels and clinical response for treatment-refractory schizophrenic patients. *Am J Psychiatry* 1995; 152: 179–82.

Case outcome: seventh interim follow-up visit (week 16)

- The patient continues to do well with regard to psychotic symptoms and denies significant depressive and anxiety symptoms. However, over the past week, she has had increasing abdominal pain, distension, and bloating
- Her last bowel movement was 4 days ago, and she denies any recent diarrhea, vomiting, fever, or chills

- She had urinary tract infection symptoms 1 week ago and was seen at an urgent care clinic where ciprofloxacin (Cipro) 500 mg twice daily was begun. She is currently on day 5 of 7 days of ciprofloxacin
- She is referred to the emergency department, given concerns for ileus
- In the emergency department, she continues to report diffuse abdominal pain without peritoneal symptoms but denies vomiting and is passing flatus
- On examination in the emergency department, her abdomen is mildly distended, but bowel sounds are present. Her vital signs are stable and laboratory studies (including a clozapine/norclozapine level at the request of her attending psychiatrist) and abdominal imaging are obtained

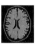

Testing: laboratory results, imaging, EKGs

ABDOMEN 2-VIEW: Bowel gas is present in a nonobstructive pattern. There is no evidence of free intraperitoneal gas, pneumatosis, abnormal calcifications, organomegaly, or abdominal mass. There is a significant amount of stool in the colon. The visualized lung bases are clear. The bones are normal.

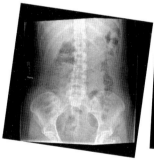
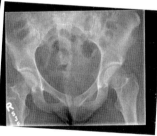

Testing: laboratory results, imaging, EKGs

	CBC	
	Value	Ref Range
WBC	12.5	4.5 – 13.0 K/mcL
RBC	5.09	4.50 – 5.30 M/mcL
HGB	15.8	13.0 – 16.0 gm/dL
HCT	44.7	37.0 – 49.0 %
MCV	87.8	78.0 – 94.0 fL
MCH	30.9	25.0 – 35.0 pg
MCHC	35.2	31.0 – 37.0 gm/dL
RDW	11.5	<14.6 %
PLATELET	235	135 – 466 K/mcL

CLOZAPINE (Clozaril)*	Value	Ref Range
CLOZAPINE	645 ng/mL	350-650 ng/mL
NORCLOZAPINE	300 ng/mL	Not established
TOTAL (Cloz+Norcloz)	945 ng/mL	Not established

* Patients dosed with 400 mg clozapine daily for 4 weeks were most likely to exhibit a therapeutic effect when the sum of clozapine and norclozapine concentrations were at least 450 ng/mL. Toxic ranges are not well established. Serum/plasma concentrations ≥1500 ng/mL (clozapine, norclozapine, and clozapine-N-oxide combined) may cause drug-induced agranulocytosis, Stevens-Johnson syndrome, seizures, hypotension, cardiovascular abnormalities, drowsiness, and death

REFERENCE: Hiemke, C., Baumann, P., Bergemann, N., et al. AGNP Consensus Guidelines for Therapeutic Drug Monitoring in Psychiatry: Update 2011. Pharmacopsychiatry Sep 2011; 44(6):195–235.

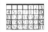

Case outcome: seventh interim follow-up visit (week 16 – continued)

- In addition to the work-up above, the emergency department physician uses focused abdominal sonography to confirm peristalsis
- Ciprofloxacin is discontinued, docusate 100 mg twice daily and polyethylene glycol 17 g daily are added, and, after discussion with the outpatient psychiatrist, the patient's clozapine dose is reduced by half for 3 days

Current medications

- Clozapine (Clozaril) 100 mg every night at bedtime
- Docusate (Colace) 100 mg twice daily
- Polyethylene glycol (Miralax) 17 g daily

Attending physician's mental notes: seventh interim follow-up (week 16)

- The patient's constipation is likely related to increased clozapine exposure. Her clozapine exposure has increased by nearly 50%, although the magnitude of the increase in her norclozapine concentration is smaller, which is pharmacokinetically consistent with the effect of adding ciprofloxacin, a potent CYP1A2 inhibitor
- Importantly, the attending physician knows that constipation should be managed aggressively in patients treated with clozapine and that prophylactic treatment should have been initiated when clozapine was begun
- Her attending physician will carefully monitor the patient over the next week to ensure that her constipation is resolving and will also monitor her psychotic symptoms, given the decrease in clozapine dose

- Regarding the dose reduction, when CYP1A2 inhibitors are used in clozapine-treated patients, the clozapine dose should be decreased by two-thirds (Meyer et al. 2016); however, in this case, given that ciprofloxacin has been discontinued by the emergency medicine physician, clozapine was decreased by only 50%

Performance in practice: confessions of a psychopharmacologist

- While practice varies in terms of when to try clozapine, this patient had failures with three second-generation antipsychotics and, as such, clozapine might have been considered earlier in her course
- Her constipation was likely precipitated by a ciprofloxacin-related increased clozapine exposure, a phenomenon that has been described in multiple case reports (Brouwers et al. 2009; Espnes et al. 2012; Sambhi et al. 2007) and in one case report contributed to fatal clozapine toxicity (Meyer et al. 2016). Some recommend that medications for constipation "commence with the first clozapine prescription for every patient, even when constipation is not a current issue" (Meyer and Stahl 2019). This should have been initiated at the time when clozapine was begun
- Regarding the interaction between clozapine and CYP1A2 inhibitors such as ciprofloxacin, ideally, this would have been noted by: (1) the prescribing clinician at the urgent care clinic, (2) a mechanism within the electronic medical record system, or (3) the dispensing pharmacy. Regardless, the attending clinician might have discussed in more detail the potential increase in plasma clozapine concentrations with some medications as well as some symptoms that might be associated with increased clozapine exposure. The attending physician could have better emphasized the need to discuss any new medications either with a pharmacist or her clinician

Take-home points

- Determining concentrations of mixed dopamine–serotonin receptor antagonists can identify nonadherence, understand metabolism, and achieve a therapeutic concentration that maximizes the treatment response likelihood
- Clozapine occupies a special place in the management of treatment-resistant schizophrenia. However, there are substantial barriers to its use, and these barriers often involve clinicians' perceptions of adverse effects, monitoring, etc.
- Prescribing clozapine requires clinicians to enroll in the clozapine REMS, a safety program required by the U.S. Food and Drug

Administration (FDA) to manage the risk of severe neutropenia associated with clozapine treatment

- The only mandatory laboratory monitoring during the first few months of clozapine treatment is the routine complete blood count (CBC) used to determine the ANC (risk of leukopenia is higher in children compared to adults). However, several clinical outcomes ought to be tracked during the first 3 months to manage signs of intolerability (Meyer and Stahl 2019) and to monitor for myocarditis, which presents predominantly during weeks 1–7 of treatment
- The patient's smoking status must be factored into any dosing and titration schedule, as nonsmokers will have plasma clozapine concentrations that are 50% greater than in smokers for any given dose (Haslemo et al. 2006)
- Clozapine is strongly antimuscarinic, with 50 mg of oral clozapine equaling the anticholinergic potency of 1 mg of benztropine in nonsmokers (de Leon 2005)
- Clozapine therapy is associated with constipation and increases the risk of ileus. Importantly, ileus risk is doubled by concurrent treatment with strongly anticholinergic agents (Nielsen and Meyer 2012). Constipation should be aggressively managed in clozapine-treated patients and general recommendations are to use docusate 100 mg twice daily or, when constipation is present, to add senna 16 mg nightly. Some clozapine-treated patients may require one medication from each class of first-line agents described in Meyer and Stahl's *Clozapine Handbook* (Meyer and Stahl 2019) for adequate relief (Table 17.3)
- Additionally, in clozapine-treated patients, bulk-forming laxatives should be avoided, given that they may worsen constipation. Finally, in any patient taking clozapine, failure to relieve constipation for 48 hours must prompt a change in treatment (e.g. dose increase, additional agent of another class, enemas, etc.)
- Finally, bacterial or viral infections may decrease CYP1A2 activity, ostensibly through inflammatory cytokine-mediated processes. In some cases, infections are associated with a tripling of clozapine concentrations. As such, therapeutic drug monitoring and serial assessment of symptoms of clozapine toxicity should be monitored during infection-related hospitalization and some recommendations suggest a 50% reduction in clozapine dose in patients hospitalized with such infections (Meyer and Stahl 2019)
- In terms of therapeutic drug monitoring, clozapine levels correlate better with efficacy than the sum of clozapine + norclozapine levels.

Ideally, a 12-hour (± 2 h) trough is obtained at steady state (i.e. after 5–7 days)
- Tracking plasma (or serum) levels is crucial to a successful clozapine trial (Meyer and Stahl 2019)
- When obtaining clozapine levels in patients treated with twice-daily regimens, make sure they hold the morning dose until the morning trough is obtained. Remember, plasma clozapine levels may fluctuate up to 30% in adherent patients, but greater fluctuations may reflect nonadherence or other pharmacokinetic-related factors (Meyer and Stahl 2019)

Table 17.3 First-line agents for constipation in clozapine-treated patients

	Mechanism	Starting dose	Maximum effective dose	Comments
Dioctyl sodium sulfosuccinate (docusate or DSS)	Anionic detergent that causes stool softening	250 mg every night at bedtime	250 mg twice daily	Commonly used despite a paucity of evidence supporting efficacy
Polyethylene glycol 3350 (PEG-3350)	Osmotic agent	17 g daily	17 g twice daily	Strong recommendation. High quality of evidence
Lactulose	Osmotic agent	30 mL daily	30 mL twice daily	Strong recommendation. Low quality of evidence
Bisacodyl	Stimulant	5 mg every night at bedtime	15 mg twice daily	Strong recommendation. Moderate quality of evidence
Sennosides	Stimulant	8.6 mg every night at bedtime	17.2 mg twice daily	Absence of controlled data

Mechanism of action moment

- Clozapine possesses numerous mechanisms of action (Figure 17.5), and its receptor pharmacology accounts for both its unique tolerability and its antipsychotic effects:
  - Clozapine only transiently reaches 60% D_2 receptor occupancy, and thus potent 5-HT$_{2A}$ antagonism may partly explain clozapine's antipsychotic efficacy
  - Weight gain may be partially associated with its potent blockade of both H$_1$ histamine and 5-HT$_{2C}$ receptors (Figure 17.5)
  - Sedation is probably linked to clozapine's potent antagonism of muscarinic M$_1$, H$_1$, and α_1-adrenergic receptors
  - Profound muscarinic blockade can also cause excessive salivation, especially at higher doses, as well as severe

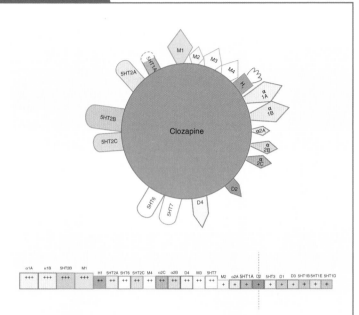

Figure 17.5 Clozapine's pharmacological icon and binding profile. This figure portrays a qualitative consensus of current thinking about the binding properties of clozapine. In addition to 5-HT$_{2A}$/D$_2$ antagonism, numerous other binding properties have been identified for clozapine, most of which are more potent than its binding at the D$_2$ receptor. It is unknown which of these contribute to clozapine's special efficacy or to its unique side effects. Adapted from *Stahl's Essential Psychopharmacology*, 2021.

  constipation that can lead to bowel obstruction, especially if administered concomitantly with other anticholinergic agents, such as benztropine (Nielsen and Meyer 2012) or other antipsychotics with potent anticholinergic properties, such as chlorpromazine
- From a kinetic standpoint, clozapine's potent 5-HT$_{2A}$ antagonism may partly explain its sustained efficacy with every night at bedtime dosing since the time course of receptor occupancy shows sustained high-level blockade throughout the day
- Clozapine has a complex metabolic pathway primarily mediated by CYP1A2. Regarding CYP1A2 substrates, clinicians should consider the importance of smoking (cigarettes or cannabis). Smoking reduces clozapine levels by 40%–50% via induction of CYP1A2 (Haslemo et al. 2006). Interestingly, however, vaping does not burn any organic matter and does not induce CYP1A2 (Meyer and Stahl 2019)

- With regard to the effects of age on clozapine metabolism, clozapine dose-to-concentration relationships vary across the lifespan, with younger patients having less clozapine exposure at a given dose compared to older patients (Figure 17.6)

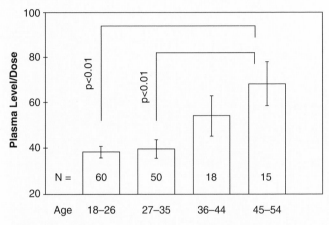

Figure 17.6 Clozapine concentrations relative to dose vary considerably and are influenced by age. Reproduced from Haring, C., et al. Dose-related plasma levels of clozapine: influence of smoking behaviour, sex and age. *Psychopharmacology (Berl)* 1989; 99(Suppl): S38-40.

Post test question

In addition to D_2 antagonism, clozapine's effect at which of the following receptors may contribute to its antipsychotic efficacy?

A. H_1
B. D_3
C. $5\text{-}HT_{2A}$
D. $5\text{-}HT_{2C}$
E. α_1

Answer: C ($5\text{-}HT_{2A}$)

Clozapine's potent $5\text{-}HT_{2A}$ effects (C) may partly explain its antipsychotic efficacy. It has no significant D_3 activity (B), and its potent blockade of both H_1 histamine (A) and $5\text{-}HT_{2C}$ receptors (D) potentially contributes to clozapine-associated weight gain. Its antagonism at α_1 (E) receptors potentially subtends the orthostatic hypotension seen with clozapine.

References

1. Brouwers, E. E. M., Söhne, M., Kuipers, S., et al. Ciprofloxacin strongly inhibits clozapine metabolism: two case reports. *Clin Drug Invest* 2009; 29(1): 59–63. https://doi.org/10.2165/0044011-200929010-00006

2. de Leon, J. Benztropine equivalents for antimuscarinic medication. *Am J Psychiatry* 2005; 162(3): 627. https://doi.org/10.1176/appi.ajp.162.3.627

3. Espnes, K. A., Heimdal, K. O., Spigset, O. A puzzling case of increased serum clozapine levels in a patient with inflammation and infection. *Ther Drug Monitor* 2012; 34(5): 489–92. https://doi.org/10.1097/FTD.0b013e3182666c62

4. Haslemo, T., Eikeseth, P. H., Tanum, L., Molden, E., Refsum, H. The effect of variable cigarette consumption on the interaction with clozapine and olanzapine. *Eur J Clin Pharmacol* 2006; 62(12): 1049–53. https://doi.org/10.1007/s00228-006-0209-9

5. Kapur, S., Remington, G., Zipursky, R. B., Wilson, A. A., Houle, S. The D2 dopamine receptor occupancy of risperidone and its relationship to extrapyramidal symptoms: a PET study. *Life Sci* 1995; 57(10): PL103–07. https://doi.org/10.1016/0024-3205(95)02037-J

6. Kapur, S., Zipursky, R., Jones, C., et al. A positron emission tomography study of quetiapine in schizophrenia: a preliminary finding of an antipsychotic effect with only transiently high dopamine D2 receptor occupancy. *Arch Gen Psychiatry* 2000; 57(6): 553–59. https://doi.org/10.1001/archpsyc.57.6.553

7. Lopez, L. V., Shaikh, A., Merson, J., Accuracy of clinician assessments of medication status in the emergency setting: a comparison of clinician assessment of antipsychotic usage and plasma level determination. *J Clin Psychopharmacol* 2017; 37(3): 310–14. https://doi.org/10.1097/JCP.0000000000000697

8. MacEwan, J. P., Forma, F. M., Shafrin, J., et al. Patterns of adherence to oral atypical antipsychotics among patients diagnosed with schizophrenia. *J Manag Care Specialty Pharm* 2016; 22(11): 1349–61. https://doi.org/10.18553/jmcp.2016.22.11.1349

9. Meyer, J. M., Proctor, G., Cummings, M. A., Dardashti, L. J., Stahl, S. M. Ciprofloxacin and clozapine: a potentially fatal but underappreciated interaction. *Case Rep Psychiatry* 2016; 2016: 5606098. https://doi.org/10.1155/2016/5606098

10. Meyer, J. M., Stahl, S. M. *The Clozapine Handbook*. Cambridge, UK: Cambridge University Press, 2019. https://doi.org/10.1017/9781108553575

11. Meyer, J. M., Stahl, S. M. *The Clinical Use of Antipsychotic Plasma Levels.* Cambridge, UK: Cambridge University Press, 2021. https://doi.org/10.1017/9781009002103

12. Nielsen, J., Meyer, J. M. Risk factors for ileus in patients with schizophrenia. *Schizophrenia Bull* 2012; 38(3): 592–98. https://doi.org/10.1093/schbul/sbq137

13. Sambhi, R. S., Puri, R., Jones, G. Interaction of clozapine and ciprofloxacin: a case report. *Eur J Clin Pharmacol* 2007; 63(9): 895–96. https://doi.org/10.1007/s00228-007-0313-5

14. Velligan, D. I., Lam, Y. W. F., Glahn, D. C., et al. Defining and assessing adherence to oral antipsychotics: a review of the literature. *Schizophrenia Bull* 2006; 32(4): 724–42. https://doi.org/10.1093/schbul/sbj075

15. Yaegashi, H., Kirino, S., Remington, G., Misawa, F., Takeuchi, H. Adherence to oral antipsychotics measured by electronic adherence monitoring in schizophrenia: a systematic review and meta-analysis. *CNS Drugs* 2020; 34(6): 579–98. https://doi.org/10.1007/s40263-020-00713-9

16. Komaryk A., Elbe D., Burgess L. Retrospective review of clozapine use in children and adolescents. *J Can Acad Child Adolesc Psychiatry* 2021; 30(1): 36–48

Case 18: Symptoms, side effects, or both? Selective serotonin reuptake inhibitor (SSRI) tolerability and physical symptoms in an anxious adolescent

The Questions: How should SSRIs be cross-titrated in adolescents? What is mechanism-based inhibition, and how does it relate to the pharmacokinetics of some SSRIs in adolescents?

The Psychopharmacological Dilemma: SSRIs are commonly associated with tremendous improvement in adolescents with anxiety and depressive disorders; however, they may be associated with side effects that require medication changes. Cross-titrating SSRIs requires an understanding of both pharmacodynamic and pharmacokinetic principles

Pretest self-assessment question

Because of mechanism-based inhibition, which of the following SSRIs has nonlinear kinetics?

A. Escitalopram (Lexapro)
B. Sertraline (Zoloft)
C. Fluvoxamine (Luvox)
D. Paroxetine (Paxil)
E. Vilazodone (Viibryd)

Answer: D (Paroxetine, Paxil)

Patient evaluation on intake

- A 13½-year-old girl with social anxiety, persistent sadness, feelings of worthlessness, difficulty with concentration, anergia, and amotivation
- She endorses initial insomnia (currently retiring to sleep at 10:30 pm and staying awake until 11:30 pm)
- Difficulty with concentration, adding that she more frequently "zones out and loses focus"
- She also experiences frequent physical symptoms, including blurry vision, constipation, dry mouth, occasional palpitations, and flushing, as well as recurrent headaches and recurrent abdominal pain
- Constant depressive symptoms and intermittent anxiety symptoms
- She endorsed depressed mood, feelings of worthlessness, difficulty with concentration, and increased appetite since beginning paroxetine and anergia but she denies suicidal ideation, intent, or plan. However, in the past, she had episodes of "wanting to die," and her father noted a pattern with regard to this. These episodes appeared to worsen contemporaneously with her menstrual cycle. Her father notes that the "amplitude of these episodes" worsens

perimenstrually. Importantly, these have improved following the initiation of an oral contraceptive

- Her anxiety has improved since beginning paroxetine (Paxil); she notes, "I feel like I don't worry as much now." However, she is still uncomfortable in groups and when talking to strangers
- She denies worries about harm happening to attachment figures, worries about harm befalling herself, including the fear of dying as well as distress associated with separation
- She experiences episodes of panic-like symptoms and has experienced these both at home and when she was away at camp, and she has taken hydroxyzine (Vistaril) on an as-needed basis for these. She notes that this has been somewhat helpful for her anxiety
- Interpersonally, she is very uncomfortable in social situations and has little interest in interacting with others – aside from a small group of individuals – and takes a rather passive, submissive stance when dealing with others. This lack of interest and initiative results in her being socially isolated, particularly with peers, avoiding most social interactions rather than running the risk of being forced to make an active commitment to a relationship. She remarks on this, "I've only opened up to like three people in my life." However, she describes an intensity and closeness in these relationships
- From an eating disorder standpoint, she has been concerned about being overweight and her appearance, and has been concerned about the appearance of certain body parts (e.g. stomach and rib cage), as well as the way in which she looks in certain clothes, including bathing suits, crop tops, and her horseback riding breeches. Further, in the sixth and seventh grades, she had more restrictive eating. Currently, she denies purging or use of laxatives, although when she was in the fifth or sixth grade, she attempted to induce vomiting but could not do so. Finally, she denies a "goal weight" and denies weighing herself regularly
- There are no obsessive compulsive disorder (OCD) symptoms
- Regarding attention-deficit hyperactivity disorder (ADHD) symptoms, she notes inattention and distractibility, and these symptoms were first noted when she was in the seventh grade. However, her current inattentive symptoms are not felt to be related to a primary diagnosis of ADHD, but rather to her affective disorder
- She has no history of aggression towards animals or theft, and has not been involved in serious violations of rules (e.g. disobeying curfews, staying out late prior to age 13, and running away from home overnight)
- There are no psychotic symptoms
- She denies any recent stressors

Psychiatric history

- Depressive and anxiety symptoms began in elementary school. She notes that initially, when these symptoms emerged, they were in the context of "bullying" during her second grade
- Her symptoms waxed and waned, although they again increased during her fourth- and fifth-grade years
- As she transitioned to middle school, during her sixth-grade year, her symptoms again worsened, and she describes feeling more isolated
- There have been intermittent episodes of Columbia-Suicide Severity Rating Scale (CSSRS) 1–2 suicidal ideation in the past, with the first being when she was in the sixth grade

Social history

- She lives with her mother, father, and two younger sisters
- At school, she reports performing well, and there is no 504 Plan or Individualized Education Plan (IEP) in place
- She owns a horse that she rides at least four to five times weekly, and during the summer and fall she competes in horse shows several times per month
- She describes a "close" relationship with her horseback riding instructor
- She is not currently engaged in any romantic relationships, although she describes liking a male peer at school. Otherwise, she describes a limited number of peer relationships
- There is no history of abuse or trauma

Medical history

- Her mother reports an uneventful pregnancy and delivery and there were no prenatal/perinatal complications
- In general, she is in good health but experienced a concussion early this year after falling from her horse while jumping. There was no loss of consciousness. Her parents report normal developmental milestones
- She is treated with an oral contraceptive and has recently begun docusate and psyllium fiber supplement for her worsening constipation

Family history

- She has a mother and father with generalized anxiety disorder, and her father has experienced two depressive episodes
- Her maternal grandmother has a history of alcohol-use disorder and coronary artery disease, as well as hypertension

- Her paternal grandfather is deceased (myocardial infarction, age 51 years)
- Maternal cousin with sudden cardiac death at age 16

Medication history

- Previously treated with escitalopram (Lexapro, 10 mg daily) with minimal improvement and was then transitioned to paroxetine which was initiated by her family practitioner at 10 mg every night at bedtime and titrated to 40 mg daily
- Paroxetine (Paxil) has been associated with weight gain and blurry vision, significant constipation, worsening palpitations, and dry mouth
- Hydroxyzine (Vistaril, 25 mg) has been used to address anxiety on an as-needed basis

Current medications

- Paroxetine (Paxil) 30 mg daily
- Docusate (Colace) 100 mg twice daily
- Psyllium fiber supplement 2 scoops twice daily
- Hydroxyzine (Vistaril) 25 mg twice daily as needed – "anxiety"
- Norgestimate-ethinyl estradiol (OrthoLo) 0.18 mg/0.215 mg daily

Psychotherapy history

- She currently works with a social worker using a cognitive behavior therapy (CBT)-based approach
- She meets with her therapist weekly and the appointments involve a brief update during the first 5 minutes of the appointment when she is seen conjointly with one of her parents
- She describes a good alliance with her therapist, but collateral information from her therapist suggests that she has been difficult to engage, and her therapist often feels that the psychotherapeutic process is somewhat superficial

Further investigation

What about additional physical symptoms and vital signs?

- Vital signs are within normal limits; her body mass index (BMI) is in the 45th percentile for age and sex and there is recent weight gain

Question

Given her current treatment, which of the following would be your next step?

- Laboratory screening for hyperthyroidism
- Pharmacogenetic testing for pharmacokinetic genes

- Obtain an electrocardiogram (EKG)
- Obtain an abdominal series (radiographs)
- Titration of paroxetine (Paxil) to 40 mg daily

Testing: laboratory results, imaging, EKGs

Complete Blood Count

Result	Value	Ref Range
WHITE BLOOD CELLS	5.51	4.5-13.5x10(3)/mcL
RED BLOOD CELL	4.33	4.1-5.10 x10(6)/mcL
HEMOGLOBIN	12.8	12.0 - 16.0 gm/dL
HEMATOCRIT	38.8	36.0 - 46.0 %
MCV	89.6	78.0 - 94.0 fL
MCH	29.6	25.0 - 35.0 pg
MCHC	33.0	31.0 - 37.0 gm/dL
RDW	12.2	<=14.6 %
PLATELET	358	135 - 466 x10(3)/mcL
LYMPHOCYTE	**32.3 (L)**	**34.0 - 42.0 %**
MONOCYTE	9.8	0 - 10.0 %
SEGMENTED NEUTROPHILS	55.4	40.0 - 62.0 %
BASOPHIL	0.5	0 - 1.0 %
Eosinophil	1.6	0 - 5.0 %
MONOCYTE ABSOLUTE	0.54	0 - 0.80 x10(3)/mcL
EOSINOPHIL ABSOLUTE	0.09	0 - 0.70 x10(3)/mcL
BASOPHIL ABSOLUTE	0.03	0 - 0.10 x10(3)/mcL
NEUTROPHIL ABSOLUTE	3.05	1.8-8 x10(3)/mcL
AUTOMATED NRBC PERCENTAGE	0.0	%
AUTOMATED NRBC ABSOLUTE	0.00	x10(3)/mcL
MPV	**9.5 (L)**	**9.6 - 11.7 fL**
IMMATURE GRANULOCYTE	**0.4 (H)**	**0 - 0.3 %**
IMMATURE GRAN ABS	0.02	0 - 0.03 x10(3)/mcL
LYMPHOCYTE ABSOLUTE	1.78	1.5 - 6.5 x10(3)/mcL

Vitamin D, 25-Hydroxy

Result	Value	Ref Range
Vitamin D, 25-Hydroxy	34	20 - 40 ng/mL

Hepatic Profile

Result	Value	Ref Range
Bilirubin Total	0.2	0.1 - 1.1 mg/dL
Bilirubin Direct	<0.1	0.0 - 0.3 mg/dL
Albumin	4.0	3.3 - 4.8 gm/dL
Globulin	3.6	gm/dl
Albumin/Globulin Ratio	1	1 - 2
Aspartate Aminotransferase	**29 (H)**	**5 - 26 unit/L**
Alanine Aminotransferase	22	<=49 unit/L
Alkaline Phosphatase	68	49 - 229 unit/L
TOTAL PROTEIN LEVEL	7.6	6.4 - 8.3 gm/dL

Basic Metabolic Panel

Result	Value	Ref Range
Sodium	138	136 - 145 mmol/L
Potassium	3.8	3.3 - 4.7 mmol/L

Chloride	102	100 - 112 mmol/L
Carbon Dioxide	24	17 - 31 mmol/L
Anion Gap	12	4 - 15 mmol/L
Blood Urea Nitrogen	7	6 - 21 mg/dL
Creatinine	0.79	0.46 - 1.00 mg/dL
Glucose	106	65 - 106 mg/dL
Calcium	9.9	8.7 - 10.8 mg/dL
Phosphorus	3.9	3.4 - 5.9 mg/dL
Magnesium	1.8	1.6 - 2.6 mg/dL

THYROID

Result	Value	Ref Range
Thyroid Stimulating Hormone	1.9	0.43 - 4.0 mcIU/mL

Testing: laboratory results, imaging, EKGs

Pharmacogenetic testing

	Genotype	Phenotype
CYP2D6	*41/*2	Normal metabolizer
CYP2C19	*17/*1	Rapid metabolizer

Testing: laboratory results, imaging, EKGs

Vent. rate	80	BPM
PR interval	150	ms
QRS duration	70	ms
QT/QTc	364/419	ms
P-R-T axes	52 52	38

Sinus rhythm with sinus arrhythmia, narrow q waves in the lateral leads

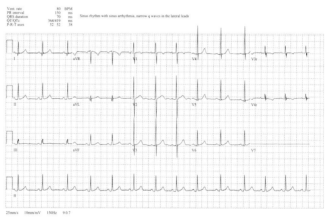

25mm/s   10mm/mV   150Hz   9.0.7

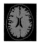

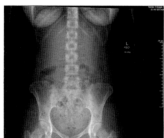

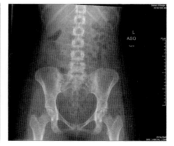

Supine and upright radiographs reveal mild constipation. There is a normal bowel gas pattern. No evidence of dilatation. The vertebral column and pelvis appear normal.

Attending physician's mental notes: initial psychiatric evaluation

- This patient has significant symptoms of major depressive disorder and social anxiety disorder, experiences symptom-limited panic attacks, and endorses myriad physical symptoms, including blurry vision, constipation, dry mouth, occasional palpitations, and flushing, as well as recurrent headaches and recurrent abdominal pain. Her physical symptoms have worsened since beginning paroxetine, although she notes that this has been helpful in terms of her social anxiety symptoms

- In terms of workup, she experiences multiple physical symptoms; some symptoms may be anticholinergically mediated (i.e. related to paroxetine) and some may be related to panic attacks or her underlying anxiety disorder (Ginsburg et al. 2006; Hughes et al. 2008). However, she has some atypical symptoms, and particularly from a cardiac standpoint, the attending physician is concerned about the family history of sudden cardiac death in a young, otherwise healthy second-degree relative and about her intermittent cardiac symptoms. His concern is amplified by some concerns that the patient has expressed about her body image, and while she denies restrictive eating and purging, he feels more comfortable obtaining some laboratory studies, including some of the laboratory studies that he might have obtained in adolescents with eating disorders (see Case 14). He is reassured by her EKG and the absence of any presyncopal symptoms, as well as exertional symptoms

- From a medication standpoint, the patient – a rapid CYP2C19 metabolizer – has previously been treated with escitalopram (Lexapro) and had minimal response. He knows that at the 15 mg dose of escitalopram, she would have had comparable, albeit slightly lower, escitalopram exposure compared to a normal CYP2C19 metabolizer (Figure 18.1) (Strawn et al. 2019, 2021). Thus, assuming adherence was reasonable, her escitalopram trial was adequate

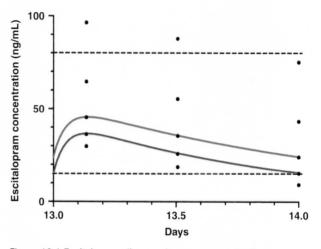

Figure 18.1 Escitalopram (Lexapro) serum concentrations, at steady state (day 13), in this adolescent who is a rapid metabolizer (blue) compared to a normal metabolizer (green). The dashed line represents proposed therapeutic range for escitalopram in adults. Data from Strawn et al. 2018.

- While some studies suggest the potential efficacy of paroxetine (Paxil) in pediatric patients with social anxiety and depressive disorders (Emslie et al. 2006; Keller et al. 2001; Wagner et al. 2004), her attending physician is concerned about paroxetine in young adolescents, given data that paroxetine is more likely to produce treatment-emergent suicidality (Cipriani et al. 2016; Dobson et al. 2019), more poorly tolerated, and more likely to produce significant anticholinergic symptoms. Additionally, her attending physician is aware of data from adults that suggest that paroxetine concentrations, even at a given dose, vary substantially (Figure 18.2) (Owens et al. 2008).
- Psychologically, her attending physician notes, based on the evaluation, that the patient wants to be seen as strong and assertive despite her inner self-doubt and frequently describes liking to be in control. The attending physician himself feels sadness as the patient describes feeling that adults would let her down and

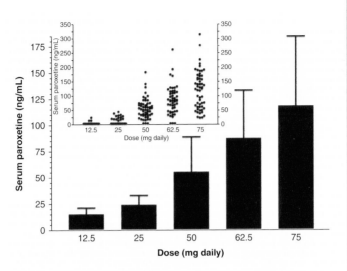

Figure 18.2 Paroxetine serum concentrations, at steady state, across multiple doses in adults as a function of dose. Mean serum concentrations (mean±SD) increased as dose increased, but, as can be seen in the inset concentrations, varied across individuals. Reproduced from Owens, M. J., et al. Estimates of serotonin and norepinephrine transporter inhibition in depressed patients treated with paroxetine or venlafaxine. *Neuropsychopharmacology* 2008; 33(13): 3201-12.

the way in which she generally tries to "handle things alone." He also notes that the patient is very concerned about being hurt, and this interferes with her ability to establish close and trusting relationships. She has a pattern of negativity and frequently fears that others will control and undermine her

- Moving forward, the attending physician is also concerned about the patient–family–clinician alliance, noting that the patient is easily offended by minor incidents and that this starts a pattern in which others behave in the way she most fears
- Further, her attending physician knows – based on her explicit comments – that she believes authority figures are not trustworthy, and she attempts to demean them. In psychopharmacology, like in psychotherapy, the therapeutic alliance is critical. Moreover, in working with children and adolescents, skill is required to maintain the alliance both with the patient and his or her family and to avoid triangulation

Question

Given her current treatment, which of the following would be your next step?

- Discontinue paroxetine (Paxil) and begin fluoxetine (Prozac) 20 mg daily
- Cross-titrate paroxetine (Paxil) to fluoxetine (Prozac)
- Augment with aripiprazole (Abilify) 2.5 mg every night at bedtime
- Titrate paroxetine (Paxil) to 60 mg every night at bedtime
- Discontinuation of paroxetine (Paxil) and trial of clomipramine (Anafranil)

Case outcome: first and second interim follow-up visits (weeks 2–4)

- At her last visit, fluoxetine (Prozac) was initiated at 20 mg daily and paroxetine (Paxil) decreased from 30 mg to 20 mg. Then 2 weeks later, fluoxetine was titrated to 40 mg daily, and paroxetine was discontinued
- Upon discontinuation of paroxetine, her fatigue and anticholinergic symptoms have improved, and she no longer reports napping
- Additionally, she notes improvement in her depressive symptoms, although she continues to feel more frustrated by interpersonal encounters and struggles with closeness and trust

Current medications

- Fluoxetine (Prozac) 40 mg every night at bedtime
- Docusate (Colace) 100 mg twice daily
- Psyllium fiber supplement (Metamucil) 1 scoop twice daily
- Hydroxyzine (Vistaril) 25 mg twice daily as needed – "anxiety"
- Norgestimate-ethinyl estradiol (OrthoLo) 0.18 mg/0.215 mg daily

Attending physician's mental notes: first and second interim follow-up visits (weeks 2–4)

- The attending physician is encouraged by her improvement and is reassured that some of her symptoms were related to paroxetine
- In considering the cross-titration from paroxetine to fluoxetine, the attending physician has some concerns given: (1) the CYP2D6 inhibition of both SSRIs, (2) the very short half-life of paroxetine, and (3) the long half-life of fluoxetine which will require several weeks to reach steady state. He is cautious in balancing the optimal period of overlap for the cross-titration, and for this reason, as well as the previously described concerns related to the alliance and the patient, he has checked in with the patient weekly during this month-long cross-titration

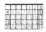

PATIENT FILE

Case outcome: third interim follow-up visit (week 8)

- She reports minimal depressive symptoms, and her Quick Inventory of Depressive Symptoms (QIDS) score is a 4 at today's visit
- She no longer reports constipation and abdominal pain, and her fiber supplement and docusate are discontinued
- The patient continues to do well academically, and her parents note that she is more engaged with friends. The patient describes less social anxiety and overall feels calmer and "not as tense." Interpersonally, she has still struggled to establish close and trusting relationships, goes to lengths to create interpersonal distance, and fears others will control and undermine her
- Her parents express their gratitude for the attending physician's work with their daughter and comment on how she has connected with him. Her mother shares that while the family was at dinner, the patient commented that she hopes her future husband is just like her attending physician – able to "understand everything about me"

Current medications

- Fluoxetine (Prozac) 40 mg every night at bedtime
- Hydroxyzine (Vistaril) 25 mg twice daily as needed – "anxiety"
- Norgestimate-ethinyl estradiol (OrthoLo) 0.18 mg/0.215 mg daily

Attending physician's mental notes: third interim follow-up visit (week 8)

- From a depression and anxiety standpoint, her attending physician is very encouraged and hopes to, in time, discontinue hydroxyzine (Vistaril)
- However, he realizes that while great strides have been made psychopharmacologically, other issues require attention. He is struck by the patient's mother's comment and the way in which the patient has idealized the treatment relationship. At this point, this could be seen as encouraging in terms of her ability to trust the clinician and develop mutuality; however, there may be a concern for over-idealization and a tendency to see the clinician as "all good." From a developmental perspective, this patient's idealization of a positive experience is common in early to mid-adolescence. The attending physician sees this as an opportunity to explore alternative psychotherapies with the patient and, following a discussion with the patient and family, makes a referral to a therapist colleague to work with the patient in interpersonal psychotherapy for adolescents (IPT-A)

311

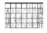

Case outcome: fourth interim follow-up visit (week 14)

- She continues to report minimal depressive symptoms, and her Quick Inventory of Depressive Symptoms score is a 6 at today's visit
- She continues to do well academically and is working in IPT-A but is still frequently disconnected from and unable to express her emotions. This has made it difficult for her to engage in a reflective psychotherapeutic process and in CBT previously
- She continues to have difficulty in close relationships

Attending physician's mental notes: fourth interim follow-up visit (week 14)

- From a depression and anxiety standpoint, her attending physician is very encouraged by her progress with regard to the absence of medication side effects and in terms of the originally targeted symptoms
- Her psychiatrist is concerned about her ongoing difficulties and struggles in psychotherapy. He considers psychological testing to obtain a clearer understanding of: (1) what makes it difficult for her to access and communicate her emotional experience and (2) how to more effectively engage her in treatment, specifically psychotherapy

Psychological testing

- The attending physician has arranged a consultation with a psychologist and, after obtaining consent and assent, discussed the patient's course with this psychologist

- The psychologist has met with the patient and family over several sessions and administered a series of tests, including the Wechsler Intelligence Scale for Children – Fourth Edition (WISC-IV), Rorschach, Thematic Apperception Test (TAT), and Minnesota Multiphasic Personality Inventory-Adolescent version (MMPI-A)

REALITY TESTING AND REASONING: The present data do not point to disordered reasoning and reality testing consistent with schizophrenic- or bipolar-spectrum illness. She can suffer profound lapses in these psychological capacities, however, under conditions of intensified emotion and when she is more on her own to make sense of things (i.e. without clear expectations, monitoring, and feedback). Specifically, her perceptions of situations and people are apt to become distorted, often when she focuses on less relevant aspects of the situation. In addition, her reasoning becomes more illogical and confused, marked by reading undue meaning into things and putting her ideas together in ways that do not make sense, leading to ill-conceived conclusions and judgments. Moreover, there is some evidence that even after the fact she does not recognize the lapses in her reasoning and judgment and, instead, views her misguided ideas as "cool" and creative.

EMOTIONAL REGULATION: This adolescent's overtly constricted demeanor and minimizing self-report belies the degree to which, internally, she is emotionally out of control and flooded. Her emotions overwhelm and over-ride her ability to use her otherwise strong verbal and thinking capacities (see "Intellectual Functioning"). Importantly, the present findings indicate that her difficulty with emotional expression is not that she is emotionally oblivious or that she lacks the emotional vocabulary to identify and differentiate among feelings. Rather, the present findings underscore that she experiences emotions with such intensity and with little sense of control that, self-protectively, she tries to cut herself off from them.

Testing highlights that her efforts to protect herself from painful and distressing feelings include consciously distancing from them; minimizing and denying them; attempting to put a superficial, positive spin on things; splitting her views of herself, others, and situations into simple black-and-white dichotomies; and viewing objectionable feelings - notably anger and aggression - as existing in others rather than herself.

EXPERIENCE OF SELF AND OTHER: The patient struggles with her self-esteem, again much more than she lets on or that one might expect based on others' views of her as intelligent and attractive. Beneath the surface, she experiences intense longings for affirmation. She has an implicit view of herself as damaged and lacking. She can be highly self-critical and self-attacking, and it is possible to speculate that one of the reasons that she avoids emotional self-reflection is that it can be acutely painful to illuminate aspects of herself that she is ashamed of. Though she is interested in people and connection, relationships are the source of considerable confusion and disappointment for her. She is apt to misread others' feelings and intentions, likely contributing to misunderstandings.

INTELLECTUAL FUNCTIONING: Her overall intellectual functioning is estimated to be in the Superior Range (General Abilities Index = 121, 92nd percentile). However, her cognitive capacities are quite uneven, with skills ranging from Superior (Verbal Comprehension Index = 123-127, 94th percentile) to Low Average (Working Memory Index = 88, 21st percentile) to Borderline (Processing Speed Index = 78, 7th percentile). For adolescents with such variability - as well as their parents and teachers - it can be highly confusing to gauge what their capacities are and what is reasonable to expect in terms of learning and performance. There is much room for misunderstanding, and often the adolescent will feel bad as areas of difficulty can be misattributed to lack of effort. Her verbal skills, including the ability to think abstractly and use common-

sense reasoning, are particularly strong. Based on the
findings above, it is possible to speculate that she
deteriorates in these abilities when stirred emotionally
and is more on her own to determine an appropriate course of
action.

Performance in practice: confessions of a psychopharmacologist

- The attending physician was perhaps too focused on the psychopharmacologic aspects of her presentation initially, although certainly these required attention both in terms of addressing side effects and improving her depressive symptoms
- However, the psychopharmacologist may have missed some of the reasons why she continued to struggle in relationships and with psychotherapy. Fortunately, psychological testing was obtained and there was an excellent collaboration between the psychologist who performed the testing and the attending physician
- Ultimately, psychological testing revealed that her residual difficulties including her struggles to engage in psychotherapy are, in large part, attributable to her profound weakness in the capacity for emotional regulation. The data from this testing clarified that it is not so much that she is incapable of being aware of and expressing emotions but, rather, that it is too painful and overwhelming to do so. The attending became aware, through the testing, that her severe difficulties regulating emotions, her style of trying to manage them (particularly attributing her own objectionable feelings to others and splitting her views into good/bad), and the vulnerability in her reasoning and reality testing suggested early borderline personality symptoms
- The attending physician, likely because of the patient's intelligence and verbal ability, had the impression that his patient was not struggling to the extent that she was. Armed with this information, he discussed alternative psychotherapeutic approaches with the patient and family

Take-home points

- Paroxetine is associated with significant tolerability concerns in pediatric populations and higher rates of treatment-emergent suicidality (Dobson et al. 2019) and should be avoided. Additionally, some pediatric pharmacokinetic data suggest that paroxetine requires three times daily dosing in youth (Findling et al. 2010)
- Paroxetine (and fluoxetine) exhibit mechanism-based inhibition of CYP2D6, which can complicate cross-titration (see Mechanism of Action Moment)

- Physical symptoms are common in pediatric patients with depressive and anxiety disorders, but should still be evaluated carefully
- Regarding antidepressant switching, several strategies have been proposed (Figure 18.3), although patient-specific factors, the presence of side effects, and drug–drug interactions between the first and second antidepressant must be considered:
  - *The direct switch* involves stopping the first antidepressant and starting a new antidepressant. This strategy may be preferred when there is a significant potential interaction between the first and second antidepressant or when there are significant side effects from the first antidepressant

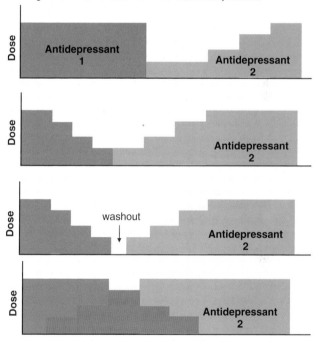

Figure 18.3 Antidepressant switching strategies. The top three figures graphically depict strategies that do not involve an overlap between the first and second antidepressants. In the bottom panel is a cross-titration strategy that involves overlap of the first and second antidepressants. In the top figure, the dose of the first antidepressant is decreased, and the second antidepressant is begun after a sufficient decrease in the dose of the first antidepressant. In the bottom panel, which represents the strategy used for this patient, the second antidepressant is added to the first antidepressant and then as the second antidepressant is titrated, the dose of the first antidepressant is decreased. This strategy minimizes the potential loss of efficacy that may have been derived from the first antidepressant.

- The taper and switch immediately involves gradually tapering the first antidepressant and starting the new antidepressant immediately after discontinuation
- The taper and switch after a washout involves gradually withdrawing the first antidepressant and then starting the new antidepressant after a washout period. This strategy may be used when there are significant interactions between the first and second antidepressant
- The cross-taper can involve tapering or maintaining the first antidepressant while beginning the new antidepressant. Alternatively, this strategy can involve beginning the new antidepressant *prior* to discontinuing the first antidepressant. This strategy may be especially useful when there was benefit from the first antidepressant, but side effects or other factors preclude continuation. This strategy is more common in pediatric practice than in adults
- Finally, even in the psychopharmacology clinic, clinicians should attend to psychological factors that are relevant to the patient's pathology and to the clinician-patient relationship. These factors often involve consideration of developmental concepts, as in the case of this patient

Mechanism of action moment

- Paroxetine differs from other SSRIs in its receptor pharmacology and pharmacokinetics
- Paroxetine has anticholinergic properties that subtend some tolerability concerns seen in this case. In addition, it has H_1 antagonism, which contributes to weight gain and sedation, with the latter potentially being beneficial in some anxious patients
- Paroxetine has weak norepinephrine transporter (NET) inhibitory properties (Figure 18.4), which could contribute to its efficacy in depression, especially at high doses
- Paroxetine inhibits nitric oxide synthase (Figure 18.4), which theoretically contributes to sexual dysfunction, especially in men
- Paroxetine is well absorbed from the gastrointestinal tract. It undergoes first-pass metabolism in the liver through a high-affinity saturable process (related to CYP2D6 activity), although other enzymes may be involved in metabolism as follows: CYP2D6 ≫ CYP3A4 > CYP1A2 > CYP2C19 > CYP3A5 (Jornil et al. 2010). CYP3A4 and CYP1A2 are most likely to be involved in paroxetine metabolism in individuals with impaired CYP2D6 activity (Jornil et al. 2010)

- In adults, paroxetine reaches steady state within 7–14 days using daily doses of 20–30 mg; however, in children and adolescents, this is shorter. For a 10 mg dose of paroxetine, the average half-life is 11 hours in children and adolescents, which is considerably shorter than the half-life reported in adults (21 hours) (Kaye et al. 1989)
- Importantly, just like in adults (Kaye et al. 1989), paroxetine exhibits nonlinear kinetics in pediatric patients (Findling et al. 1999, 2006)
- Paroxetine is a strong CYP2D6 inhibitor, which influences its own metabolism leading to phenoconversion (see Case 4). In other words, a normal CYP2D6 metabolizer taking paroxetine is converted to an intermediate metabolizer and an intermediate metabolizer taking paroxetine is converted to a poor metabolizer, and so on
- Paroxetine is notorious for causing withdrawal reactions upon sudden discontinuation, with symptoms such as akathisia, restlessness, gastrointestinal symptoms, dizziness, and tingling, especially when suddenly discontinued from long-term high-dose treatment. This is possibly due not only to serotonin receptor (SERT) inhibition, since all SSRIs can cause discontinuation reactions, but also to anticholinergic rebound and potentially to mechanism-based inhibition (see Two-minute tutorial). Importantly, children (to a lesser extent) and adolescents may be more susceptible to these effects since the half-life of paroxetine is considerably shorter in pediatric patients compared to adults (Findling et al. 1999)

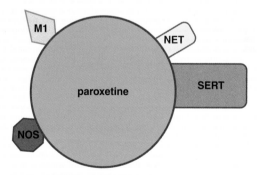

Figure 18.4 Paroxetine. In addition to serotonin reuptake inhibition, paroxetine has mild anticholinergic actions (M$_1$), which can be calming or possibly sedating; weak norepinephrine transporter (NET) inhibition, which may contribute to further antidepressant actions; and inhibition of the enzyme nitric oxide synthase (NOS), which may contribute to sexual dysfunction). Reproduced from *Stahl's Essential Psychopharmacology*, 2021.

PATIENT FILE

Two-minute tutorial: mechanism-based inhibition

- Mechanism-based inhibition is best known as a phenomenon associated with fluoxetine and paroxetine. It generally involves the activation of a substrate medication by a cytochrome into a reactive metabolite, which binds to the enzyme (typically at the active site), resulting in irreversible persistent loss of enzyme activity (Deodhar et al. 2020)
- The cytochrome must degrade the substrate for inhibition to proceed. As more drug is metabolized, more complexes snarl the active sites, increasing inhibition over time before it reaches a plateau. As such, mechanism-based inhibition is saturable (Deodhar et al. 2020)
- Given that a competing substrate (including the drug itself) cannot remove an irreversible inhibitor from the enzyme, the binding is locked so permanently that such irreversible enzyme inhibition is sometimes called the work of a "suicide inhibitor" since the enzyme essentially commits suicide by binding to the irreversible inhibitor (Figure 18.5). Consequently, enzyme activity cannot be restored unless another molecule of the enzyme is synthesized

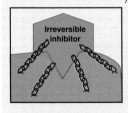
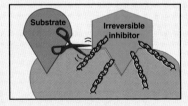

Figure 18.5 Mechanism-based inhibition. Some medications, such as paroxetine and fluoxetine, are inhibitors of CYP2D6. Shown here is an irreversible inhibitor of an enzyme, depicted as binding to the enzyme with chains (left). A competing substrate (including the drug itself) cannot remove an irreversible inhibitor from the enzyme, depicted as scissors unsuccessfully attempting to cut the chains off the inhibitor (right). The binding is locked so permanently that such irreversible enzyme inhibition (aka mechanism-based inhibition) is sometimes called the work of a "suicide inhibitor," since the enzyme essentially commits suicide by binding to the irreversible inhibitor. Enzyme activity cannot be restored unless another molecule of enzyme is synthesized by the cell's DNA. Reproduced from *Stahl's Essential Psychopharmacology*, 2021.

- In the case of paroxetine, paroxetine-derived reactive metabolites are produced at the active site of the CYP2D6 enzyme, which thwarts CYP2D6 catalytic activity, as described above. During titration, the concentration of CYP2D6 inhibitor (paroxetine) increases, which increases the CYP2D6 inhibition. Consistent with this, in a pharmacokinetic study of paroxetine in children and adolescents, Findling and colleagues demonstrated that pediatric patients with greater CYP2D6 activity produce more paroxetine-related heme-reactive metabolites within the active site on the CYP2D6 enzyme and have greater CYP2D6 inhibition. As such, paroxetine clearance decreases as the dose increases in children and adolescents (Figure 18.6) (Findling et al. 2006)

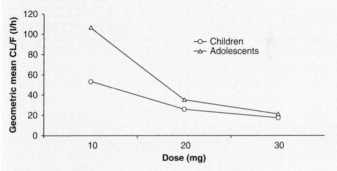

Figure 18.6 Relationship of paroxetine oral clearance and daily dose in pediatric patients. Reproduced from Findling et al. Multiple dose pharmacokinetics of paroxetine in children and adolescents with major depressive disorder or obsessive–compulsive disorder. *Neuropsychopharmacology* 2006; 31: 1274–85.

- Mechanism-based inhibition has important implications for paroxetine discontinuation. As paroxetine is titrated from 20 mg to 30 mg daily, it starts inhibiting its own metabolism, and plasma concentrations double. Importantly, as the paroxetine dose is decreased, the same process occurs – in reverse. That is, as the paroxetine dose is decreased, it stops inhibiting its own metabolism and is thus more rapidly metabolized by CYP2D6. Then, whoosh! Its concentrations rapidly decline, giving way to withdrawal symptoms far greater than with the standard SSRI

Post test question

Because of mechanism-based inhibition, which of the following SSRIs has non-linear kinetics?

A. Escitalopram (Lexapro)
B. Sertraline (Zoloft)
C. Fluvoxamine (Luvox)
D. Paroxetine (Paxil)
E. Vilazodone (Viibryd)

Answer: D (Paroxetine, Paxil)

Paroxetine (D), like fluoxetine, exhibits mechanism-based inhibition, a process that involves the activation of paroxetine by CYP2D6 into a reactive metabolite, which binds to the enzyme at the active site, resulting in irreversible persistent loss of enzyme activity (Deodhar et al. 2020). This results in nonlinear kinetics. Escitalopram (A) and sertraline (B) are primarily metabolized by CYP2C19, although CYP2B6 plays a role in sertraline metabolism as well. Importantly, neither escitalopram, sertraline, nor fluvoxamine (C) exhibit mechanism-based inhibition.

References

1. Cipriani, A., Zhou, X., del Giovane, C., et al. Comparative efficacy and tolerability of antidepressants for major depressive disorder in children and adolescents: a network meta-analysis. *Lancet* 2016; 388(10047): 881–90. https://doi.org/10.1016/S0140-6736(16)30385-3
2. Deodhar, M., al Rihani, S. B., Arwood, M. J., et al. Mechanisms of CYP450 inhibition: understanding drug-drug interactions due to mechanism-based inhibition in clinical practice. *Pharmaceutics* 2020; 12(9): 846. https://doi.org/10.3390/pharmaceutics12090846
3. Dobson, E. T., Bloch, M. H., Strawn, J. R. Efficacy and tolerability of pharmacotherapy for pediatric anxiety disorders: a network meta-analysis. *J Clin Psychiatry* 2019; 80(1): 17r12064. https://doi.org/10.4088/JCP.17r12064
4. Emslie, G. J., Wagner, K. D., Kutcher, S., et al. Paroxetine treatment in children and adolescents with major depressive disorder: a randomized, multicenter, double-blind, placebo-controlled trial. *J Am Acad Child Adolesc Psychiatry* 2006; 45(6): 709–19. https://doi.org/10.1097/01.chi.0000214189.73240.63

5. Findling, R. L. How (not) to dose antidepressants and antipsychotics for children. *Current Psychiatry* 2007; 6(6): 79-83

6. Findling, R. L., Nucci, G., Piergies, A. A., et al. Multiple dose pharmacokinetics of paroxetine in children and adolescents with major depressive disorder or obsessive-compulsive disorder. *Neuropsychopharmacology* 2006; 31: 1274–85. https://doi.org/10.1038/sj.npp.1300960

6. Findling, R. L., Reed, M. D., Myers, C., et al. Paroxetine pharmacokinetics in depressed children and adolescents. *J Am Acad Child Adolesc Psychiatry* 1999; 38(8): 952–59. https://doi.org/10.1097/00004583-199908000-00010

7. Ginsburg, G. S., Riddle, M. A., Davies, M. Somatic symptoms in children and adolescents with anxiety disorders. *J Am Acad Child Adolesc Psychiatry* 2006; 45(10): 1179–87. https://doi.org/10.1097/01.chi.0000231974.43966.6e

8. Hughes, A. A., Lourea-Waddell, B., Kendall, P. C. Somatic complaints in children with anxiety disorders and their unique prediction of poorer academic performance. *Child Psychiatry Hum Dev* 2008; 39(2): 211–20. https://doi.org/10.1007/s10578-007-0082-5

9. Jornil, J., Jensen, K. G., Larsen, F., Linnet, K. Identification of cytochrome P450 isoforms involved in the metabolism of paroxetine and estimation of their importance for human paroxetine metabolism using a population-based simulator. *Drug Metab Disposition* 2010; 38(3): 376–85. https://doi.org/10.1124/dmd.109.030551

10. Kaye, C. M., Haddock, R. E., Langley, P. F., et al. A review of the metabolism and pharmacokinetics of paroxetine in man. *Acta Psychiatr Scand* 1989; 80(350 S): 60–75. https://doi.org/10.1111/j.1600-0447.1989.tb07176.x

11. Keller, M. B., Ryan, N. D., Strober, M., et al. Efficacy of paroxetine in the treatment of adolescent major depression: a randomized, controlled trial. *J Am Acad Child Adolesc Psychiatry* 2001; 40(7): 762–72. https://doi.org/10.1097/00004583-200107000-00010

12. Owens, M. J., Krulewicz, S., Simon, J. S., et al. Estimates of serotonin and norepinephrine transporter inhibition in depressed patients treated with paroxetine or venlafaxine. *Neuropsychopharmacology* 2008; 33(13): 3201–12. https://doi.org/10.1038/npp.2008.47

13. Strawn, J. R., Poweleit, E. A., Ramsey, L. B. CYP2C19-guided escitalopram and sertraline dosing in pediatric patients: a pharmacokinetic modeling study. *J Child Adolesc*

Psychopharmacol 2019; 29(5): 340–47. https://doi.org/10.1089/cap.2018.0160

14. Strawn, J. R., Poweleit, E. A., Uppugunduri, C. R. S., Ramsey, L. B. Pediatric therapeutic drug monitoring for selective serotonin reuptake inhibitors. *Front Pharmacol* 2021; 12: 749692. https://doi.org/10.3389/fphar.2021.749692

15. Wagner, K. D., Berard, R., Stein, M. B., et al. A multicenter, randomized, double-blind, placebo-controlled trial of paroxetine in children and adolescents with social anxiety disorder. *Arch Gen Psychiatry* 2004; 61(11): 1153–62. https://doi.org/10.1001/archpsyc.61.11.1153

Appendix 1

FDA-Approved Serotonin Norepinephrine, Dopamine Reuptake Inhibitor Medications in Children and Adolescents

Class	Medication	Age (years)							
		6	7	8	9	10	11	12	13-17
SSRI	Citalopram	NONE							
	Escitalopram	NONE							MDD
				GAD					
	Fluoxetine			OCD					
		NONE		MDD					
	Fluvoxamine	NONE		OCD					
	Paroxetine	NONE							
	Sertraline	OCD							
	Vilazodone	NONE							
	Vortioxetine	NONE							
SNRI	Duloxetine			GAD					
	Desvenlafaxine	NONE							
	Venlafaxine	NONE							
Atypical antidepressant	Bupropion	NONE							
	Mirtazapine	NONE							
	Trazodone	NONE							

Appendix 2

FDA-Approved Dopamine Receptor Antagonist and Mixed Dopamine Serotonin Receptor Antagonist Medications in Children and Adolescents

Class	Medication	Age (years)							
		6	7	8	9	10	11	12	13–17
Mixed Dopamine Serotonin Receptor Antagonists	Asenapine					BP, mixed or manic episodes (10–17)			
	Aripiprazole								Schizophrenia
						BP, mixed or manic episodes (10–17)			
		Irritability associated with autism spectrum disorder (6–17)							
		Tourette's syndrome (6–17)							
	Lurasidone								Schizophrenia
						BP, major depressive episodes (10–17)			
	Olanzapine								Schizophrenia
									BP, mixed or manic episodes (13–17)
						BP, depressive episodes, adjunctive (10–17)			
	Paliperidone							Schizophrenia	
	Quetiapine Quetiapine XR								Schizophrenia
						BP, mixed or manic episodes (10–17)			
	Risperidone								Schizophrenia (13–17)
						BP, mixed or manic episodes (10–17)			
		Irritability associated with autism spectrum disorder (5–17)							
		6	7	8	9	10	11	12	13–17
Dopamine Receptor Antagonists	Chlorpromazine								Schizophrenia
									intractable singultus (adolescents)
		ODD with severe behavioral problems or other disruptive behavioral disorders, or ADHD with "excessive motor activity with accompanying conduct disorders"							
		Severe agitation in hospitalized pediatric patients (5–12 years)							
		Adjunctive treatment of tetanus (6 months – adult)							

Appendix 3

Stature for Age and Weight for age Chart for Boys Aged 2–20

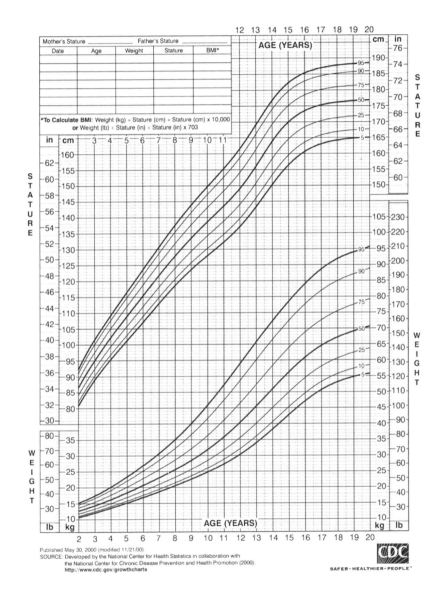

Published May 30, 2000 (modified 11/21/00)
SOURCE: Developed by the National Center for Health Statistics in collaboration with
the National Center for Chronic Disease Prevention and Health Promotion (2000).
http://www.cdc.gov/growthcharts

SAFER · HEALTHIER · PEOPLE™

Appendix 4

Stature for Age and Weight for age Chart for Girls Aged 2–20

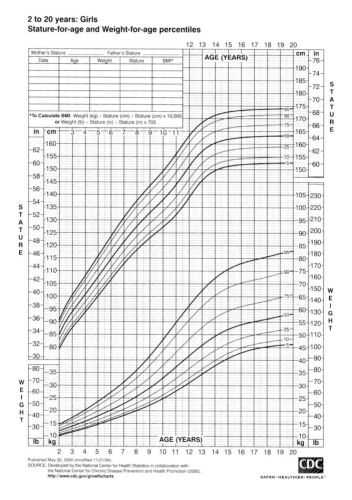

2 to 20 years: Girls
Stature-for-age and Weight-for-age percentiles

Appendix 5

Pediatric Respiratory Rates. Fleming, S., Thompson, M., Stevens, R., Heneghan, C., Plüddemann, A., Maconochie, I., Tarassenko, L., Mant, D., Normal ranges of heart rate and respiratory rate in children from birth to 18 years of age: a systematic review of observational studies. *Lancet.* 2011 Mar 19; 377(9770): 1011–8.

Age Range	1st centile	10th centile	25th centile	Median	75th centile	90th centile	99th centile
0–3 months	25	34	40	43	52	57	66
3–6 months	24	33	38	41	49	55	64
6–9 months	23	31	36	39	47	52	61
9–12 months	22	30	35	37	45	50	58
12–18 months	21	28	32	35	42	46	53
18–24 months	19	25	29	31	36	40	46
2–3 years	18	22	25	28	31	34	38
3–4 years	17	21	23	25	27	29	33
4–6 years	17	20	21	23	25	27	29
6–8 years	16	18	20	21	23	24	27
8–12 years	14	16	18	19	21	22	25
12–15 years	12	15	16	18	19	21	23
15–18 years	11	13	15	16	18	19	22

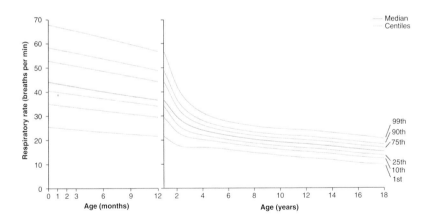

Appendix 6

Pediatric Heart Rates. Adapted from Fleming, S., Thompson, M., Stevens, R., Heneghan, C., Plüddemann, A., Maconochie, I., Tarassenko, L., Mant, D. Normal ranges of heart rate and respiratory rate in children from birth to 18 years of age: a systematic review of observational studies. *Lancet* 2011; 377(9770): 1011–8.

Age Range	1st centile	10th centile	25th centile	Median	75th centile	90th centile	99th centile
0–3 months	107	123	133	143	154	164	181
3–6 months	104	120	129	140	150	159	175
6–9 months	98	114	123	134	143	152	168
9–12 months	93	109	118	128	137	145	161
12–18 months	88	103	112	123	132	140	156
18–24 months	82	98	106	116	126	135	149
2–3 years	76	92	100	110	119	128	142
3–4 years	70	86	94	104	113	123	136
4–6 years	65	81	89	98	108	117	131
6–8 years	59	74	82	91	101	111	123
8–12 years	52	67	75	84	93	103	115
12–15 years	47	62	69	78	87	96	108
15–18 years	43	58	65	73	83	92	104

"Birth" refers to the immediate neonatal period.

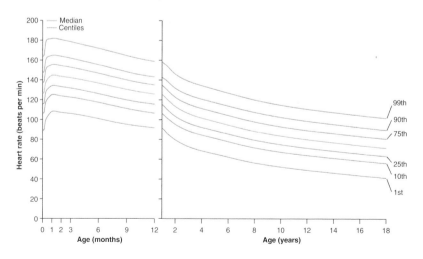

Appendix 7

Normal blood pressure in children: 50th to 90th percentiles.

Age	Systolic pressure, mmHg	Diastolic pressure, mmHg
Infant, 6 months	87–105	53–66
Toddler, 2 years	95–105	53–66
School age, 7 years	97–112	57–71
Adolescent, 15 years	112–128	66–88

The median (50th percentile) systolic blood pressure for children older than 1 year may be approximated by the following formula: 90 mmHg + (2 x age in years).

The lower limit (5th percentile) of systolic blood pressure can be estimated with this formula: 70 mmHg + (2 x age in years).

Adapted from the Report of the Second Task Force on Blood Pressure Control in Children–1987. Task Force on Blood Pressure Control in Children. National Heart, Lung, and Blood Institute, Bethesda, Maryland. *Pediatrics* 1987; 79: 1.

Appendix 8

Therapeutic Threshold, Point of Futility, AGNP/ASCP Laboratory Alert Level, and Average Oral Concentration–Dose Relationships for Antipsychotic Medications in Adults.

Antipsychotic	Therapeutic Threshold (ng/mL)	Point of Futility (ng/mL)	AGNP/ASCP Laboratory Alert Level (ng/mL)	Oral Concentration/ Dose Relationship [a]
Amisulpride	100	550–700	Not reported	Females: 0.60 Males: 0.46
Aripiprazole	110	500	1000	11.0
Asenapine (sublingual)	1.0	(Based on maximal licensed dose of 10 mg sublingual twice daily)	10	5 mg twice daily: 0.15 10 mg twice daily: 0.20
Asenapine (transdermal) [b]	1.0	(Based on maximal licensed dose of 7.8 mg/24 hrs)	10	0.53
Brexpiprazole	36	(Based on maximal licensed dose of 4 mg every night at bedtime)	280	CYP2D6 EM: 18 CYP2D6 IM: 46
Cariprazine [c]	5.6	(Based on maximal licensed dose of 6 mg every night at bedtime)	40 [c]	1.91
Chlorpromazine	3–30	100	600	0.06
Clozapine	350	1000	1000	Female Smoker: 0.80 Female Nonsmoker: 1.32 Male Smoker: 0.67 Male Nonsmoker: 1.08
Flupenthixol (cis isomer)	0.43	3.0	15	0.20
Fluphenazine	1.0	4.0	15	Smoker: 0.06 Nonsmoker: 0.08 – 0.10
Haloperidol	2.0	18	15	0.78
Loxapine	3.8	18.4	20	0.22
Lurasidone [d]	7.2	(Based on maximal licensed dose of 160 mg with an evening meal)	120	0.18
Olanzapine	23	150	100	Smoker: 1.43 Nonsmoker: 2.0
Paliperidone	20	90	120	4.09
Perphenazine	0.81	5.0	5	CYP2D6 EM: 0.04 CYP2D6 PM: 0.08
Risperidone (active moiety) [e]	15	112	120	7.0
Thiothixene	1.0	12	Not reported	Smoker: 0.04 Nonsmoker: 0.05
Trifluoperazine	1.0	2.3	Not reported	Unknown
Zuclopenthixol	2.0	9.0	Not reported	0.65

CYP: cytochrome P450; **EM:** extensive metabolizer; **IM:** intermediate metabolizer; **PM:** poor metabolizer

[a] Multiply by the conversion factor to obtain 12-hr trough levels in ng/mL for patients receiving all or most of their dose at bedtime. These mean values apply to patients not exposed to metabolic inhibitors or inducers, and who are extensive metabolizers for the relevant enzymes. Due to extensive population variation for most 12-hr trough levels, low levels may not reflect poor adherence. A second data point on the same dose will be of significant help in differentiating kinetic and adherence issues (see Chapter 4).

[b] Although the lowest transdermal formulation dose of 3.8 mg/24 hrs provides equivalent asenapine exposure to the sublingual dose of 5 mg twice daily (as calculated by the AUC), the trough levels for the sublingual dose are lower due to higher peak:trough variation. This conversion factor of 0.53 is for the transdermal dose (per 24 hrs). **Example:** 3.8 mg/24 rs x 0.53 = 2.0 ng/mL.

c The values provided for cariprazine do not include the metabolites. At steady state on 6 mg/d the active moiety is: cariprazine 28%, DCAR 9%, and DDCAR 63%.[1] However, very few laboratories have cariprazine assays, and none report the metabolites at present. Should this change, the active moiety values represented will be 4-fold higher. For example, the steady state cariprazine level on 6 mg/d is 11.2 ng/mL, but the active moiety level will be approximately 40 ng/mL. The rationale behind the AGNP/ASCP laboratory alert level of 40 ng/mL is not clearly delineated in the paper.[3]

d The concentration:dose relationships for lurasidone are based on 12-hr trough values obtained at steady state (day 9 or later) and with lurasidone administered within 30 minutes of an evening meal of at least 350 kcal. This does not include the active metabolite ID-14283 (exohydroxylurasidone), which comprises 25% of the active moiety, but whose levels are not reported by commercial laboratories presently.[4]

e The risperidone active moiety is the sum of risperidone + 9-OH risperidone levels

References

1. FDA Center for Drug Evaluation and Research (2015). Cariprazine Pharmacology/Toxicology NDA Review and Evaluation.

2. Periclou, A., Willavize, S., Jaworowicz, D., et al. (2019). Relationship between plasma concentrations and clinical effects of cariprazine in patients with schizophrenia or bipolar mania. *Clin Transl Sci*,

3. Schoretsanitis, G., Kane, J. M., Correll, C. U., et al. (2020). Blood levels to optimize antipsychotic treatment in clinical practice; a joint consensus statement of the American Society of Clinical Psychopharmacology (ASCP) and the Therapeutic Drug Monitoring (TDM) Task Force of the Arbeitsgemeinschaft für Neuropsychopharmakologie und Pharmakopsychiatrie (AGNP). *J Clin Psychiatry* 81, doi:10.4088/JCP.4019cs13169.

4. Findling, R. L., Goldman, R., Chiu, Y. Y., et al. (2015). Pharmacokinetics and tolerability of lurasidone in children and adolescents with psychiatric disorders. *Clin Ther* 37, 2788–2797.

Case Studies Index

Locators in **bold** refer to tables; those in *italics* to figures

Broad classes/drug types are indexed below; for specific drugs *see* drug index

Abnormal Involuntary Movement Scale (AIMS) 128
accommodation, SSRI-refractory anxiety 4
activation syndromes, SSRI-related *21*, *29*; *see also* mania (SSRI-induced)
   clinical approaches 20
   clinical reflections 25
   family history 18
   follow-ups (1st) 20
   follow-ups (2nd) 22–23
   medical history 18
   medication 18, *19*
   medication mechanisms of action **26–28**, 27–29, *28*
   medication metabolism 22
   medication pharmacogenetics 29–30
   medication pharmacokinetics *23*, *24*
   patient descriptions/evaluations 17, *19*
   post test self-assessment question 30–31
   pretest self-assessment question 17
   psychiatric history/evaluations 17, 19–20
   psychotherapy history 18
   social history 18–19
   take-home points 25
   test results 22
   tips/pearls of wisdom 25–26
   treatment-related weight gain *24*
acute kidney injury 189
ADHD *see* attention deficit hyperactivity disorder
adherence to medication 283, *283*, 294–96
   adolescence
   sleep architecture 249–50
   SSRI concentrations *182*
adolescent case studies *see* anorexia nervosa; anxiety; bipolar disorder; cannabis-related drug interactions; insomnia

disorder; mania (SSRI-induced); obsessive-compulsive disorder; SSRIs (discontinuation); major depressive disorder; schizophrenia
adrenergic uptake inhibitors *see* α-adrenergic agonists
adverse effects of medication *282*
affective spectrum, SSRI-induced mania *70*
age of onset, bipolar disorder *140*
aggression, ASD in a child 259–60, 265, 273
akathisia 29, 58
alcohol use disorder 151
α-adrenergic agonists 229–30
   ADHD in a child 111–15
   concentration in relation to CYP2D6 metabolism *168*
   mechanisms of action 42–43, *254*, *255*
   pharmacology/binding profile *166*
   plasma concentration–time curves 112
   prefrontal cortex effects *167*
   PTSD with ADHD 41, *42*
amygdala 9, *42*, 42–43
anorexia nervosa, adolescent
   clinical approaches 194, 196
   family history 185
   follow-ups (1st) 193–94
   follow-ups (2nd) 194–95
   follow-ups (3rd) 195–96
   follow-ups (4th) 196
   hospitalization 192–93
   medical examinations in eating disorders **197**
   medical history 185
   medication 185
   medication effects *200*
   medication mechanisms of action 198–99
   medication plasma concentration–time curves *199*
   patient descriptions/evaluations 185–86, 187–88, **190–92**

anorexia nervosa, adolescent (cont.)
post test self-assessment question 200–1
pretest self-assessment question 185
psychiatric history/evaluations 185, 189–90
psychotherapy history 185
refeeding syndrome risks **190**, 197–98
social history 185
take-home points 196–97
test results **188–89**, **193**, **195**
tips/pearls of wisdom 198
anticholinergic symptoms
antipsychotics 295, 296–97
histamine antagonists *242*
SSRIs 317–18, *318*
tricyclic antidepressants 86, 87, 89, 90
antidepressant switching strategies *316*,
316–17; *see also* SSRIs; tricyclic
antidepressants
antidiuretics 227–28
mechanisms of action *230*, 230
sublingual formulation vs. tablets *229*
antihistamines 241, *242*, *243*, 248
antihypertensives 95, 111–12, 115–16
antipsychotics; *see also* second-generation
antipsychotics
mechanisms of action 132–33, 165
pharmacology/binding profile *133*, *166*
anxiety in adolescence, SSRI tolerability/side
effects
antidepressant switching strategies *316*,
316–17
clinical approaches 304–5, 310
clinical reflections 315
constipation 306
family history 301
follow-ups (1st and 2nd) 310
follow-ups (3rd) 311
follow-ups (4th) 312
mechanism-based inhibition *319*, 319–20
medical history 301
medication 301, 304, 310, 311
medication clearance relative to dosage *320*
medication mechanisms of action 317–18, *318*
medication serum concentrations *308*, *309*
patient descriptions/evaluations 301–2, 304
pharmacogenetic testing **306**
post test self-assessment question 321
pretest self-assessment question 301
psychiatric history/evaluations 301, 307–9

psychological testing 312–14
psychotherapy history 301
social history 301
take-home points 315–17
test results **305–6**
anxiety in adolescence, treatment-resistant
clinical approaches 4–5
clinical reflections 8
family history 2
follow-ups (1st) 5
follow-ups (2rd) 6
follow-ups (3rd) 6–7
follow-ups (4th) 7
medical history 2, 3
medication 3
medication interactions 11, *12*, *13*
medication mechanisms of action 9, *10*, *11*
medication responses *9*, 11, *12*
patient descriptions/evaluations 1, 3–4
post test self-assessment question 13–14
pretest self-assessment question 1
psychiatric history/evaluations 2, 4
psychotherapy history 3
social history 3
take-home points 7–8
tips/pearls of wisdom 9
ASD *see* autism spectrum disorder
attention deficit hyperactivity disorder (ADHD),
child
clinical approaches 102, 105
developmental neurophysiology *108*,
108–10, *109*
educational history 96
family history 97
follow-ups (1st) 103–5
follow-ups (2nd) 105–6
follow-ups (3rd) 107
intelligence testing 97–99, **98**
medical history 97
medication 97, **102–3**
medication mechanisms of action *110*, 110–15
neuronal signal distribution *114*
neuropharmacology of ADHD *115*, 115
patient descriptions/evaluations 95, 97, 102
plasma concentration–time curves 112
post test self-assessment question 115–16
pretest self-assessment question 95
psychiatric history/evaluations 96, 101
social history 97

take-home points 107–8
test results 103, *104*
attention-deficit hyperactivity disorder, with
    PTSD *see* posttraumatic stress disorder
    combined with ADHD
attention-deficit hyperactivity disorder, with tics
    see Tourette syndrome
atypical antipsychotics *see* second-generation
    antipsychotics
autism spectrum disorder (ASD), side effects
    of SGAs 276
    clinical approaches 264
    clinical reflections 271
    family history 259
    follow-ups (1st) 265–66
    follow-ups (2nd) 266
    follow-ups (3rd) 267, 269–71
    follow-ups (4th to 6th) 271
    genetic work-up 275–76
    medical history 259
    medication 259, 261
    medication effects on BMI *267*
    medication mechanisms of action 274–75
    medication pharmacology/binding profile *270*
    medication responses *265*
    medication switching *273*
    patient descriptions/evaluations 259–60,
        261–63
    pharmacogenetic testing **268**, *272*
    post test self-assessment question 276
    pretest self-assessment question 259
    prolactin release *275*
    psychiatric history/evaluations 259, 264
    psychotherapy history 259
    Scales of Independent Behavior-Revised
        262–63
    social history 259
    take-home points 272
    test results 267, **268**–**69**
    tips/pearls of wisdom 273
    Weschler Intelligence Scale for Children
        261–**62**, 262
autoimmune disease **126**, 159
avoidance, social anxiety disorder 3, 4, 8

BEARS Sleep Screening Tool (B=Bedtime
    Issues, E=Excessive Daytime Sleepiness,
    A=Night Awakenings, R=Regularity and
    Duration of Sleep, S=Snoring) **234**–**35**

bedwetting *see* nocturnal enuresis
benzodiazepines (BZDs)
    benefits/response to 11
    mechanisms of action 9, *10*, *11*
    medication interactions 11, *12*, *13*
    medication responses *12*
binding profiles *see* pharmacology/binding
    profile
bipolar disorder, medication dosage in
    adolescents; *see also* mania (SSRI-
    induced)
    age of onset for diagnosis *140*
    BID vs. TID dosage regimes 151–52
    clinical approaches 140, 142
    family history 138
    follow-ups (1st) 140–41
    follow-ups (2nd) 142–46
    illness details 149–51
    lithium *vs.* placebo *146*
    medical history 138
    medication 138, 139
    medication mechanisms of action *148*, 148–49
    Monte Carlo simulations, concentration-dose
        147
    mood symptoms *150*
    patient descriptions/evaluations 137
    pharmacokinetic clearance modeling *148*
    post test self-assessment question 152
    pretest self-assessment question 137
    psychiatric history/evaluations 137–38, 139
    psychotherapy history 138
    routine medication monitoring **144**, 146
    social history 139
    take-home points 146–47
    test results **143**
BMI (body mass index) *see* weight gain
bowel function *see* constipation
bullying 301
BZDS *see* benzodiazepines

caffeine exposure
    insomnia disorder in an adolescent 239–40,
        240
    nocturnal enuresis in a child *225*
cannabis-related drug interactions
    clinical approaches 208, 211, 212
    clinical reflections 213
    dopamine synthesis capacity in the striatum
        210

caffeine exposure (cont.)
educational outcomes in cannabis users *210*
endogenous cannabinoid system *217*, 217–19
family history 203
follow-ups (1st) 209–10
follow-ups (2nd) 211
follow-ups (3rd) 212
medical history 203
medication 203, 204
medication effects *216*
medication mechanisms of action 215–17
mesolimbic dopamine pathway *218*
monoamine/GABAergic/glutamatergic
signaling *214*
N-acetylcysteine trial *213*
patient descriptions/evaluations 203, 205
plasma concentration–time curves *206*, *208*
post test self-assessment question 219–20
pretest self-assessment question 203
psychiatric history/evaluations 203, 205–8
psychotherapy history 203
social history 203
take-home points 213–15
THC effects **207**
THC exposure *207*
tips/pearls of wisdom 215
CBT *see* cognitive behavior therapy
Child and Adolescent Service Intensity
Instrument (CASII) 69
Child Yale-Brown Obsessive Compulsive Scale
(CY-BOCS) 79, 80–81
child case studies *see* activation syndromes;
attention-deficit hyperactivity disorder;
autism spectrum disorder; nocturnal
enuresis; posttraumatic stress disorder;
Tourette syndrome
children
sleep architecture 249
SSRI concentrations *182*
circadian rhythms
in depression *239*; *see also* insomnia
disorder
diurnal variation in urine production *231*
medication mechanisms of action *251*, 251–52
CNS (central nervous system) stimulants; *see
also* α-adrenergic agonists
mechanisms of action *110*, 110–15, *114*
neuropharmacology *115*

cognitive behavior therapy (CBT)
insomnia disorder in an adolescent 241
SSRI discontinuation in adolescents *181*
complete blood count, SSRI side effects **305–6**
compliance with medication 283, *283*, 294–96
constipation
SGAs **296**
SSRIs 306
Coping Cat psychotherapy intervention 19
cortisol dynamics, ADHD with PTSD *44*
COVID-19 pandemic 233
cyclic adenosine monophosphate (cAMP) *114*,
115, 115
CYP2C19 (cytochrome P450 2C19) metabolism
drug clearance 25–26, *26*
effects of SSRIs 21, *22*, 29–30
CYP2D6 (cytochrome P450 2D6) metabolism
MDD *59*, *60*
Tourette syndrome *168*

delusions 122, 127, 279–80
depression 66; *see also* major depressive
disorder
sleep/wake cycles *239*
developmental milestones, delayed
autism spectrum disorder 259
early-onset schizophrenia 121
Tourette syndrome 155
developmental neurophysiology, ADHD 108–10
brain circuits *109*
brain maturation/onset of psychiatric
disorders *108*
diagnostic criteria *see* DSM-5 criteria
disinhibition 259
dopamine/dopaminergic system
cannabis-related drug interactions *210*
CNS stimulants *110*, *114*
effects of caffeine exposure *240*
reward systems *218*
side effects of SGAs *275*
dopamine–serotonin receptor antagonists *see*
second-generation antipsychotics
DSM-5 (Diagnostic and Statistical Manual of
Mental Disorders) criteria
ADHD 35, 223
anorexia nervosa 189
bipolar disorder 149
major depressive disorder 49, 203

nocturnal enuresis 225
sleep disorder 160
Tourette syndrome 163
drugs *see* medication

early-onset schizophrenia, adolescence
clinical approaches 122, 126, 128, **129**
family history 121
follow-ups (1st) 123
follow-ups (2nd) 126–28, **128**
follow-ups (3rd) 128–30, **129**
follow-ups (4th) 131
medical history 120–21
medication mechanisms of action 132–33
medication pharmacology/binding profile *133*
patient descriptions/evaluations 119, 121–22
post test self-assessment question 134
pretest self-assessment question 119
psychiatric history/evaluations 120, 122
psychotherapy history 120
social history 121
take-home points 132
test results 123–24, **124**–**25**, **126**, **128**
eating disorders *see* anorexia nervosa
educational history, ADHD in a child 96
educational outcomes, cannabis users *210*
endocannabinoid system *217*, 217–19
enuresis *see* nocturnal enuresis
Epworth sleepiness scale **237**
exposure work, child and adolescent anxiety 6
extrapyramidal symptoms (EPS) 127–28, 132

Family-to-Family Program (National Alliance on
Mental Illness) 279
family-based therapy 185, 193
family history *see under specific cases*
5-HT *see* serotonin
Fluid Reasoning Index (FRI), WISC-5 99
fragile X syndrome 259, 264, 272

GABA$_A$ (gamma aminobutyric acid sub-type A)
receptors 9, *10*
GABAergic signaling, drug interactions *214*
General Ability Index (GAI), WISC-5 97–99
generalized anxiety disorder (GAD) 3, 4, 13, 19,
61; *see also* anxiety
genetics *see* pharmacogenetics
glutamatergic signaling, drug interactions *214*

hallucinations 122, 127, 279
headaches 138, 228, 267, 301
herbal supplements 126
hippocampus atrophy, ADHD with PTSD 45
histamine 1 receptor antagonists 241, *242*,
243, 248
hyperbolic discontinuation, SSRIs 180
hypotension 298
hypothalamic pituitary adrenal (HPA) axis *45*

individualized education plans (IEPs) 72, 259
infections, Tourette syndrome 158
insomnia 35–36; *see also* posttraumatic stress
disorder
insomnia disorder, adolescence 233
BEARS Sleep Screening Tool **234**–**35**
caffeine exposure 239–40, *240*
circadian rhythms, effect of depression *239*
clinical approaches 241, 244, 246
Epworth Sleepiness Scale **237**
family history 233
follow-ups (1st) 241–42
follow-ups (2nd) 243–44
follow-ups (3rd) 244–45
follow-ups (4th) 245–46
follow-ups (5th) 247
medical history 233
medication 233, *242*, *243*
medication mechanisms of action *251*,
251–52, *254*, *255*
patient descriptions/evaluations 233, 236–37
post test self-assessment question 256
pretest self-assessment question 233
psychiatric history/evaluations 233–34,
238–41
psychotherapy history 233
sleep architecture in adolescence 249–50
sleep architecture in childhood 249
social history 233
social jet lag 239
take-home points 248–49
test results **237**–**38**, 246–47
tips/pearls of wisdom 250
intelligence testing, ADHD 97–99, **98**
intellectual disability 259, 264, 276
interpersonal psychotherapy (IPT) 38, 54,
65–66, 120, 196, 311
iron studies, insomnia disorder **238**, **247**

kidney disease 151, 279

laboratory tests *see under specific cases* (test results)

major depressive disorder (MDD), treatment resistant
  clinical approaches 54, 57
  CYP2D6 phenotype *59*, *60*
  family history 49
  follow-ups (1st) 54–55
  follow-ups (2nd) 55–58
  follow-ups (3rd) 58
  medical history 49
  medication 49, 50
  medication plasma concentration–time curves *60*
  patient descriptions/evaluations 49, 51–53
  phenoconversion 59
  post test self-assessment question 60–61
  pretest self-assessment question 49
  psychiatric history/evaluations 49, 54
  psychotherapy history 49
  social history 49
  take-home points 58–59
  tips/pearls of wisdom 59
mania, SSRI-induced 69; *see also* activation syndromes; bipolar disorder
  affective spectrum/mood disorders continuum *70*
  clinical approaches 68
  family history 66
  follow-ups (1st) 67–68
  follow-ups (2nd) 68–70
  follow-ups (3rd) 71–72
  medical history 66
  medication 66, 71–72, 73–74
  medication mechanisms of action 74
  medication pharmacology/binding profile 75
  medication plasma concentration time curves *73*
  patient descriptions/evaluations 65–67
  post test self-assessment question 75
  pretest self-assessment question 65
  psychiatric history/evaluations 66, 67
  psychotherapy history 66
  social history 66
  take-home points 72–73
  tips/pearls of wisdom 73–74

MDD *see* major depressive disorder
mechanism-based inhibition, SSRIs *319*, 319–20
medication dosage *see* bipolar disorder (medication dosage)
medication interactions *see* cannabis-related interactions
medication side effects *see* side effects
medication withdrawal *see* SSRIs, discontinuation
mesolimbic dopamine pathway, reward systems *218*
methyl tetrahydrofolate reductase (*MTHFR*) gene 284
mindfulness-based therapies 138
mixed dopamine–serotonin receptor antagonists *see* second-generation antipsychotics
mixed symptoms, mood disorders continuum *70*
monoamine signaling, drug interactions *214*; *see also* dopamine; norepinephrine; serotonin
Monte Carlo simulations, drug concentrations *147*; *see also* bipolar disorder (medication dosage)
mood disorders continuum, SSRI-induced mania *70*
mood stabilizers 138, 139; *see also* bipolar disorder (medication dosage)
  mechanisms of action *148*, 148–49
  pharmacokinetics *147*
movement disorders 29, 58, 246, 247
movement ratings, early-onset schizophrenia **129**
MRI scanning, early-onset schizophrenia 123–24
MTHFR (methyl tetrahydrofolate reductase) gene 284

National Alliance on Mental Illness (NAMI) 279
nausea 3, 41, 138, 203
NDRIs *see* norepinephrine–dopamine reuptake inhibitors
neuronal signal distribution, ADHD in a child *114*
neutropenia 294–95
nocturnal enuresis, child 230
  caffeine exposure *225*
  clinical approaches 225

diurnal variation in urine production *231*
family history 224
follow-ups (1st) 226
medical history 224
medication 224
medication effects *229*
medication mechanisms of action *230*, 230
medication responses **226**
patient descriptions/evaluations 223, 224–25
post test self-assessment question 231
pretest self-assessment question 223
psychiatric history/evaluations 223, 225
social history 224
take-home points 227
tips/pearls of wisdom 227–30
non-adherence *see* adherence to medication
norepinephrine; see also SNRIs
  CNS stimulants *110*, *114*, *115*
  PTSD with ADHD *42*, 43–45, *44*
  receptors *253*
norepinephrine–dopamine reuptake inhibitors
    (NDRIs)
  effects on prefrontal cortex and striatum *216*
  mechanisms of action 215–17

obsessive-compulsive disorder, adolescence
  clinical approaches 82–83, 85–86
  family history 78, *82*
  follow-ups (1st) 83–84
  follow-ups (2nd) 85–86
  follow-ups (3rd) 87–88
  medical history 78
  medication 78, 79, *85*
  medication mechanisms of action 89–90
  medication receptor pharmacology *90*
  medication responses *91*
  patient descriptions/evaluations 77–78, 79,
    80–81
  post test self-assessment question 91
  pretest self-assessment question 77
  psychiatric history/evaluations 78, 81–82
  psychotherapy history 78
  social history 78
  take-home points 88–89, *89*
  test results 84, **86**
  tips/pearls of wisdom 90
  treatment outcomes *82*
omega-3 fatty acid supplementation
  bipolar disorder 67

schizophrenia 122, 126, 127, 131
  SSRI-induced mania 72
opioid antagonists
  effects on ventral tegmental area *200*
  mechanisms of action 198–99
  plasma concentration–time curves *199*
oral contraceptives 138, 301, 302
orthostatic hypotension 298

Patient Health Questionnaire-9 (PHQ-9) 51–52
pediatrics *see* adolescent case studies; child
    case studies
Personality Assessment Inventory for
    Adolescents (PAI-A) 53
pharmacogenetics
  SGAs **268**, *272*
  SSRIs 29–30, **306**
pharmacokinetics
  mood stabilizers *148*
  SSRIs *23*, *24*, *26*, 179, *320*, 321
pharmacology/binding profiles
  α-adrenergic agonists *166*
  antipsychotics *133*, *166*
  NDRIs *166*
  SGAs *74*, *270*, *297*
phenoconversion 59
plasma concentration–time curves
  α-adrenergic agonists 112
  opioid antagonists *199*
  SGAs *73*
  SSRIs *206*, *208*
polycystic ovarian syndrome 75
posttraumatic stress disorder (PTSD)
    combined with ADHD
  clinical approaches 38
  family history 37
  follow-ups (1st) 38–39
  follow-ups (2nd) 39–40
  follow-ups (3rd) 40
  HPA axis stress response *45*
  medical history 36, 37
  medication 36, 37
  medication mechanism of action 42–43
  medication responses *42*
  noradrenergic hyperactivity *42*
  norepinephrine and cortisol dynamics
    43–45, *44*
  patient descriptions/evaluations 35, 37
  post test self-assessment question 45

posttraumatic stress disorder (PTSD)
combined with ADHD (cont.)
pretest self-assessment question 35
psychiatric history/evaluations 35–36, 37
psychotherapy history 37
social history 37
take-home points 40–41
tips/pearls of wisdom 41
PRACTICE acronym, PTSD 38–39
prefrontal cortex
α-adrenergic agonists *167*
norepinephrine–dopamine reuptake
inhibitors *216*
Processing Speed Index (PSI), WISC-5 99
prolactin release, side effects of SGAs *275*
psychosis *see* early-onset schizophrenia;
schizophrenia
psychotherapy *see under specific cases*
PTSD *see* posttraumatic stress disorder

Quick Inventory of Depressive Symptoms
(QUIDS -SR) 51–52

receiver operating characteristic (ROC) curves,
SGAs 291
re-feeding syndrome **190**, 197–98; *see also*
anorexia nervosa
relapses *181*; *see also* SSRI discontinuation
renal disease 151, 279
reward systems, mesolimbic dopamine
pathway *218*

safety concerns *see* suicidal ideation
Scales of Independent Behavior-Revised
(SIB-R) **262**–**63**
schizophrenia, treatment-resistant; *see also*
early-onset schizophrenia
clinical approaches 284, 285, 289
clinical reflections 294
constipation **296**
family history 279
follow-ups (1st) 285–87
follow-ups (2nd to 4th) 287–88
follow-ups (5th) 288–89
follow-ups (6th) 289–91
follow-ups (7th) 291–94
medical history 279
medication 279, 281, 287, 288, 293
medication adherence *283*, 294–96

medication checklist for initiation **286**
medication dosage relative to serum
concentration *289*, *298*
medication mechanisms of action 296–98
medication outpatient titration values **286**
medication pharmacology/binding profile
297
medication responses 291
medication responses and adverse effects
282
patient descriptions/evaluations 279–80, 282
post test self-assessment question 298
pretest self-assessment question 279
psychiatric history/evaluations 279, 282–83
psychotherapy history 279
social history 279
take-home points 294–96
test results **284**–**85**, **290**, **292**–**93**
second-generation antipsychotics (SGAs); *see
also* autism spectrum disorder (side-
effects of SGAs)
adherence to medication *283*, 294–96
adverse effects *282*
checklist for initiation **286**
constipation **296**
CYP2D6 phenotype *59*
dosage relative to serum concentration *289*,
298
mechanisms of action 74, 274–75, *275*,
296–98
outpatient titration values **286**
pharmacology/binding profile *74*, *270*, *297*
plasma concentration–time curves *60*
receiver operating characteristic curves 291
SSRI-induced mania 71–72, *73*–*74*
sedation (side effect) 3, 6, 23, 69–70, 133,
166, 296, 317
sedatives *see* benzodiazepines
selective serotonin reuptake inhibitors *see*
SSRIs
serotonin–norepinephrine reuptake inhibitors
(SNRIs) *9*
separation anxiety *9*
serotonin, effects of SGAs *275*; *see also* SSRIs
sexual dysfunction 317, *318*
SGAs
see second-generation antipsychotics
side effects of medication; *see also* activation
syndromes; anxiety in adolescence;

autism spectrum disorder; mania;
    sedation; weight-gain
SGAs *267*, *275*, **296**
SSRIs 306
sleep architecture; *see also* insomnia disorder
    adolescence 249–50
    childhood 249
sleep disorders 160; *see also* insomnia
    disorder
sleep hygiene 39
SNRIs (serotonin–norepinephrine reuptake
    inhibitors) *9*
social anxiety disorder 1, 3, 4, 8, *9*, 185, 301,
    307–9
social jet lag 239; *see also* insomnia disorder
socioeconomic status 151
somatodendritic α-2 receptors *255*
SSRIs (selective serotonin reuptake inhibitors)
    177–78; *see also* activation syndromes;
    anxiety; cannabis-related drug
    interactions; mania (SSRI-induced)
    concentrations in children and adolescents
        182
    CYP2C19 metabolism *24*, *176*
    CYP2D6 phenotype *59*
    mechanism-based inhibition *319*, 319–20
    mechanisms of action **26–28**, 27–29, *28*,
        181, 317–18
    metabolism *22*
    pharmacogenetics 29–30, **306**
    pharmacokinetics *23*, *24*, *26*, *320*, 321
    plasma concentration–time curves *24*, *176*,
        177, *206*, *208*
    PTSD with ADHD 39
    responses to *9*, *91*
    serum concentrations *308*, *309*
    weight gain, treatment-related *24*
    withdrawal pharmacokinetics/
        pharmacodynamics 179; *see also below*
SSRIs, discontinuation in adolescents
    clinical approaches 177
    CYP2C19 metabolism *176*
    family history 174
    follow-ups 177–78
    medical history 174
    medication 174
    medication concentrations in children and
        adolescents *182*
    medication mechanisms of action 181

medication plasma concentration–time
    curves *176*, *177*
patient descriptions/evaluations 173, 174
post test self-assessment question 183
pretest self-assessment question 173
psychiatric history/evaluations 173–74,
    175
psychotherapy history 174
relapses *181*
social history 174
take-home points 178–79
test results 175
tips/pearls of wisdom 180
withdrawal pharmacokinetics/
    pharmacodynamics 179
stimulants *see* CNS (central nervous system)
    stimulants
stress response *45*; *see also* posttraumatic
    stress disorder
striatum
    cannabis-related drug interactions *210*
    norepinephrine–dopamine reuptake
        inhibitors *216*
    substance abuse *see* cannabis-related drug
        interactions
suicidal ideation
    anorexia nervosa 185, 198
    bipolar disorder 138
    early-onset schizophrenia 121–22

therapeutic drug monitoring **86**, 90, 147, *182*,
    295–96
Tourette syndrome, child
    clinical approaches 160
    CYP2D6 metabolism *168*
    developmental milestones 155
    family history 155
    follow-ups (1st) 160–61
    follow-ups (2nd) 161–62
    follow-ups (3rd) 162–63
    follow-ups (4th) 163
    medical history 155
    medication 155, 157, **161**
    medication effects *167*
    medication mechanisms of action 165–67
    medication pharmacology/binding profile *166*
    parental resources 169
    patient descriptions/evaluations 155, 157–58
    post test self-assessment question 168

Tourette syndrome, child (cont.)
  pretest self-assessment question 155
  psychiatric history/evaluations 155, 159–60
  psychotherapy history 155
  rating scales **158–59**, 158, **163**
  take-home points 163–64
  test results 162
  tips/pearls of wisdom 165
Tourette's Impairment – Child self report
  158–59, 158, **163**
transcranial magnetic stimulation (TMS) 4–5
trauma *see* posttraumatic stress disorder
treatment-resistant anxiety *see* anxiety
treatment-resistant depression *see* major
  depressive disorder
treatment-resistant schizophrenia *see*
  schizophrenia
tricyclic antidepressants
  mechanisms of action 89–90
  metabolism of *88*
  receptor pharmacology *90*
  therapeutic drug monitoring **86**; *see also*
    obsessive compulsive disorder

urine production, diurnal variation *231*; *see
  also* nocturnal enuresis

Vanderbilt ADHD Rating Scale 99
vasodilators, mechanisms of action 252, *254*
ventral tegmental area (VTA), opioid
  antagonists *200*
Verbal Comprehension Index (VCI), WISC-5 98
vesicular monoamine transporter 2 (VMAT2)
  253
Visual-Spatial Index (VSI), WISC-5 99
vitamin D deficiency **190–92**

weight gain, treatment-related 23, *24*, *267*;
  see also autism spectrum disorder (side
  effects of SGAs)
weight loss 7, 51, 105, **190**, 194; *see also*
  anorexia nervosa
Weschler Intelligence Scale for Children
  (WISC-V) 97–99, **261–62**
withdrawal from medication *see* SSRIs
  (discontinuation)
Working Memory Index (WMI), WISC-5 99

Drugs Index

Locators in **bold** refer to tables; those in *italics* to figures

Abilify *see* aripiprazole
acetaminophen 138, 139
acetylcysteine 212, 213–15, *213*
Adderall *see* amphetamine salts
Adnasia XR *see* methylphenidate
albuterol 279
amitryptiline 224
amphetamine salts 105–6, 155, 168, 264
Anafranil *see* clomipramine
Aptensio XR *see* methylphenidate
arginine vasopresssin (AVP) 229–30
aripiprazole 20, 57, 59, *60*, 70, 77, 91, 121,
    128, 137, 139, 140–41, 150, 155, 160–61,
    162–64, 168, 203, 213–15, 219–20, 259,
    269–74, 276, 279, 310
armodafinil 85–86
asenapine 65, 68–70, 71–72, 73–74, 75, 150,
    285
ashwagandha 126
atomoxetine 102, 155, 157, 160–61, 162–63,
    166–68, 211–12
atorvastatin 121
Azstarys *see* serdexmethylphenidate

benztropine 128, 296–97
bisacodyl 295
bromocriptine 269–71
bupropion 3–4, 208, 211–12, 215–17

carbamazepine 65, 75, 150
Catapres *see* clonidine
cetirizine 2, 3
chloral hydrate 241
chlorpromazine 296–97
ciprofloxacin 293
citalopram 22–23, 29–30, 38–45, 213–15,
    219–20
clomipramine 77, 83, 84–87, 89–90, 91, 310
clonazepam 13–14, 20

clonidine 18, 19, 42–43, 107–8, 110–15,
    160–63, 233–34, 241–42, 250, 259, 261
clozapine 65, 75, 119, 121, 279, 284–98
Clozaril *see* clozapine
Colace *see* docusate
Concerta *see* methylphenidate (OROS
    formulation)
Contempla XR *see* methylphenidate
Cozaar *see* losartan
Crestor *see* rosuvastatin
Cymbalta *see* duloxetine
cyproheptadine 194

Daytrana *see* methylphenidate
DDAVP *see* desmopressin
Depakote *see* divalproex
Desaryl *see* trazodone
desmethylclomipramine *see* norclomipramine
desmopressin 223, 225–26, 227–30, *230*,
    231
desvenlafaxine 223, 231
dexmethylphenidate 36, 37, **102–3**
diazepam 155, 168
diphenhydramine 241–42, 243–44, 250
divalproex 3, 65, 67, 75, 138, 150
docusate 85–86, 293–95, 301, 304, 310
drospirenome 139
duloxetine 1, 4–5, 13–14, 20, 49, 60–61, 77,
    91, 105–6

Effexor *see* venlafaxine
Emsan *see* selegeline
escitalopram 13–14, 20, 22–23, *24*, 25–26,
    29–30, 49, 57, 126, 137–38, 142, 178–79,
    213–15, 219–20, 269–71, 301, 307–8,
    321
ethinyl estradiol 139

fexofenadine 66

fluoxetine 3–4, 39, 49, 54–61, 67–70, 78, 88,
    120, 150, 179, 180, 183, 185, 194, 203,
    213–15, 219–20, 223, 231, 233–34, 241,
    243–46, 285, 310–11, 315–17
fluvoxamine 78, 79, 82–83, 88, 301, 321
Focalin *see* dexmethylphenidate

Glucophage XR *see* metformin
guanfacine 1, 13–14, 17, 30–31, 38, 42–43,
    102, 105–6, 107–8, 110–15, 264

Haldol *see* haloperidol
haloperidol 119, 160–61, 164
hydroxyzine 18, 19, 20, 301–2, 304, 310–11

iloperidone *273*
imipramine 39, 77, 91, 223, 225–26, 227, 231
Inderal *see* propranolol
Intuniv *see* guanfacine
Invega *see* paliperidone

Jornay *see* methylphenidate

Kapvay *see* clonidine
Klonopin *see* clonazepam

lactulose 295
lamotrigine 150
Lexapro *see* escitalopram
lithium 137, 140–41, 142, **143**, 143–149, 151–52
loratadine 97
losartan 279
lurasidone 70, 150, 165, *273*
Luvox *see* fluvoxamine

melatonin 18, 36, 37, 38, 39, 45, 49, 50, 54,
    155, 157, 233, 244–46, 248, 251–52, 256,
    259, 264
MetadateCD *see* methylphenidate
Metamucil *see* psyllium fiber supplement
metformin 66, 72, 121, **129**, 130, 132, 279
methylphenidate 91, 97, 99, 102, **102–3**,
    103–6, 107–8, 110–15
methylphenidate (OROS formulation) 101, 155,
    168, 259
Minipress *see* prazosin
Miralax *see* polyethylene glycol
mirtazapine 241, 244–46, 250

Moban *see* molindone
molindone 119

N-acetylcysteine (NAC) 122, 212, 213–15, *213*
naltrexone 185, 196, 198–99, 200–1, *200*, 208
norclomipramine 85–87, 89
norgestimate-ethinyl estradiol 304, 310–11

olanzapine 150, 185, 193–96, 200–1
OrthoLo *see* norgestimate-ethinyl estradiol
oxcarbazepine 150
oxytocin 233, 256

paliperidone 119, 126–28, 131, 132–33, 259,
    269–71, *273*, 276, 285
paroxetine 35, 45, 49, 60–61, 185, 194, 200–1,
    211–12, 301–2, 304–5, 308, 310–11,
    315–21
Paxil *see* paroxetine
perphenazine 126
pimozide 164
polyethylene glycol 293–95
prazosin 35, 38–45
Pristiq *see* desvenlafaxine
propranolol 35, 45
Prozac *see* fluoxetine
psyllium fiber supplement 301, 304, 310

quetiapine 3, 35, 45, 66, 67, 68, 150, 279
Quillichew *see* methylphenidate
Quillivant *see* methylphenidate

ramelteon 233, 256
Revia *see* naltrexone
Risperdal *see* risperidone
risperidone 82–83, 132–33, 150, 259, 264–65,
    269–74, 276, 279, 280–82, 284–86
Ritalin LA *see* methylphenidate
rosuvastatin 279

Saphris *see* asenapine
selegeline 185, 200–1
sennosides 295
serdexmethylphenidate **102–3**
Seroquel *see* quetiapine
sertraline 3, 5, 8, 22–23, 29–30, 38, 39, 88, 174–
    79, 181, *182*, 203, 205–6, 208, 209–10,
    211–12, 213–15, 219–20, 301, 321

Strattera *see* atomoxetine
suvorexant 233, 244–46, 256

Tegratol *see* carbamazepine
Tenex *see* guanfacine
THC (tetrahydrocannabinol) *207*, **207**
Tofranil *see* imipramine
topiramate **129**, 130
trazodone 54, 55, 243–44, 250
Trintillix *see* vortioxetine

Valium *see* diazepam
venlafaxine 49, 54, 60–61, 77, 91

Viibryd *see* vilazodone
vilazodone 203, 219–20, 301, 321
viloxazine 224, 225, 229–30
Vistaril *see* hydroxyzine
vortioxetine 259, 276

Wellbutrin *see* bupropion

ziprasidone 165, *273*
Zoloft *see* sertraline
zolpidem 241, 244–46, 249
Zyprexa *see* olanzapine
Zyrtec *see* cetirizine